# Contemporary Cardiology

**Series Editor**
Peter P. Toth, Ciccarone Center for the Prevention of Cardiovascular Disease
Johns Hopkins University School of Medicine
Baltimore, MD, USA

For more than a decade, cardiologists have relied on the Contemporary Cardiology series to provide them with forefront medical references on all aspects of cardiology. Each title is carefully crafted by world-renown cardiologists who comprehensively cover the most important topics in this rapidly advancing field. With more than 75 titles in print covering everything from diabetes and cardiovascular disease to the management of acute coronary syndromes, the Contemporary Cardiology series has become the leading reference source for the practice of cardiac care.

Margarita Pena · Anwar Osborne
W. Frank Peacock

Editors

# Short Stay Management of Chest Pain

Second Edition

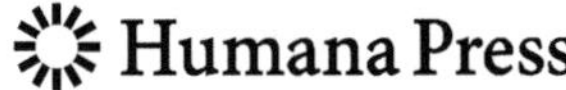 Humana Press

*Editors*
Margarita Pena
School of Medicine
Wayne State University
Grosse Pointe Park, MI, USA

Anwar Osborne
School of Medicine
Emory University
Decatur, GA, USA

W. Frank Peacock
Baylor College of Medicine
Houston, TX, USA

ISSN 2196-8969　　　　　　ISSN 2196-8977　(electronic)
Contemporary Cardiology
ISBN 978-3-031-05522-5　　ISBN 978-3-031-05520-1　(eBook)
https://doi.org/10.1007/978-3-031-05520-1



This Humana imprint is published by the registered company Springer Nature Switzerland AG
The registered company address is: Gewerbestrasse 11, 6330 Cham, Switzerland

# Preface

There is a medical school adage that says, "More than half of what you learn in medical school will be obsolete in 10 years." In the field of chest pain, this 10-year time is far too long, because the world seems to shift almost annually. This text will hopefully serve as a guide for healthcare providers who have chosen to focus their efforts on the short-term management of this population. While this text shares many new and updated facets in this field, finding and presenting them was only possible because of the giants of the field on whose shoulders we stand. The editors would like to thank some of the most important people in our lives, Daniel Morris, Marco and Clemencia Peña, Lisa Osborne, Dorothy Osborne, and Gretchen Cochran. We are forever grateful for their love and support. We hope that this book is of service to the human condition in sharing the most current knowledge on this subject. However, despite all of these advances we present here, heart disease remains the leading killer of humans on earth. There is so much more work to do.

<table>
<tr><td>Grosse Pointe Park, MI, USA</td><td>Margarita Pena</td></tr>
<tr><td>Decatur, GA, USA</td><td>Anwar Osborne</td></tr>
<tr><td>Houston, TX, USA</td><td>W. Frank Peacock</td></tr>
</table>

# Contents

# Contributors

**Maria Aini, MD** Clinical Operations, Department of Emergency Medicine, Thomas Jefferson University Hospital, Philadelphia, PA, USA

**Mani M. Alavi** Department of Emergency Medicine, University of Texas, Southwestern Medical Center, Dallas, TX, USA

**Edris Aman, MD** Division of Cardiovascular Medicine, Cardiology and Internal Medicine, UC Davis Medical Center, Sacramento, CA, USA

**Ezra A. Amsterdam, MD** Division of Cardiovascular Medicine, Cardiology and Internal Medicine, UC Davis Medical Center, Sacramento, CA, USA

**Kristin Aromolaran, MD, MBA** Department of Emergency Medicine, Emory University School of Medicine, Atlanta, GA, USA

**Christopher Baugh** Department of Emergency Medicine, Brigham and Women's Hospital, Harvard Medical School, Boston, MA, USA

**DaMarcus Baymon** Department of Emergency Medicine, Brigham and Women's Hospital, Harvard Medical School, Boston, MA, USA

**Natalie Bracewell** Division of Cardiovascular Medicine, University of Florida College of Medicine, Gainesville, FL, USA

**Donatella Brisinda, MD, PhD** Fondazione Policlinico Universitario A. Gemelli IRCCS, Università Cattolica del Sacro Cuore, Rome, Italy

Biomagnetism and Clinical Physiology International Center (BACPIC), Rome, Italy

**Christopher Caspers, MD** Ronald O. Perelman Department of Emergency Medicine, NYU Langone Health, New York, NY, USA

**Robert Christianson** Clinical Chemistry Labs, University of Maryland, Baltimore, MD, USA

**Shahriar Dadkhah** University of Illinois at Chicago, Chicago, IL, USA

**Matthew DeLaney, MD** Department of Emergency Medicine, University of Alabama at Birmingham, Birmingham, AL, USA

**Deborah B. Diercks** Department of Emergency Medicine, University of Texas, Southwestern Medical Center, Dallas, TX, USA

**Riccardo Fenici, MD** Biomagnetism and Clinical Physiology International Center (BACPIC), Rome, Italy

**Laura Goyack, MD** Department of Emergency Medicine, University of Alabama at Birmingham, Birmingham, AL, USA

**Michael A. Granovsky** LogixHealth, Bedford, MA, USA

**Ahmed Kazem, DO** Division of Internal Medicine, Henry Ford Hospital, Detroit, MI, USA

**Svadharma Keerthi** School of Medicine, Emory University, Decatur, GA, USA

**Vijaya Arun Kumar, MD, MPH** Department of Emergency Medicine, Wayne State University, Detroit, MI, USA

**Yue Jay Lin, MD** Ronald O. Perelman Department of Emergency Medicine, NYU Langone Health, New York, NY, USA

**Muhammad Majid, MD** Division of Cardiovascular Medicine, Cardiology and Internal Medicine, UC Davis Medical Center, Sacramento, CA, USA

**James McCord, MD, FACC** Wayne State University, Detroit, MI, USA
Division of Cardiology, Henry Ford Heart and Vascular Institute, Detroit, MI, USA

**Quinten Meadors** Department of Emergency Medicine, Emory University School of Medicine, Atlanta, GA, USA

**Kushal Nandam** Emory University, Atlanta, GA, USA

**Brian O'Neil, MD, FACEP, FAHA** Department of Emergency Medicine, Wayne State University, Detroit, MI, USA

**Anwar Osborne** School of Medicine, Emory University, Decatur, GA, USA

**Jaron Raper, MD** Department of Emergency Medicine, University of Alabama at Birmingham, Birmingham, AL, USA

**Michael Ross** Emory University, Atlanta, GA, USA

**Korosh Sharain** Mayo Clinic, Rochester, MN, USA

**Peter Smars, MD** Emergency Medicine Department, Mayo Clinic, Rochester, USA

**Damian Stobierski, MD** Ronald O. Perelman Department of Emergency Medicine, NYU Langone Health, New York, NY, USA

**Jason P. Stopyra, MD, MS** Department of Emergency Medicine, Wake Forest University School of Medicine, Winston-Salem, NC, USA

**Natasia Terry, MD, MBA** Department of Emergency Medicine, Emory University School of Medicine, Atlanta, GA, USA

**Sandhya Venugopal, MD** Division of Cardiovascular Medicine, Cardiology and Internal Medicine, UC Davis Medical Center, Sacramento, CA, USA

**Yitzchak Weinberger, MD** Ronald O. Perelman Department of Emergency Medicine, NYU Langone Health, New York, NY, USA

**Matthew Wheatley** Department of Emergency Medicine, Emory University School of Medicine, Atlanta, GA, USA

**David E. Winchester** Cardiology Section, Malcom Randall VAMC, Gainesville, FL, USA

# Epidemiology and Demographics of Coronary Artery Disease

Shahriar Dadkhah and Korosh Sharain

## 1   A Brief History of Coronary Artery Disease

Coronary artery disease (CAD) has plagued mankind for thousands of years. In fact, recent computed tomography imaging studies of mummies over 4000 years old identified vascular atherosclerosis in a large number who had an average age of death of 43 years [1]. However, the description of coronary atherosclerosis is much more recent and dates back just centuries. Leonardo da Vinci was one of the first to describe vascular atherosclerosis in the late fifteenth century stating "vessels in the elderly, through thickenings of the tunics, restrict the transit of the blood [2]." Over 200 years later, in 1772 William Heberden is credited with the first description of angina [2, 3]:

> Those who are afflicted with it are seized, while they are walking, and more particularly when they walk soon after eating, with a painful and most disagreeable sensation in the breast which seems as if it would take their life away if it were to increase or to continue. The moment they stand still, all this uneasiness vanishes.

The connection between angina and CAD was made by Edward Jenner in the late eighteenth century, after a patient of his who described angina was found to have ossified coronary arteries on autopsy [2]. It was not until the nineteenth century that Rudolph Virchow described his famous triad of thrombosis and provided the early theories of the development of atheroma which remain relevant today [2] (see Fig. 1 for current understanding of the development of coronary atherosclerosis and myocardial infarction). In 1910, Obrastzow and Straschesko, two Russian clinicians described clinical acute myocardial infarction (MI) in a living patient confirmed

S. Dadkhah (✉)
University of Illinois at Chicago, Chicago, IL, USA

K. Sharain
Mayo Clinic, Rochester, MN, USA



M. Pena et al. (eds.), *Short Stay Management of Chest Pain*, Contemporary Cardiology, https://doi.org/10.1007/978-3-031-05520-1_1

Our understanding of the pathophysiology of coronary artery disease is multifactorial and continues to evolve. A key initiator is injury or dysfunction of the endothelium caused by hypertension, dyslipidemia, smoking, or other inflammatory processes. This injury in turn increases the expression of endothelial adhesion molecules and causes release of chemoattractant cytokines which attract circulating leukocytes to the area of injury. These two processes lead to adherence of leukocytes to the endothelial surface and eventual migration into the intima where lipids are phagocytosed by macrophages to form foam cells and fatty streaks, the earliest morphologic changes of atherosclerosis. Through complex communication mechanisms, endothelial smooth muscle cells then migrate to the intima and proliferate with eventual alterations and remodeling of the extracellular matrix of the artery. Accumulation of lipids and other materials can form a necrotic core which if disrupted can expose the blood to procoagulants causing occlusive thrombosis and acute myocardial infarction.

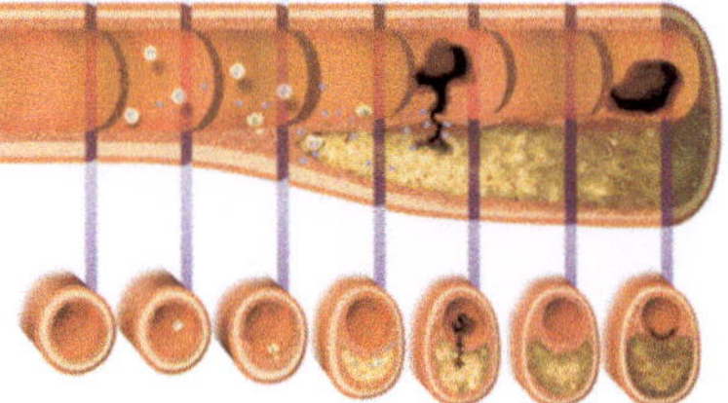

Figure courtesy of Libby P. *Circulation*. 2001;104:365-372.

**Fig. 1** Brief pathophysiology of coronary artery disease

later on autopsy [2, 3]. Just 2 years later, James Herrick established the use of electrocardiography to diagnose MI and the role of bed rest for management [2–4].

The twentieth century saw a boom in the understanding and diagnosis of CAD with the discovery of lipoproteins, the advent of cardiac catheterization by Werner Forssmann in 1929, selective coronary angiography by Mason Sones in 1958, and identification of risk factors associated with CAD through the Framingham Heart Study [2, 5]. Additionally, the treatment of CAD with medical therapy through clinical trials and the development of coronary artery stents were paramount in the late twentieth century.

Despite the advances in our understanding of CAD in regard to diagnosis, management, and prevention, cardiovascular diseases (CVD), and specifically coronary heart disease (CHD), remain the leading causes of death in the twenty-first century.

## 2 History of Coronary Artery Disease Epidemiology

The study of epidemiology is vital in identifying the connections which exist between lifestyle, environment, and disease, thus providing knowledge of the factors, distribution, and pathology of the particular disease. A notable shift in the study of epidemiology occurred in the mid-twentieth century when epidemiological studies began to include chronic noncommunicable diseases such as lung cancer and CAD [6]. Prior to that, epidemiology studies largely focused on infectious diseases as they were easier to diagnose. On the other hand, noncommunicable diseases like CAD were much more difficult to diagnose and understand as they had long latency periods [6, 7]. In order to understand CAD, a paradigm shift in the approach to disease was warranted, one that required the understanding of disease as the outcome of numerous compounding factors, often habitual in nature, and that were chronic rather than acute [6].

Coronary artery disease was the consequence of multiple "risk" factors with unpredictable onset and disease progression resulting in atherosclerotic lesions which could not be observed in the living patient. In fact, a diagnosis of CAD in the beginning of the twentieth century could only be made postmortem. Therefore, it was difficult to truly assess the prevalence and mortality of CAD, although even at that time it was estimated that approximately one in five deaths in the United Kingdom were due to atherosclerotic heart disease [6]. Additionally, such factors of risk or "risk factors" (which was a term that was not well established until the early 1960s) were not always present in patients with disease [6]. Thus, the implementation of prospective cohort studies by the Framingham Study sought to better understand CAD epidemiology.

The Framingham study, which investigated heart disease epidemiology, was designed in 1947 as a longitudinal study intended to perform long-term follow-up of a population of individuals without known heart disease and assess the progression of CAD in order to study the natural history of coronary heart disease (CHD) [6]. Risk factor epidemiology emerged from the CAD methodology of epidemiology which, unlike prior noncommunicable disease epidemiology studies, identified multiple risk factors for a single disease [6]. Coronary artery disease epidemiologists incorporated the multiple risk factor concept that the insurance industry had used for years previously [6]. Over the ensuing years, factors including hypercholesterolemia, hypertension, use of tobacco, and physical activity were identified to impact risk of CAD although a causal link was not established due to study design until the 1980s [6].

Since then, numerous studies have been performed that have evaluated the natural history and epidemiology of CAD providing clinicians with the tools to better diagnose, treat, and even prevent CVD and CAD.

## 3 Total Cardiovascular Disease Statistics

### 3.1 Prevalence

According to the most updated 2020 America Heart Association (AHA) heart disease and stroke statistics, the prevalence of CVD (including CHD, heart failure, stroke, and hypertension) in the United States (US) is approximately 121.5 million or 48% of adults $\geq$20 years of age (Fig. 2), which accounts for almost one out of every two adults $\geq$20 years of age [8, 9]. The prevalence of CVD is lower in women, those with a bachelor's degree or higher, and those who are employed [9].

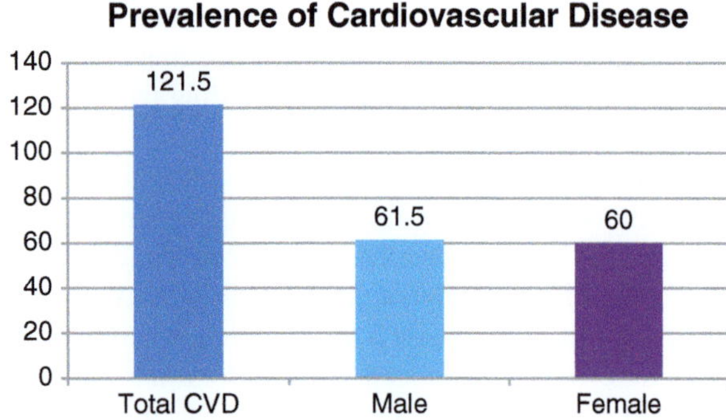

**Fig. 2** Prevalence of cardiovascular disease by sex in the US in adults ≥20 years of age (data presented in millions). *CVD* = cardiovascular disease, *US* = United States. Data extracted from the American Heart Association heart disease and stroke statistics—2020 update [9]



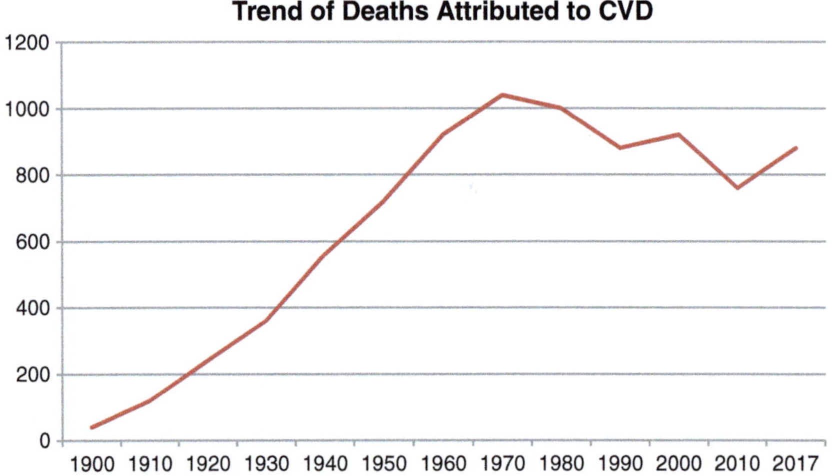



**Fig. 3** General trend of deaths attributed to CVD in the US between 1900–2017. Deaths are presented in the thousands. *CVD* = cardiovascular disease. Data extracted from the American Heart Association heart disease and stroke statistics—2020 update [9]

### 3.2 Mortality

Globally, CVD is the leading cause of death, and in 2017, approximately 17.8 million deaths were attributed worldwide to CVD, which is a 21% increase compared to a decade prior [9].

According to the Centers for Disease Control and Prevention, CVD remains the leading cause of death in the US accounting for one in four deaths [8]. Deaths attributable to CVD increased from the 1900s to the 1980s where it declined in 2010; however, recently there has been an increase (Fig. 3) [9]. Although the absolute number of CVD deaths continues to increase, the age standardized death rate has decreased by approximately 15% from 2007 to 2017 [9]. In 2016, over 1000 CVD-related deaths occurred daily with the highest mortality rates in non-Hispanic blacks (Fig. 4) [9].

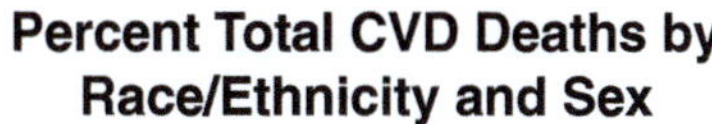
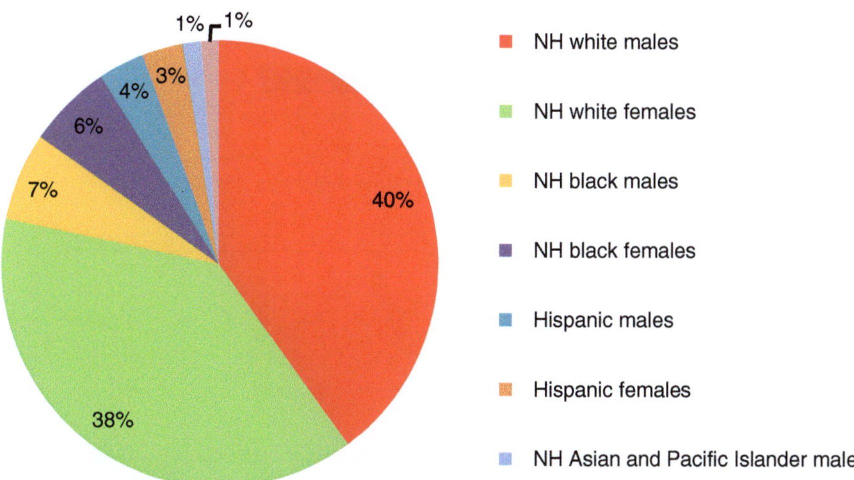



**Fig. 4** Percent total CVD death by race/ethnicity and sex in the US. *CVD* cardiovascular disease, *NH* = non-Hispanic. Data extracted from the American Heart Association heart disease and stroke statistics—2020 update [9]

**Fig. 5** Mortality associated with cardiovascular disease by sex in the US. *CVD* = cardiovascular disease, *US* = United States. Data extracted from the American Heart Association heart disease and stroke statistics—2020 update [9]

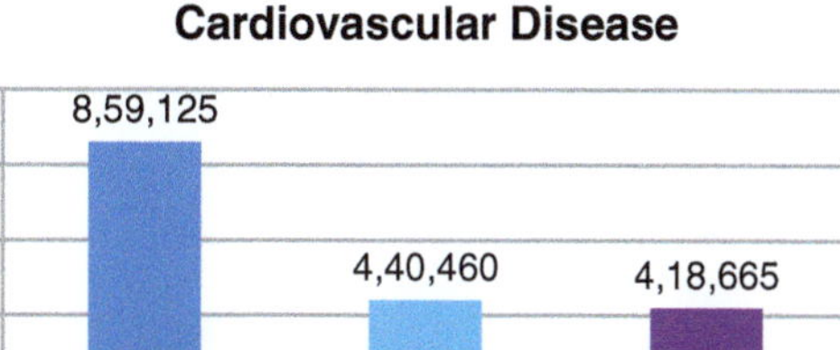



A common misconception is that cardiovascular diseases do not affect females as it does males. This could not be further from the truth (Fig. 5). Cardiovascular diseases claimed the lives of approximately 420,000 American females in 2017; by comparison, breast cancer took the lives of just over 42,000 American females. For comparison, Fig. 6 illustrates the other top causes of death in the US. Of note, the data presented in Fig. 6 is based on 2017 data and does not take into account deaths caused by the 2020 Coronavirus disease 19 (COVID-19) pandemic, which at the time of writing this chapter accounted for approximately 350,000 deaths (per report, it was the third leading cause of death at the current time) [8].

Regionally, the highest CVD-related mortality rates are in Louisiana, Mississippi, Alabama, and Oklahoma, and the lowest rates are in Minnesota, Colorado,

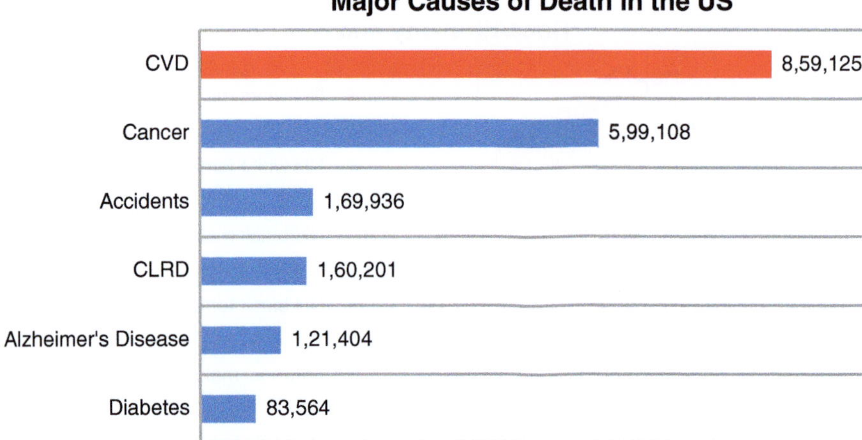



**Fig. 6** Major causes of death in the US (total number) per 2017 data. *CLRD* = chronic lower respiratory disease, *CVD* = cardiovascular disease. Data extracted from the American Heart Association heart disease and stroke statistics—2020 update [9]

Massachusetts, and Hawaii [9]. CVD mortality is higher with lack of insurance and lower socioeconomic status.

The estimated direct and indirect cost of CVD is approximately $220 billion.

## 4　Coronary Artery Disease Statistics

### *4.1　Prevalence*

Heart disease caused by CAD or CHD accounts for almost half of all causes of heart disease and remains the leading cause of death in the US in those over age 35 years (Fig. 7) [9]. Approximately 18.2 million Americans ≥20 years old have CHD (9.4 million males and 8.8 million females). For comparison, the population of the four most populated cities in the US combined is approximately 18 million (New York City, Los Angeles, Chicago, and Houston). The prevalence of CHD is 6.7% of US adults ≥20 years of age (7.4% for males and 6.2% for females) with the highest prevalence among blacks (Fig. 8).

The prevalence of CHD has decreased over time based on autopsy studies in US military personnel. Autopsy confirmed that CHD in soldiers in the Korean War in the 1950s was approximately 77%, while it was 8.5% in soldiers who died from 2001 to 2011, although the majority of the soldiers were male [10, 11].

Globally, it is estimated that 126.5 million people have CHD, which is almost a 75% increase between 1990 and 2017, with highest prevalence in North Africa, the Middle East, and Eastern Europe.

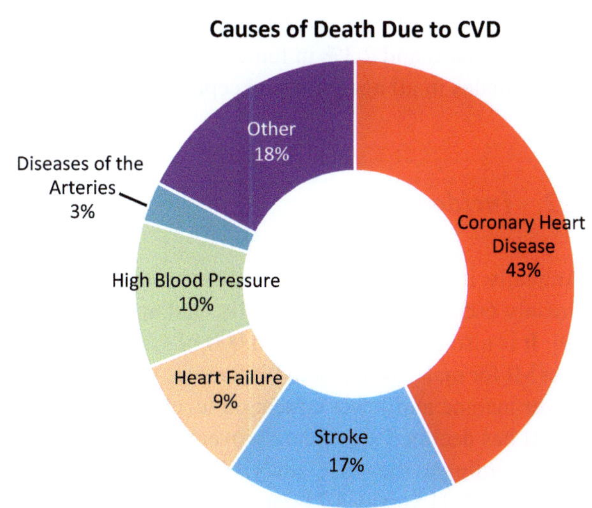



**Fig. 7** Causes of death attributed to CVD by percent. *CVD =* cardiovascular disease. Data extracted from the American Heart Association heart disease and stroke statistics—2020 update [9]

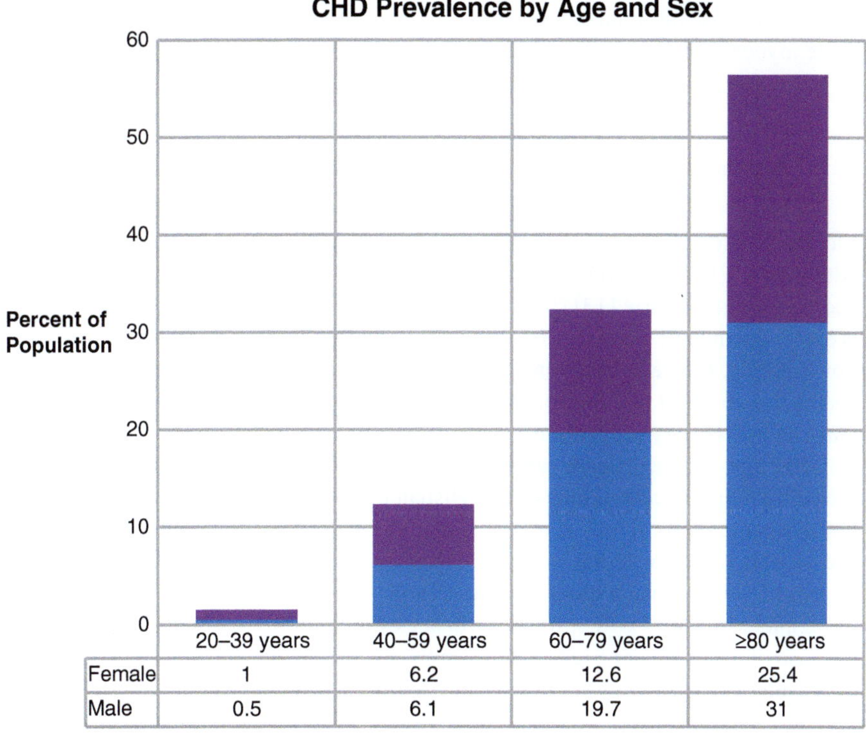



| | 20–39 years | 40–59 years | 60–79 years | ≥80 years |
|---|---|---|---|---|
| Female | 1 | 6.2 | 12.6 | 25.4 |
| Male | 0.5 | 6.1 | 19.7 | 31 |

**Fig. 8** Coronary heart disease prevalence (in percent) by age and sex in the United States. *CHD =* coronary heart disease. Data extracted from the American Heart Association heart disease and stroke statistics—2020 update [9]

In regard to MI, the overall prevalence is 3.0% in US adults ≥20 years of age (4.0% in males and 2.3% in females). Interestingly, males have a higher prevalence than females in all age groups except the 20–39 year age group [9].

## 4.2  Incidence

Annually, it is estimated that 805,000 Americans will have an MI. Of these, approximately 605,000 are first time MIs, and approximately 200,000 are recurrent MI's [9]. It is also estimated that 170,000 of these MIs will be silent. The average age at first MI for males is 65.6 and for females is 72.0. The incidence of MI increases with lower income and lower education level. However, there is suggestion that the rate of MI has declined significantly over time [9].

According to the ARIC study, clinically recognized MI was higher in whites than in blacks (5.04 versus 3.24 per 100 person-years) [12].

Interestingly, the rate of MI as a primary diagnosis decreased, while the rate of MI as a secondary diagnosis increased (this may be due to increased type 2 events or acute myocardial injury in response to acute illness rather than type 1 events or acute myocardial injury) [9].

## 4.3  Mortality

Mortality associated with CHD was 541,008, and MI mortality was 149,028 [9]. Although CVD and CHD remain leading causes of death, mortality from MI has decreased significantly [13] (by over 50% over the last 25 years). Fortunately, there is also a downward trend in CHD mortality, and this trend is predicted to continue. For example, between 2007 and 2017, there was a 10% decline in the number of deaths due to CHD [9]. Reasons for this trend largely are due to therapy (both primary and secondary prevention).

CHD age-adjusted death rates were highest in non-Hispanic black males followed by non-Hispanic white males, Hispanic males, non-Hispanic black females, non-Hispanic white females, and Hispanic females [9]. Additionally, survival and life expectancy after an MI is higher in whites than in blacks (7.4% vs. 5.7%) and improved with higher socioeconomic area [9]. Unfortunately, approximately 35% of people with CHD will suffer a coronary event and approximately 14% will die because of the coronary event. Interestingly, over 75% of CHD deaths occurred out of hospital [9].

The estimated direct and indirect cost of CHD and MI combined is approximately $21 billion and accounts for two of the top ten most expensive conditions treated in the US.

Mortality from CAD is expected to increase in developing countries due to economic and societal changes that occur with advanced development [14, 15]. The risk of development of CAD is said to increase with the transition of rural, agrarian, economically underdeveloped to urbanized, industrialized modern societies [14, 15]. Modernization leads to a more sedentary lifestyle, diets higher in calories, and psychosocial stresses [15]. It was found that a population of Japanese people (Japan being a low risk CAD location) who immigrated to the US acquired an incidence of CAD that was similar to those native to the US [14]. Higher life expectancy, changes in diet, lifestyle, and environment may be to blame [15]. India, China, and the United States are among the countries with the highest deaths attributed to CAD [14].

See Fig. 9 for a quick overview of relevant statistics related to CVD and CAD.

## 5 Risk Factors Associated with CAD

Epidemiological studies have provided the medical community with determinants of CAD. Approximately 90% of patients with CAD have at least one major modifiable risk factor such as hypertension, physical inactivity, smoking, hyperlipidemia, obesity, dietary factors, and regular alcohol use [16]. See Fig. 10 for a brief list of

**Fig. 9** Cardiovascular disease fast stats. *CVD* = cardiovascular disease, *MI* = myocardial infarction, *US* = United States

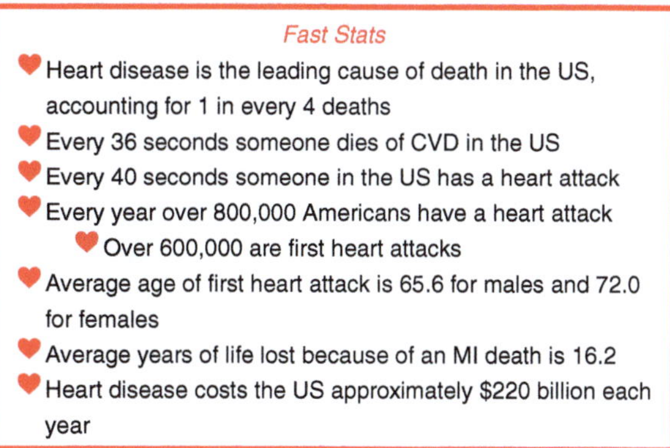


**Fig. 10** Brief list of risk factors associated with CVD and CHD. *CHD* = coronary heart disease, *CVD* = cardiovascular disease

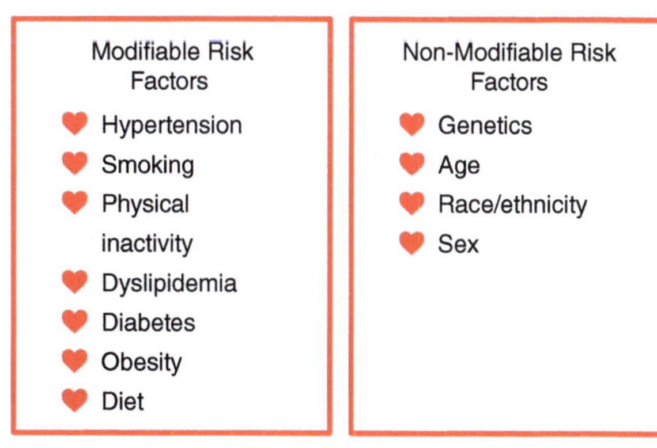

risk factors associated with CAD. The more risk factors a person has, the higher the risk of CVD and CAD [16]. The following section is a brief discussion regarding some common CAD risks factors.

## 5.1 Hypertension

The prevalence of hypertension (defined as a blood pressure greater than or equal to 130/90 mmHg) was 46% or 116.4 million adults (58.7 million males and 57.7 million females), which translates to roughly one in three Americans [9]. However, it is estimated that 35% of adults are unaware that they have hypertension [9]. There is a doubling of mortality from CHD and stroke for every 20/10 mmHg increase in blood pressure [17].

## 5.2 Physical Inactivity

Physical inactivity is another major risk factor of CAD. Physical inactivity increases risk of CAD by up to twofold [9]. Based on self-reporting, the prevalence of physical inactivity among adults has declined from 40.2% in 2005 to 25.9% in 2017 [9]. However, the prevalence of high school students meeting the recommended physical activity goal of $\geq$60 minutes of moderate to vigorous activity 7 days a week was 26.1% with girls meeting this goal half as likely as boys [9]. Additionally, 19.5% of girls and 11.0% of boys report that they do not participate in $\geq$60 min of any kind of physical activity in the prior week. Of note, these data are based on 2017 data, prior to implementation of the virtual learning environment due to the COVID-19 pandemic.

## 5.3 Smoking/Tobacco Use

Smokers are 2–3 times more likely to develop CHD than nonsmokers [18]. Smoking just one cigarette per day carries a greater than expected risk of developing CHD. In fact, smoking just one cigarette per day carries half the risk of smoking 20 cigarettes per day, thus there is no safe level of smoking in regard to CVD risk [18]. However, 27.1% of high school students and 7.2% of middle school students admit to using tobacco products with highest rates in non-Hispanic whites [9]. Although the rates of smoking have decreased by 50% since the 1960s, currently the prevalence for smoking in adults $\geq$18 years of age is 34.1 million or 14% of the adult population [8]. The highest rates of smoking are in males, those aged 45–64 years, non-Hispanic American Indians/Alaska Natives, lower education level, lower income, and those who are divorced/separated/widowed [8]. Approximately 90% of people that use cigarettes daily begin before age 18 years [8].

The most commonly used tobacco product in adolescents is now electronic cigarettes which has increased from 1.5% to 20.8% from 2011 to 2018 (although the CVD risks associated with electronic cigarettes are not known at this time) [9]. Quitting smoking at any age does significantly lower mortality from diseases related to smoking including CVD [9, 18].

## *5.4   Overweight and Obesity*

Obesity is an independent risk factor for CHD, and over 80% of patients with CHD are overweight or obese [19]. The hazard ratio for CHD in adults with obesity ranges between 2 and 3 [9]. The prevalence of obesity in adults increased significantly (30.5% in 1999) to 38.3% in 2018 (36% of males and 40.4% of females). The highest rates in males are in Hispanics and in females are in non-Hispanic blacks. Obesity correlates with CHD, diabetes mellitus (DM), hypertension, hyperlipidemia, and sleep-disordered breathing which can all worsen CVD.

In adolescents aged 12–19 years, the prevalence of obesity (defined as BMI ≥95th percentile for age) is 20.6% with lowest rates in non-Hispanic Asians. Longitudinal studies have identified that adolescents with obesity carry a significantly increased risk of CHD-related death as adults with a hazard ratio of 4.9 compared to adolescents at the lowest BMI quartile [9].

## *5.5   Hyperlipidemia*

It is estimated that 92.8 million Americans have total blood cholesterol ≥200 mg/dL, which is about 38.2% of the adult population with an increasing trend [9]. Females had higher prevalence of total cholesterol ≥200 mg/dL (40.4% vs 35.4% in males) and the mean LDL-C for adults ≥20 years of age was 112.1 mg/dL and for HDL was 54.2 mg/dL [9].

## *5.6   Diabetes*

Diabetes mellitus doubles the risk of CHD [8]. It is estimated that 26 million adults have diagnosed DM, 9.4 million have undiagnosed DM and 91.8 million have prediabetes [9]. Additionally, 1.5 million new cases of diabetes were diagnosed in adults in 2015 [9]. Worldwide, the trend of diabetes is increasing [9].

## 6  Conclusion

Despite the wealth of knowledge gained through epidemiological studies of CVD and CHD, there is still much work to do as CVD and CHD remain the leading causes of death. We must continue to push community education and awareness programs. In fact, the median time from cardiac symptom onset to hospital arrival has not improved significantly (45% presented within first 2 hours of symptoms between 2001 and 2003 compared to 48% between 2009 and 2011) [9]. Additionally, it is unknown what the consequences of the COVID-19 pandemic will have on CVD and CHD rates going forward. There is data suggesting that the delay in cardiac symptom to first medical contact has increased as a result of fears related to contracting COVID-19 [20, 21]. Additionally, there is concern that patients may be avoiding health care all together, suffering MIs at home. Only time will tell as to the longer term cardiovascular sequelae of COVID-19. As we continue to monitor the distribution of CAD in populations, epidemiology will provide us with even better insights into such devastating disease worldwide.

## References


1. Thompson RC, Allam AH, Lombardi GP, et al. Atherosclerosis across 4000 years of human history: the Horus study of four ancient populations. Lancet. 2013;381(9873):1211–22.
2. Gotto AM. Some reflections on arteriosclerosis: past, present, and future: presidential address. Circulation. 1985;72(1):1–17.
3. Hajar R. Coronary heart disease: from mummies to the 21st century. Heart Views. 2017;18(2):68–74.
4. Herrick JB. Clinical features of sudden obstruction of the coronary arteries. JAMA. 1912;59(23):2015–20.
5. Nabel EG, Braunwald E. A tale of coronary artery disease and myocardial infarction. NEJM. 2012;366(1):54–63.
6. Oppenheimer GM. Profiling Risk: the emergency of coronary heart disease epidemiology in the United States (1947-70). Int J Epidemiol. 2006;35:720–30.
7. Lynch J, Smith GD. A life course approach to chronic disease epidemiology. Annu Rev Public Health. 2005;26:1–35.
8. CDC website. https://www.cdc.gov. Accessed 28 December 2020.
9. Benjamin EJ, Muntner P, Alonsoa A, et al. Heart disease and stroke statistics – 2019 update: a report from the American Heart Association. Circulation. 2019;139:56–8.
10. Joseph A, Ackerman D, Talley JD, et al. Manifestations of coronary atherosclerosis in young trauma victims—an autopsy study. JACC. 1993;22(2):459–67.
11. Webber BJ, Sequin PG, Burnett DG, et al. Prevalence of and risk factors for autopsy-determined atherosclerosis among US service members, 2001-2011. JAMA. 2012;308(24):2577–83.
12. Zhang ZM, Rautaharju P, Prineas RJ. Race and sex differences in the incidence and prognostic significance of silent myocardial infarction in the atherosclerosis risk in communities (ARIC) study. Circulation. 2016;133(22):2141–8.
13. Gerber Y, Weston SA, Jiang R, et al. The changing epidemiology of myocardial infarction in Olmsted County, Minnesota, 1995-2012. Am J Med. 2015;128:144–51.
14. Tyroler HA. Coronary heart disease epidemiology in the 21st century. Epidemiol Rev. 2000;22(1):7–13.

15. Sanchis-Gomar F, Perez-Quilis C, Leischik R, et al. Epidemiology of coronary heart disease and acute coronary syndrome. Ann Transl Med. 2016;4(13):256.
16. Yusuf S, Hawken W, Ounpuu S, et al. Effect of potentially modifiable risk factors associated with myocardial infarciton in 52 countries (the INTERHEART study): case-control study. Lancet. 2004;364:937–52.
17. Lewington S, Clarke R, Qizilbash N, et al. Age-specific relevance of unusual blood pressure to vascular mortality: a meta-analysis of individual data for one million adults in 61 prospective studies. Lancet. 2002;360:1903–13.
18. Hacksaw A, Morris JK, Boniface S, et al. Low cigarette consumption and risk of coronary heart disease and stroke: meta-analysis of 141 cohort studies in 55 study reports. BMJ. 2018;360:j5855.
19. Ades PA, Savage PD. Obesity in coronary heart disease: an unaddressed behavioral risk factor. Prev Med. 2017;104:117–9.
20. Abdelaziz H, Abdelrahman A, Nabi A, et al. Impact of COVID-19 pandemic on patients with ST-segment elevation myocardial infarction: insights form a Britich cardiac center. Am Heart J. 2020;226:45–8.
21. Tam CCF, Cheung KS, Lam S, et al. Impact of coronavirus disease 2019 (COVID-19) outbreak on ST-segment elevation myocardial infarction care in Hong Kong, China. Circ Cardiovasc Qual Outcomes. 2020;13:1–3.

# The Financial Impact of Acute Coronary Syndromes

**DaMarcus Baymon and Christopher Baugh**

## 1 Introduction

For decades, mitigating the financial impact of patients presenting to the emergency department (ED) with chest pain has been a vexing task for the healthcare system. Chest pain is the second most common presenting complaint in the ED, comprising up to 5% of the 139 million annual visits in 2017 [1]. A plethora of diagnoses ranging from benign to life threatening, such as musculoskeletal pain, gastroesophageal reflux disease, pneumonia, pneumothorax, myocardial ischemia, aortic dissection, and many others all share the common symptom of chest pain. Assessing for, confirming, or adequately excluding a diagnosis of acute coronary syndrome (ACS) from this wide variety of possibilities while also avoiding unnecessary testing or hospitalization has been a ubiquitous challenge faced by many emergency physicians.

ACS encompasses three diagnoses of myocardial ischemia and infarction including unstable angina, non-ST segment elevation myocardial infarction (NSTEMI), and ST segment elevation myocardial infarction (STEMI). Type 1 myocardial infarction occurs when an atherosclerotic plaque ruptures, leading to a threatened endothelium with associated inflammation, adhesive cellular molecules, and intracoronary thrombosis [2]. The other type of myocardial infarction relevant in the ED is type 2, which is myocardial infarction due to a supply demand mismatch, usually secondary to a primary event such as hypotension or tachyarrhythmia. Evaluation of ACS entails eliciting a description of the

D. Baymon · C. Baugh (✉)
Department of Emergency Medicine, Brigham and Women's Hospital, Harvard Medical School, Boston, MA, USA
e-mail: CBAUGH@bwh.harvard.edu



M. Pena et al. (eds.), *Short Stay Management of Chest Pain*, Contemporary Cardiology, https://doi.org/10.1007/978-3-031-05520-1_2

15

discomfort, review of existing risk factors for coronary artery disease (CAD), electrocardiograph (ECG), cardiac biomarkers, and symptom management. Thirty-day mortality for ACS ranges from 2% to 11%; therefore, proper diagnostic work-up is crucial [3]. Once ACS is diagnosed or strongly suspected, emergency physicians admit patients to the hospital, and subsequent costs are driven by the duration of inpatient admission, further diagnostics such as cardiac imaging or stress testing, and treatments. Treatments include pharmacological interventions such as anti-anginal and antithrombotic pharmacologic therapies and, if indicated, invasive procedures such as percutaneous coronary intervention (PCI) and coronary artery bypass grafting (CABG) [3].

ACS evaluations should be prompt but can be costly. The ACS evaluation tools previously described are not benign and can come with a risk of death. A delay in a proper ACS diagnosis can also come with long-term morbidity secondary to compromised cardiac function, leading to heart failure due to delays in stabilizing ongoing infarcts. However, many patients without clear evidence of ACS demonstrated during the ED evaluation exist within a zone of uncertainty, with questionable benefit of further hospitalization and cardiac testing. Targeting specific interventions to reduce avoidable healthcare resource use (and thus cost) as it relates to ACS investigation includes cardiac biomarkers, validated risk stratification scores, and advanced cardiac imaging or stress testing. ED observation units (EDOUs) have been employed to provide a setting of care for this subsequent evaluation, which extends the window for data collection beyond a typical ED visit. Patients who have reassuring test results and a stable or improved clinical course in an EDOU can be sent home without the need for inpatient admission. This practice decreases the cost without sacrificing the quality of patient care due to the significantly reduced length of stay typically achieved in a dedicated EDOU that leverages a chest pain protocol in those patients with an ACS risk too high to allow for a routine ED discharge.

Furthermore, novel diagnostic tools recently introduced in the United States, such as high-sensitivity troponin assays first approved for use by the Food and Drug Administration in 2017, allow for a larger portion of patients with chest pain to be safely evaluated with cycling of cardiac biomarkers as rapidly as 1 h apart. More widespread adoption of evidence-based accelerated diagnostic protocols (ADPs) used to shift eligible patients out of inpatient hospital areas into an EDOU or earlier discharge home from the ED in eligible patients reduces avoidable hospitalizations and their associated healthcare costs while also providing reassurance for patients that their chest pain is extremely unlikely to be caused by myocardial ischemia.

## 2  Frequency/Burden of Disease of ACS by Demographics

ACS affects about 16 million Americans [4]. The prevalence of ACS in men is 2–2.5 times more than women with increasing prevalence from 0.75%, 6%, 16%, and 28% in the 20-39, 40–59, 60–79, and 80+ age group, respectively [5].

Although men are more likely to experience ACS, women have been shown to have worse outcomes, such as increase in hospital readmission and a 4% increase in mortality in some studies [6]. Similar to differences seen with age, women tend to have more atypical symptoms upon presentation and higher readmission rates for recurrent anginal symptoms after invasive cardiac angiography [6, 7]. Female gender has also been shown to be an independent predictor of 30-day mortality even in young females [8]. Readmission rates increase the burden on the cost of ACS and repeat ED visits for a missed diagnosis [8]. In a study that looked at gender differences in approximately 50,000 patients in British Columbia, women with ACS trended toward higher ages and had more comorbid conditions such as diabetes, hypertension, and hyperlipidemia [9]. In the USA, if a patient has two or more risk factors, their lifetime risk for ACS is about 40% for men and 20% for women [10].

Age is an important risk factor for ACS due to increasing comorbidities associated with age and poorer outcomes [11]. Along with additive comorbidities, our aging populations have worse outcomes due to other risk factors such as atypical presentations of their ACS and a higher likelihood of underlying cognitive impairment that may contribute to delays in seeking care or difficulty in providing a clear history [11]. Due to the aging Baby Boom generation, from 2010 to 2040, the population of 65 years of age is expected to double from 40 to 80 million [12]. This projected increase is predicted to increase coronary healthcare cost by approximately $50 billion USD; therefore, innovating and adopting breakthroughs in the evaluation of possible ACS is imperative to maintain high-quality care while controlling cost [12].

In addition to the costs associated with an index hospitalization, readmission rates have been a target of payer-driven efforts to reduce cost and improve the discharge planning process. In 2010, the Centers for Medicare and Medicaid Services (CMS) created a program which penalized hospitals for increased 30-day readmissions following several specific diagnoses, including myocardial infarction [13]. From 2009 to 2013, the 10–20% readmission rate of patients with acute myocardial infarction led to an extra $1 billion USD increase in hospital costs [14].

ACS also disproportionately affects ethnic minority groups. For example, from 2007 to 2010 among African American males, the prevalence of ACS was 45% compared to 36% for white males [15]. In the USA, racial minorities, such as African Americans, tend to be disproportionately affected by ACS due to lack of access to healthcare and health insurance [16]. Additionally, African American patients tend to have more comorbid conditions such as diabetes mellitus and hypertension that further increase their risk [16]. Similar trends related to ACS were found among Latinx patients as well [5, 16]. Latinx patients were also found to have rates of obesity and diabetes of 48% and 23% compared to the rates 38% and 15% of Caucasian patients, respectively [5, 16]. Certain Asian populations have a higher or minimal risk of ACS based on a combination of genetic predisposition and comorbid conditions [17]. Understanding racial and ethnic differences related to ACS is crucial as these differences translate to variable outcomes, readmission rates, and repeat ED visits.

## 3  Costs of ACS

The USA has been consumed by healthcare costs for years, and strategies to decrease those costs continue to be an important topic of scrutiny as it increasingly crowds out other essential areas of government and personal spending. As of 2018, the USA currently spends approximately 18% of its gross domestic product on healthcare, which estimates to $4 trillion USD, with a third of spending seen as wasteful [18, 19]. For every American, the USA spends on average $11,000–12,000 USD per capita on healthcare (Fig. 1) [18]. Switzerland spends about $8000 USD per capita on healthcare, making it the second highest global healthcare spender [20]. By 2027, healthcare costs are expected to increase to $6 trillion USD at a growth rate of about 5–6% per year [21]. About 33% of healthcare costs can be attributed to hospital inpatient care services while physician services encompass 20% (Fig. 2) [22].

Cardiovascular disease is one of the most common diagnoses encountered in the ED every year. An estimated 8 million patients visit the ED each year with chest pain, making it the second most common chief complaint [23]. Of those 8 million, less than 10% receive a final diagnosis of ACS [23, 24]. ACS diagnostic and

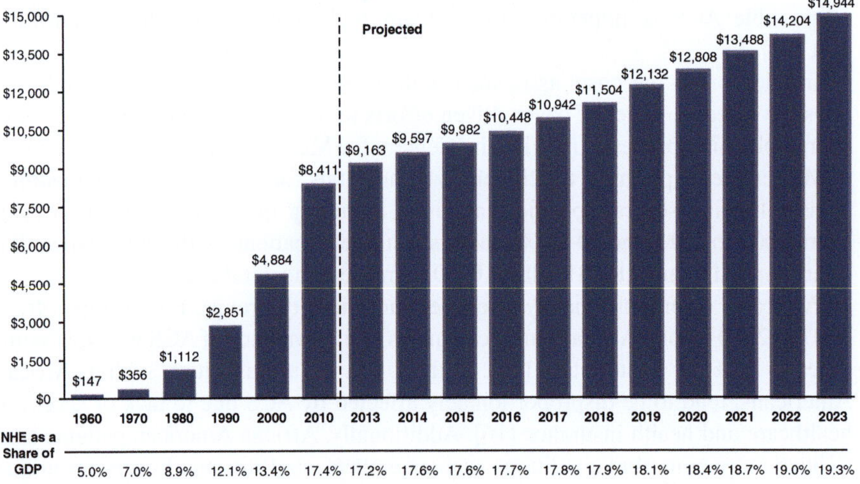


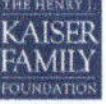


**Fig. 1** Total healthcare expenditures through 2023. Kaiser Family Foundation, National Health Expenditures per Capita, 1960–2023, published March 2014, accessed December 29, 2020

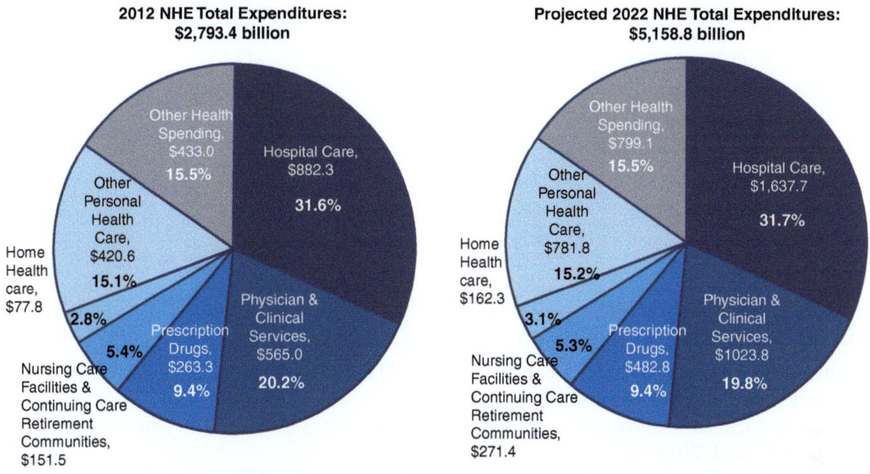


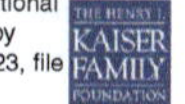


**Fig. 2** Distribution of national health expenditures. Kaiser Family Foundation, Trends in HealthCare Costs and Spending, March 2014, accessed December 29, 2020

treatment care cost $150-200 billion USD annually, a majority of the cost is due to hospitalization and equipment, physician services, and pharmacological therapies (Table 1) [5, 25]. Per patient, the total cost of ACS treatment ranges from $23,000 to 32,000 USD [26]. The total 1-year cost was highest for patients undergoing CABG, followed by patients who receive PCI and then those who are medically managed [26]. The cost of ED ACS evaluations are about $10–13 billion USD per year [27]. From 2009 to 2014, a cohort in Switzerland found 33% of patients hospitalized with ACS also had one or more other acute illnesses contributing to their need for hospitalization, which increased their associated costs of treatment [28]. For example, one study in 2015 found that individuals with comorbid atrial fibrillation and/or heart failure experienced $8000–21,000 USD more in hospital costs compared to those with ACS alone [29]. Another study in the same year found that comorbid atrial fibrillation increased hospital costs related to ACS by 40% [30]. A study in Asia analyzed predictors of high cost of ACS treatment and found associations between previous hospitalizations within 90 days, male gender, age, and income [31].

**Table 1** Costs of cardiac care in the United States 2020

|  | HD[a] | Stroke | Hypertensive disease[b] | Other circulatory conditions[c] | Total CVD |
|---|---|---|---|---|---|
| Direct costs[d] |  |  |  |  |  |
| Hospital inpatient stays | 59.4 | 17.4 | 7.9 | 12.8 | 97.5 |
| Hospital ED visits | 6.3 | 0.8 | 1.3 | 1.0 | 9.4 |
| Hospital outpatient or office-based provider visits | 22.6 | 2.4 | 13.7 | 7.9 | 46.6 |
| Home health care | 11.1 | 6.6 | 8.2 | 1.6 | 27.5 |
| Prescribed medicines | 10.0 | 0.8 | 20.2 | 1.8 | 32.8 |
| Total expenditures | 109.4 | 28.0 | 51.3 | 25.1 | 213.8 |
| Indirect costs[e] |  |  |  |  |  |
| Lost productivity/mortality | 109.3 | 17.5 | 4.6 | 6.1 | 137.5 |
| Grand totals | 218.7 | 45.5 | 55.9 | 31.2 | 351.3 |

Numbers do not add to total because of rounding. CVD indicates cardiovascular disease. *ED* emergency department; *HD* heart disease

Estimated direct and indirect costs (in billions of dollars) of CVD and stroke, United States, average annual, 2014–2015

This table lists the estimated direct and indirect costs from 2014 to 2015 of specific cardiovascular diseases and stroke including categories for hospital inpatient stays, emergency department visits, hospital outpatient or office-based provider visits, home health care, prescribed medicine, and lost productivity and mortality

Sources: Unpublished National Heart, Lung, and Blood Institute tabulation using Household Component of the MEPS for direct costs (average annual 2014–2015) [6]. Indirect mortality costs are based on 2014–2015 counts of deaths by the National Center for Health Statistics and an estimated present value of lifetime earnings furnished for 2014 by Wendy Max (Institute for Health and Aging, University of California. San Francisco. April 4. 2018) and inflated to 2015 from change in worker compensation reported by the US Bureau of Labor Statistics [5]

[a]This category includes coronary HD, heart failure, part of hypertensive disease, cardiac dysrhythmias, rheumatic HD; cardiomyopathy, pulmonary HD, and other or ill-defined HDs

[b]Costs attributable to hypertensive disease are limited to hypertension without HD

[c]Other circulatory conditions include arteries, veins, and lymphatics

[d]Medical Expenditure Panel Survey (MEPS) healthcare expenditures are estimates of direct payments for care of a patient with the given disease provided during the year, including out-of-pocket payments and payments by private insurance, Medicaid, Medicare, and other sources. Payments for over-the-counter drugs are not included. These estimates of direct costs do not include payments attributed to comorbidities. Total CVD costs are the sum of costs for the 4 diseases but with some duplication

[e]The Statistics Committee agreed to suspend presenting estimates of lost productivity attributable to morbidity until a better estimating method can be developed. Lost future earnings of people who died in 2015–2016, discounted at 3%

## 4 Cost Analysis of Risk Stratification Tools

Many tools have been employed to identify low-risk patients such as the HEART score and pathway, the Emergency Department Assessment of Chest pain Score (EDACS), a new accelerated diagnostic protocol (ADAPT), and the Vancouver Chest Pain Rule [32, 33]. These rules identify patients who are either safe for discharge or need further work-up. Patients with an acute myocardial infarction as identified as an STEMI or NSTEMI, intractable chest pain highly concerning for unstable angina, malignant arrhythmias, cardiogenic shock, or rising troponin on serial measurement with significant delta values require inpatient hospitalization without a safe opportunity for a more efficient and less costly disposition.

In those without a dangerous diagnosis confirmed during the initial ED work-up, unstructured clinical gestalt as the only driver of disposition and further care typically lead to highly variable care that is not evidence based with a risk of unnecessary hospitalization and testing. Use of these decision rules can lead to a decrease in hospital admissions that correlates with lower costs. As our understanding of ACS has advanced and new diagnostic tools have become available, the decision rules have become more refined and easier to use, thus improving their adoption and ability to reduce unnecessary care costs. A study from 2015 found that an ADP saved $334 USD per patient compared to 90-day follow-up costs to the routine care group [34]. In-hospital costs were similar in both the groups [34]. In 2017, a level 1 trauma center with an average hospital cost of $2800 USD per day found that implementation of the HEART score decreased hospital admission by over 20% and saved the institution over $1 million USD [27]. Another study of 270 patients found a $200–250 USD per patient savings with the implementation of the HEART score upon ED presentation, particularly when stratified into dichotomous low- and high-risk groups [35]. This difference was largely driven by a decrease in cost from cardiac diagnostics [35]. In the Netherlands, cost analysis estimated that implementation of the HEART score could save $40 million USD while also minimizing the adverse outcomes in patients discharged from the ED [36]. The risk–benefit in cost analysis must consider the risk of missed MACE, typically with a 30-day follow-up window from the index ED visit.

The various scoring algorithms that are available to clinically evaluate a patient with chest pain come with a certain miss rate percentage to balance against the benefit of cost savings. In 2016, a study in the United Kingdom compared the HEART score and the thrombolysis in myocardial infarction (TIMI) score and found a savings of $28,000 USD with the HEART score and $80,000 USD with the TIMI score [37]. The savings difference was met with a 30-day MACE miss rate of <1% with the HEART score and 3% using the TIMI score [37]. Over the last couple of decades, novel risk stratification tools have started to overcome the routine use of TIMI among emergency physicians, as these newer tools were developed in patients more similar to those commonly encountered in the ED and have compared favorably with regard to the proportion of patients that can be classified as low risk with an appropriately low 30-day risk of MACE.

## 5   Emergency Department Observation Units

Over the past few decades, one of the most innovative strategies employed to mitigate hospital costs related to chest pain is the EDOU. EDOUs by definition are a dedicated space where patients managed in observation status (an outpatient billing status) are cohorted together to receive further diagnostics and treatments in order to determine their need for subsequent inpatient admission. EDOUs are also typically run by ED staff and located within or adjacent to the ED; however, some units are distant from the ED due to a lack of available nearby space. A minority of observation units are run by hospitalists or post-procedure staff and may be called by a different name. Chest pain observation units first emerged in the 1980s and were the first use case for today's EDOUs [38]. Starting in the 1990s, research helped to establish the cost advantages of EDOU use in eligible patients who would have otherwise been hospitalized on inpatient services [39]. EDOUs that leverage evidence-based protocols enable providers to deliver care efficiently and less costly without jeopardizing patient safety.

When patients present to the ED with chest pain, their likelihood for admission is based on their overall risk of a major adverse cardiac event (MACE) after discharge. In the literature, patients with a risk of MACE of less than 2% have been characterized as low risk and safe for discharge; nevertheless, variable care still results in the admission of many low-risk patients [28]. From 2008 to 2013, a study of 50,000 patients revealed those with two negative cardiac biomarker values, a nonischemic ECG, and normal vital signs were not likely to benefit from inpatient admission [40]. Although findings exist to support the lack of benefit of admission for low-risk patients, providers often still admit these patients, due to the risk of malpractice from data showing a 2–10% missed ACS rate [41]. About 20% of malpractice claims against emergency physicians are due to a missed ACS event [41]. The initial ECG is only 50% sensitive for ACS and many hospitals around the country use cardiac biomarkers with varying sensitivity and specificity. This variability can lead to over-use of resources and thus increased cost of avoidable hospitalizations. A strategy to reduce avoidable hospitalizations and address physician concern over missed ACS events led to the creation of the EDOUs. Protocol-driven observation units, defined units with clear inclusion and exclusion criteria, evidence-based testing and treatments, and a clear timeline and criteria for a home versus inpatient admission decision have been shown to decrease cost and length of stay and provide quality patient care when compared to inpatient admission [42, 43]. Ideally, more than 75% of patients should be discharged within 15 h and accumulate into a savings of about $1500 per patient for all medical conditions [44, 45]. Chest pain is typically the most common condition managed in an EDOU, but the total cost savings across all conditions is estimated to be $4.6 million USD and $8.5 billion USD hospital care and national healthcare cost, respectively; 2.4 million inpatient admissions would also be avoided [44, 45].

EDOUs ideally serve as areas for patients who have no ongoing recurrence of their symptoms, a nonconcerning ECG, negative or adynamic serial cardiac biomarkers, and a risk for ACS too high to allow a safe discharge home based on the data gathered from the ED visit alone. The advent of EDOUs allows for continuous throughput from the ED while saving inpatient beds for individuals with more acute or complex medical conditions clearly requiring inpatient care. Occupancy for EDOUs rarely reaches 100% until the late evening and overnight hours due to predictable bed turnover and patient arrival patterns [44]. The average length of stay in an EDOU should be less than 24 h with an associated 20% rate of subsequent inpatient admission [44].

Hospital costs have largely been driven by inpatient admissions, and EDOUs help drive costs down by distributing eligible patients to less intense settings of care with more efficient staffing ratios while also reducing length of stay by avoiding inpatient admission altogether for about 80% of visits. When comparing inpatient and EDOU cost of ACS evaluation, savings range from $151 to $567 USD per patient [44]. Furthermore, observation stays not only reduce hospital costs but, contrary to a common misperception, are also likely to reduce patient out-of-pocket costs. For example, among Medicare beneficiaries undergoing a short-stay hospitalization, 94% of those managed in observation status experienced an out-of-pocket cost lower than the alternative of a Part A inpatient deductible payment [34, 46]. As shown in Fig. 3, another way to illustrate this cost savings is comparing the expected out-of-pocket cost of just over $700 USD for an observation stay due to the Medicare Part B observation co-insurance cost versus over $1500 USD for a short inpatient stay, largely driven by the Medicare Part A inpatient deductible cost [34, 46]. This finding of lower patient expenses for observation stays has also been seen among patients with commercial insurance and the addition of a secondary payer, which is present among ~85% of Medicare beneficiaries [27, 47]. Exceptions to these examples include patients who are readmitted as inpatients within a 60-day spell of

| SERVICE | INPATIENT | OBSERVATION |
| --- | --- | --- |
| **Facility fees** | Patient pays Part A deductible: $1,408<br><br>Medicare Part A pays Diagnosis Related Group (DRG) 313: $4,183 (pre deductible $2,775) | Patient pays 20% of C-APC 8011: $440.67<br><br>Medicare pays 80% of C-APC 8011: $1,762.68 |
| **Professional fees**<br><br>Initial evaluation<br>Subsequent evaluation<br>Discharge evaluation<br>ECG interpretation x3<br>Stress test interpretation | Patient pays 20% of fees: $107.03<br>Medicare Part B pays 80%: $428.11<br><br>CPT 99223: $206.07<br>CPT 99223: $106.10<br>CPT 99239: $108.99<br>CPT 99010 x3: $25.98<br>CPT 78492: $88 | Patient pays 20% of fees: $75.27<br>Medicare Part B pays 80%: $301.08<br><br>CPT 99220: $188.39<br>-<br>CPT 99217: $73.98<br>CPT 93010 x3: $25.98<br>CPT 78492: $88 |
| **Medications** | Patient pays $0<br>Medicare Part A pays DRG payment | Patient pays entire cost: $207<br>Medicare Part B pays $0 |
| **Laboratory** | Patient pays $0<br>Medicare Part A pays DRG payment | Patient pays $0<br>Medicare Part B pays C-APC payment |
| **Facility Diagnostics**<br>Cardiac monitoring x48h<br>Nuclear perfusion stress test<br>ECG x3 | Patient pays $0<br>Medicare Part A pays DRG payment | Patient pays $0<br>Medicare Part B pays C-APC payment |
| **Total Payments**<br><br><br>**Total Revenue** | Patient: $1,515.03<br>Medicare Part A: $2,775<br>Medicare Part B: $428.11<br><br>Hospital: $4,183<br>Professional: $535.14 | Patient: $722.94<br>Medicare Part A: $0<br>Medicare Part B: $2,063.76<br><br>Hospital: $2,410.35<br>Professional: $376.35 |
| **TOTAL COST** | $4,718.14 | $2,786.70 |

**Fig. 3** Comparison of medicare out-of-pocket expenses for ED observation and inpatient cost in ACS evaluation

illness, which excludes the need to pay the Part A deductible again [34, 46]. In addition, self-administered medications (e.g., patient home medications) and time spent in observation status do not count toward the 3-day stay typically required for a Medicare benefit to cover post-discharge skilled nursing facility services [34, 46]. Although avoiding unnecessary admission is the goal, EDOU care should not be offered for patients with ACS who need inpatient admission or deemed too high risk despite inpatient boarding or overcrowding.

In 2012, there were 1.5 million observation stays from Medicare patients with a 4-year growth of 8% from 2010 to 2014, but growth decreased from 2016 to 2017 by 1.2% [48]. In 2012, inpatient stays decreased by 3%, but increased slightly by 0.7% from 2016 to 2017 [49]. EDOUs have been shown to decrease hospital admissions by 17–44%, leading to a potential annual savings of $9 billion USD a year for the healthcare system overall [49]. From 2006 to 2016, the chest pain inpatient admission rate declined from 19% in 2006 to 3.9% in 2016; associated inpatient hospitalization costs declined from $10.4 billion (2006–2008) to $6.2 billion (2012–2014) [50]. This inpatient cost savings were likely largely driven by a shift from inpatient care to outpatient care, including the use of EDOUs [50].

ACS costs alone total about $75–150 billion USD annually and account for 800,000 to 1.2 million US hospital discharges [22, 51]. Up to 75% of ACS costs are related to hospital readmissions [23]. In 2009, 1.2 million patients were hospitalized due to ACS and the cost of productivity loss estimated at $80 billion USD [22, 26, 51]. Productivity loss is defined as healthcare-related absence from work due to chronic illness, sick days, or personal time off. The productivity loss also varied by the intervention type (e.g., medical management vs. PCI vs. CABG), with patients undergoing CABG having the highest annual productivity loss of about $18,000 USD [26]. One year short-term disability was $9400 USD and $6000 USD for PCI and medically managed patients, respectively [26]. In 2015, about 50% of patients who experienced a new coronary event would have a recurrence that same year [26]. These recurrences account for 40–45% of the healthcare costs related to ACS [26]. ACS is further stratified by patient income. Low- and high-income families were billed at similar rates for cardiovascular care, while low-income families experienced a loss of higher proportions of the income due to medical treatment, which resulted in a 20–40% loss of their post subsistence income [52].

In the USA, out-of-pocket costs for individuals with known cardiovascular disease was $2200 USD, and nearly half of the cost was due to medications [52]. A multicenter trial showed that patients had difficult time accessing prescriptions after an ACS event due to hospital cost and, therefore, suffered from recurrent angina and higher rates of cardiac re-hospitalization [39]. From 1998 to 2009, the Medical Expenditure Panel Survey also found that individuals with ACS could lose about on average $5000-6000 USD per year while seeking medical treatment [26]. Therefore, interventions to decrease ACS cost from a hospital level could also significantly impact patients on an individual financial level.

## 6  Novel ACS Evaluation Innovation Cost Analysis

The diagnostic evaluation of ACS has evolved to provide more sensitivity and specificity in differentiating patients who are at low or high risk. After an ACS evaluation, determining the proper risk stratification imaging tool to use comes with challenges as well (Fig. 4). The advent of high-sensitivity troponins (hs-Tn)) has allowed clinicians to detect a measurable troponin value in more than 50% of all patients and defines an abnormally elevated troponin value, suggesting myocardial injury above a 99th percentile cut point. In 2019, a study of 32,000 patients found those presenting within 2 h of symptom onset with a change in serially measured troponin level, or delta troponin, of less than 5 ng/L had a 99.5% negative predictive value for ACS [53]. Also, Peacock et al. found out of 1300 patients, those with a hs-TnI of less than 19 ng/L had a 30-day adverse event rate of less than 1%, further increasing the safety profile of hs-TnI [54]. An Australian study found that use of hs-Tn saved $1300 USD per patient with a $108,000 USD saving per adverse event avoided [55]. Jülicher et al. found that patients under the hs-TnI algorithm saved $113–147 USD per patient and decreased hospital length of stay by a mean of 6.2 h [56]. Note that given the value of serial or delta troponin measurements with

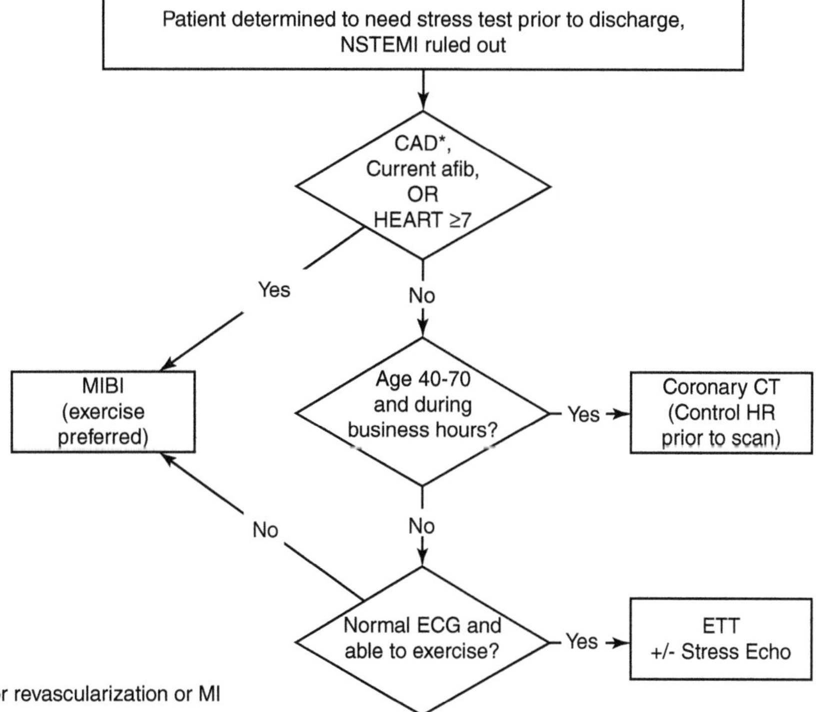


**Fig. 4** Algorithm for determining proper cardiac imaging risk-stratification testing

high-sensitivity assays versus contemporary assays, the volume of troponin testing typically increases after adoption of a high-sensitivity assay, so there is usually a marginal increase in the lab costs associated with more troponin sampling. When the hs-TnI was combined with the ADAPT score and delta detection limit, savings increased to $486 USD per patient while increasing diagnostic accuracy from 90% to 94% [56]. An example of an ADP with the use of a hs-Tn is found in Fig. 5.

Another diagnostic advance developed to evaluate ACS includes coronary computerized tomography angiography (coronary CTA). The cost of coronary CTA based on Medicare reimbursement is $466 USD with an additional $300 USD for medical work-up after incidental findings from the coronary CTA [57]. The cost of PCI is approximately $2770 USD [57]. Use of coronary CTA has risen in recent years to replace functional imaging in those with stable chest pain or without known CAD. Studies show that coronary CTAs have a >95% sensitivity and specificity, and individuals with coronary CTA scores of zero had a 12-year survival of 99% [58]. Patients with low-risk chest pain with the use of an early coronary CTA algorithm with and without an EDOU stay had a decrease in length of stay by 10 and 15 h, respectively [59]. There was a cost difference from $7500 USD for standard care compared to $6100 USD and $4300 USD for early coronary CTA algorithm with and without an observation, respectively [59]. In 2010, Halpern et al. found a false-negative rate of 2.5% and $800 USD savings per patient in those with a positive

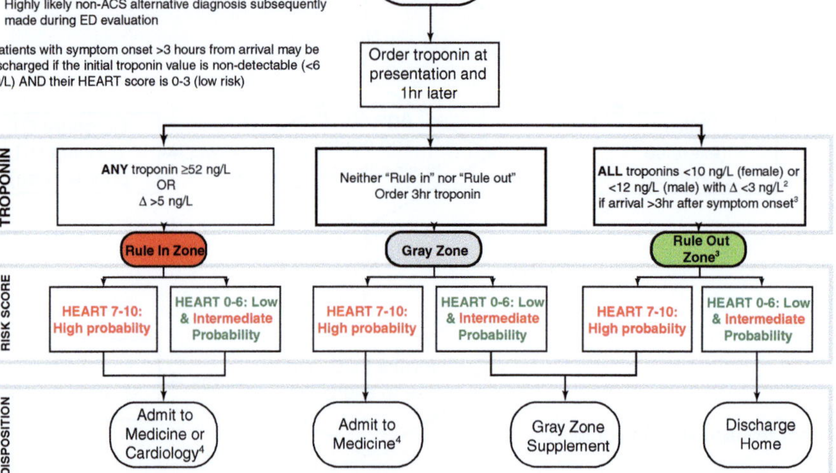


**Fig. 5** Brigham and Women's Hospital Emergency Department ADP for ACS evaluation

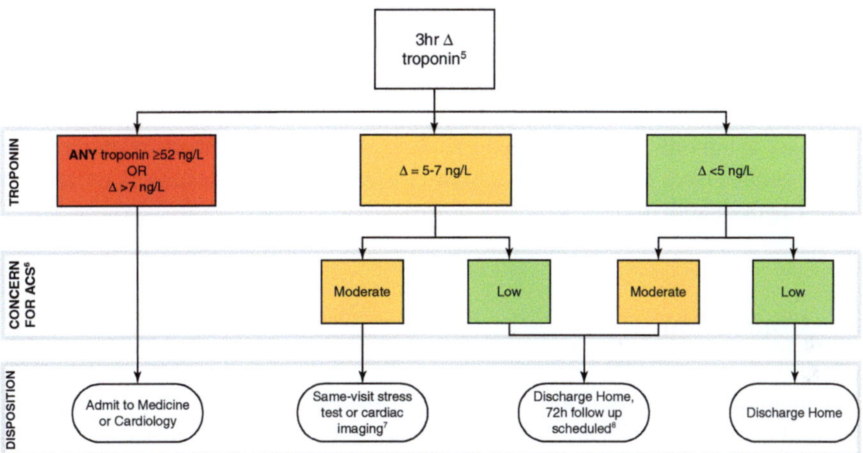


**Fig. 5** (continued)

stress who underwent coronary CTA instead of PCI [60]. When using CAD prevalence of 30–50% based on age, coronary CTA had a cost-effective threshold of $50,000 USD using quality-adjusted life-year (QALY)) [57]. Min et al. found that in populations with high incidences of coronary artery disease, PCI is more cost-effective [57]. There is also conflicting data regarding the necessity of PCI after coronary CTA vs. single photon emission computed tomography (SPECT) and the cost-effectiveness. These studies were not stratified by patient risk of coronary disease after initial evaluation.

Further novel approaches such as a coronary magnetic resonance (CMR) and coronary SPECT are being used to evaluate patients for ACS. The cost of coronary SPECT and CMR is $774 USD and $860 USD, respectively [57, 61]. In Germany, Bold et al. showed CMR to have $1256 USD savings per case when compared to SPECT [62]. In Australia and the UK, CMR followed by a positive exercise stress test was cost-effective of a minimum $40,000 USD per QALY gained [63, 64]. SPECT cost-effectiveness is still under active investigation. Another novel imaging modality under current investigation is 90-s magnetocardiogram (MCG). MCG involves analysis of magnetic fields of the heart similarly to the ECG P, QRS, and T wave patterns [65]. MCG has been shown to find abnormal mapping patterns in 72% of patients ultimately diagnosed with CAD despite a normal ECG and echocardiogram [66]. Early studies on MCG in a small ED population show that MCG may have a negative predictive value of 89–92% in evaluation of ACS [65]. This technology could help shorten EDOU length of stay by having 24/7 access to advanced cardiac imaging/testing that could be performed and interpreted by ED staff, similar to point of care ultrasound. This shortened length of stay would potentially drive down cost and increase patient flow through the ED.

Although these imaging modalities are available, they may not save money if performed on patients at too low risk to have a pre-test probability of coronary disease to justify the expense. Patients are also at risk for increased radiation exposure and spend additional time in the hospital since most of these tests are not available 24/7. Therefore, patients presenting to the ED outside of early morning hours (and at many hospitals, at any time on weekends or holidays) need to stay overnight to get the test. Discharge with expedited testing may be an option for patients with resolved symptoms, but they need excellent access to outpatient resources, and some studies have demonstrated a high no-show rate when testing is deferred to post-ED discharge [67].

## 7 Conclusion

Technological advances in the evaluation of patients presenting to the ED with a clinical concern for ACS are constantly evolving. Given the prevalence of coronary disease in the USA and the frequency of ED visits related to chest pain, the costs to the healthcare system and patients associated with their evaluation and treatment are quite high compared to other conditions. As budgetary pressures surrounding healthcare spending continue to escalate, the significance of these costs and strategies to safely control them will continue to be of supreme importance. From 2007 to 2017, cardiovascular mortality decreased to 233 from 260 per 100,000 although cardiovascular-associated diagnoses increased by 28.5% from 485.6 million to 621 million globally [68]. Therefore, the evaluation of ACS will only increase to mirror the larger population of surviving patients with coronary disease [68]. A majority of these patients will interact with the ED; therefore, tools targeted for safe and efficient evaluation of ACS in the ED yield tremendous quality and economic benefits.

Novel and more accurate approaches to evaluating ACS in the ED will improve the quality of care delivered, allocate resources efficiently, and provide cost reductions that are necessary to keep up the increasing demands on the healthcare system. Appropriate use of tools such as ADPs, high-sensitivity troponin assays, EDOUs, and advanced cardiac imaging are the step in the right direction to tackle a proper and efficient ACS evaluation.

## References


1. FastStats - Emergency Department Visits. Centers for Disease Control and Prevention. 2020. https://www.cdc.gov/nchs/fastats/emergency-department.htm. Accessed December 23, 2020.
2. Sandoval Y, Thygesen K, Jaffe AS. The universal definition of myocardial infarction. Circulation. 2020;141(18):1434–6. https://doi.org/10.1161/circulationaha.120.045708.

3. Kumar A, Cannon CP. Acute coronary syndromes: diagnosis and management, Part II. Mayo Clin Proc. 2009;84(11):1021–36. https://doi.org/10.4065/84.11.1021.

4. Singh A. Acute coronary syndrome. StatPearls. 2020. https://www.ncbi.nlm.nih.gov/books/NBK459157/. Accessed December 15, 2020.

5. Virani SS, Alonso A, Benjamin EJ, et al. Heart disease and stroke statistics—2020 update: a report from the American Heart Association. Circulation. 2020;141(9):757. https://doi.org/10.1161/cir.0000000000000757.

6. Canto JG, Rogers WJ, Goldberg RJ, et al. Association of age and sex with myocardial infarction symptom presentation and in-hospital mortality. JAMA. 2012;307(8):199. https://doi.org/10.1001/jama.2012.199.

7. Oosterhout REMV, Boer ARD, Maas AHEM, Rutten FH, Bots ML, Peters SAE. Sex differences in symptom presentation in acute coronary syndromes: a systematic review and meta-analysis. J Am Heart Assoc. 2020;9:014733. https://doi.org/10.1161/jaha.119.014733.

8. Ricci B, Cenko E, Vasiljevic Z, et al. Acute coronary syndrome: the risk to young women. J Am Heart Assoc. 2017;6(12):007519. https://doi.org/10.1161/jaha.117.007519.

9. Izadnegahdar M, Mackay M, Lee MK, et al. Sex and ethnic differences in outcomes of acute coronary syndrome and stable angina patients with obstructive coronary artery disease. Circulation. 2016;9(2):002483. https://doi.org/10.1161/circoutcomes.115.002483.

10. Sanchis-Gomar F, Perez-Quilis C, Leischik R, Lucia A. Epidemiology of coronary heart disease and acute coronary syndrome. Ann Transl Med. 2016;4(13):256. https://doi.org/10.21037/atm.2016.06.33.

11. Alexander DS, Philip DB, John K, Nigel D, Christopher PG. Acute coronary syndromes: an old age problem. J Geriatr Cardiol. 2012;9(2):192–6. https://doi.org/10.3724/sp.j.1263.2012.01312.

12. Odden MC, Coxson PG, Moran A, Lightwood JM, Goldman L, Bibbins-Domingo K. The impact of the aging population on coronary heart disease in the United States. Am J Med. 2011;124(9):10. https://doi.org/10.1016/j.amjmed.2011.04.010.

13. Wadhera RK, Yeh RW, Maddox KEJ. The hospital readmissions reduction program — time for a reboot. N Engl J Med. 2019;380(24):2289–91. https://doi.org/10.1056/nejmp1901225.

14. Wang H, Zhao T, Wei X, Lu H, Lin X. The prevalence of 30-day readmission after acute myocardial infarction: a systematic review and meta-analysis. Clin Cardiol. 2019;42(10):889–98. https://doi.org/10.1002/clc.23238.

15. Go AS, Mozaffarian D, Roger VL, et al. Heart disease and stroke statistics—2014 update. Circulation. 2014;129(3):28. https://doi.org/10.1161/01.cir.0000441139.02102.80.

16. Graham G. Racial and ethnic differences in acute coronary syndrome and myocardial infarction within the United States: from demographics to outcomes. Clin Cardiol. 2016;39(5):299–306. https://doi.org/10.1002/clc.22524.

17. Lanza GA. Ethnic variations in acute coronary syndromes. Heart. 2004;90(6):595–7. https://doi.org/10.1136/hrt.2003.026476.

18. Shrank WH, Rogstad TL, Parekh N. Waste in the US health care system. JAMA. 2019;322(15):1501. https://doi.org/10.1001/jama.2019.13978.

19. Historical. CMS. https://www.cms.gov/Research-Statistics-Data-and-Systems/Statistics-Trends-and-Reports/NationalHealthExpendData/NationalHealthAccountsHistorical. Accessed December 15, 2020.

20. Sawyer B, Cox C. How does health spending in the U.S. compare to other countries? 2018. https://www.healthsystemtracker.org/chart-collection/health-spending-u-s-compare-countries/. Accessed December 22, 2020.

21. National Health Expenditure Projections 2018-2027. 2020. https://www.cms.gov/Research-Statistics-Data-and-Systems/Statistics-Trends-and-Reports/NationalHealthExpendData/Downloads/ForecastSummary.pdf. Accessed December 15, 2020.

22. Kamal R. How has U.S. spending on healthcare changed over time? 2020. https://www.healthsystemtracker.org/chart-collection/u-s-spending-healthcare-changed-time/. Accessed December 22, 2020.

23. Miller C, Granger C. Evaluation of emergency department patients with chest pain at low or intermediate risk for acute coronary syndrome. UpToDate. https://www.uptodate.com/contents/evaluation-of-emergency-department-patients-with-chest-pain-at-low-or-intermediate-risk-for-acute-coronary-syndrome. Accessed December 15, 2020.

24. Ko DT, Dattani ND, Austin PC, et al. Emergency department volume and outcomes for patients after chest pain assessment. Circulation. 2018;11(11):004683. https://doi.org/10.1161/circoutcomes.118.004683.

25. Canivell S, Muller O, Gencer B, et al. Prognosis of cardiovascular and non-cardiovascular multimorbidity after acute coronary syndrome. PLoS One. 2018;13(4):0195174. https://doi.org/10.1371/journal.pone.0195174.

26. Turpie AGG. Burden of disease: medical and economic impact of acute coronary syndromes. Am J Manag Care. 2006;2006:S430–4.

27. Zhao Z, Winget M. Economic burden of illness of acute coronary syndromes: medical and productivity costs. BMC Health Serv Res. 2011;11(1):35. https://doi.org/10.1186/1472-6963-11-35.

28. Yau AA, Nguyendo LT, Lockett LL, Michaud E. The HEART pathway and hospital cost savings. Crit Pathw Cardiol. 2017;16(4):126–8. https://doi.org/10.1097/hpc.0000000000000124.

29. Kea B, Manning V, Alligood T, Raitt M. A review of the relationship of atrial fibrillation and acute coronary syndrome. Curr Emerg Hospl Med Rep. 2016;4(3):107–18. https://doi.org/10.1007/s40138-016-0105-2.

30. Ii RP, Nair K, Ghushchyan V. Indirect and direct costs of acute coronary syndromes with comorbid atrial fibrillation, heart failure, or both. Vasc Health Risk Manag. 2014;25:72331. https://doi.org/10.2147/vhrm.s72331.

31. Jan S, Lee SW-L, Sawhney JPS, et al. Predictors of high-cost hospitalization in the treatment of acute coronary syndrome in Asia: findings from EPICOR Asia. BMC Cardiovasc Disord. 2018;18(1):139. https://doi.org/10.1186/s12872-018-0859-4.

32. Borawski JB, Graff LG, Limkakeng AT. Care of the patient with chest pain in the observation unit. Emerg Med Clin North Am. 2017;35(3):535–47. https://doi.org/10.1016/j.emc.2017.03.003.

33. Stopyra J, Snavely AC, Hiestand B, et al. Comparison of accelerated diagnostic pathways for acute chest pain risk stratification. Heart. 2020;106(13):977–84. https://doi.org/10.1136/heartjnl-2019-316426.

34. Asher E, Reuveni H, Shlomo N, et al. Clinical outcomes and cost effectiveness of accelerated diagnostic protocol in a chest pain center compared with routine care of patients with chest pain. PLoS One. 2015;10(1):0117287. https://doi.org/10.1371/journal.pone.0117287.

35. Weinstock MB, Weingart S, Orth F, et al. Risk for clinically relevant adverse cardiac events in patients with chest pain at hospital admission. JAMA Intern Med. 2015;175(7):1207. https://doi.org/10.1001/jamainternmed.2015.1674.

36. Riley RF, Miller CD, Russell GB, et al. Cost analysis of the history, ECG, age, risk factors, and initial troponin (HEART) pathway randomized control trial. Am J Emerg Med. 2017;35(1):77–81. https://doi.org/10.1016/j.ajem.2016.10.005.

37. Poldervaart JM, Reitsma JB, Backus BE, et al. Effect of using the HEART score in patients with chest pain in the emergency department. Ann Intern Med. 2017;166(10):689. https://doi.org/10.7326/m16-1600.

38. Nieuwets A, Poldervaart JM, Reitsma JB, et al. Medical consumption compared for TIMI and HEART score in chest pain patients at the emergency department: a retrospective cost analysis. BMJ Open. 2016;6(6):e010694. https://doi.org/10.1136/bmjopen-2015-010694.

39. Field JL. Economics of chest pain centers: what really matters? Clin Ther. 1995;14:68.

40. Barr R. Society of chest pain centers heart attack care in the United States. Crit Pathw Cardiol. 2011;10(4):193–4. https://doi.org/10.1097/hpc.0b013e3182347e66.

41. McCarthy BD, Beshansky JR, D'Agostino RB, et al. Missed diagnoses of acute myocardial infarction in the emergency department: results from a multi-center study. Ann Emerg Med. 1993;22:579–82.

42. Sun BC, McCreath H, Liang LJ, et al. Randomized clinical trial of an emergency department observation syncope protocol versus routine inpatient admission. Ann Emerg Med. 2014;64:167–75.
43. Ross MA, Hockenberry JM, Mutter R, Barrett M, Wheatley M, Pitts SR. Protocol-driven emergency department observation units offer savings, shorter stays, and reduced admissions. Health Aff. 2013;32(12):2149–56. https://doi.org/10.1377/hlthaff.2013.0662.
44. Baugh CW, Venkatesh AK, Bohan JS. Emergency department observation units: a clinical and financial benefit for hospitals. Health Care Manag Rev. 2011;36:28–37.
45. Baugh CW, Venkatesh AK, Hilton JA, Samuel PA, Schuur JD, Bohan JS. Making greater use of dedicated hospital observation units for many short-stay patients could save $3.1 billion a year. Health Aff. 2012;31:2314–23.
46. Doyle BJ, Ettner SL, Nuckols TK. Supplemental insurance reduces out-of-pocket costs in medicare observation services. J Hosp Med. 2016;11(7):502–4. https://doi.org/10.1002/jhm.2588.
47. Adrion ER, Kocher KE, Nallamothu BK, Ryan AM. Rising use of observation care among the commercially insured may lead to total and out-of-pocket cost savings. Health Aff. 2017;36(12):2102–9. https://doi.org/10.1377/hlthaff.2017.0774.
48. Hospital inpatient and outpatient services. MedPAC. 2019. http://www.medpac.gov/docs/default-source/reports/mar19_medpac_ch3_sec.pdf. Accessed December 15, 2020.
49. Wright S. Memorandum report: hospitals' use of observation stays and short inpatient stays for medicare beneficiaries, OEI-02-12-00040. Department of Health and Human Services, Office of Inspector General. 2013.
50. Aalam AA, Alsabban A, Pines JM. National trends in chest pain visits in US emergency departments (2006–2016). Emerg Med J. 2020;37(11):696–9. https://doi.org/10.1136/emermed-2020-210306.
51. Ii RP, Ghushchyan V, Bos JVD, et al. The cost of inpatient death associated with acute coronary syndrome. Vasc Health Risk Manag. 2016;13:94026. https://doi.org/10.2147/vhrm.s94026.
52. Khera R, Valero-Elizondo J, Okunrintemi V, et al. Association of out-of-pocket annual health expenditures with financial hardship in low-income adults with atherosclerotic cardiovascular disease in the United States. JAMA Cardiol. 2018;3(8):729. https://doi.org/10.1001/jamacardio.2018.1813.
53. Bularga A, Lee KK, Stewart S, et al. High-sensitivity troponin and the application of risk stratification thresholds in patients with suspected acute coronary syndrome. Circulation. 2019;140(19):1557–68. https://doi.org/10.1161/circulationaha.119.042866.
54. Peacock WF, Baumann BM, Bruton D, et al. Efficacy of high-sensitivity Troponin T in identifying very-low-risk patients with possible acute coronary syndrome. JAMA Cardiol. 2018;3(2):104. https://doi.org/10.1001/jamacardio.2017.4625.
55. Kaambwa B, Ratcliffe J, Horsfall M, et al. Cost effectiveness of high-sensitivity troponin compared to conventional troponin among patients presenting with undifferentiated chest pain: a trial based analysis. Int J Cardiol. 2017;238:144–50. https://doi.org/10.1016/j.ijcard.2017.02.141.
56. Jülicher P, Greenslade JH, Parsonage WA, Cullen L. The organisational value of diagnostic strategies using high-sensitivity troponin for patients with possible acute coronary syndromes: a trial-based cost-effectiveness analysis. BMJ Open. 2017;7(6):e013653. https://doi.org/10.1136/bmjopen-2016-013653.
57. Min JK, Gilmore A, Budoff MJ, Berman DS, O'Day K. Cost-effectiveness of coronary CT angiography versus myocardial perfusion SPECT for evaluation of patients with chest pain and no known coronary artery disease. Radiology. 2010;254(3):801–8. https://doi.org/10.1148/radiol.09090349.
58. Nakanishi R, Budoff MJ. A new approach in risk stratification by coronary CT angiography. Forensic Sci. 2014;2014:1–10. https://doi.org/10.1155/2014/278039.

59. May JM, Shuman WP, Strote JN, et al. Low-risk patients with chest pain in the emergency department: negative 64-MDCT coronary angiography may reduce length of stay and hospital charges. Am J Roentgenol. 2009;193(1):150–4. https://doi.org/10.2214/ajr.08.2021.
60. Halpern EJ, Savage MP, Fischman DL, Levin DC. Cost-effectiveness of coronary CT angiography in evaluation of patients without symptoms who have positive stress test results. Am J Roentgenol. 2010;194(5):1257–62. https://doi.org/10.2214/ajr.09.3209.
61. Hegde VA, Biederman RW, Mikolich JR. Cardiovascular magnetic resonance imaging—incremental value in a series of 361 patients demonstrating cost savings and clinical benefits: an outcome-based study. Clin Med Insights. 2017;11:117954681771002. https://doi.org/10.1177/1179546817710026.
62. Boldt J, Leber AW, Bonaventura K, et al. Cost-effectiveness of cardiovascular magnetic resonance and single-photon emission computed tomography for diagnosis of coronary artery disease in Germany. J Cardiovasc Magn Reson. 2013;15(1):30. https://doi.org/10.1186/1532-429x-15-30.
63. Kozor R, Walker S, Parkinson B, et al. Cost-effectiveness of cardiovascular magnetic resonance in diagnosing coronary artery disease in the Australian Health Care System. Heart Lung Circ. 2020;30(3):380–7. https://doi.org/10.1016/j.hlc.2020.07.008.
64. Walker S, Girardin F, Mckenna C, et al. Cost-effectiveness of cardiovascular magnetic resonance in the diagnosis of coronary heart disease: an economic evaluation using data from the CE-MARC study. Heart. 2013;99(12):873–81. https://doi.org/10.1136/heartjnl-2013-303624.
65. Pena ME, Pearson CL, Goulet MP, et al. A 90-second magnetocardiogram using a novel analysis system to assess for coronary artery stenosis in Emergency department observation unit chest pain patients. IJC Heart Vasc. 2020;26:100466. https://doi.org/10.1016/j.ijcha.2019.100466.
66. Li Y, Che Z, Quan W, Yong R. Diagnostic outcomes of magnetocardiography in patients with coronary artery disease. Int J Clin Exp Med. 2015;8(2):2441–6.
67. Madsen T, Mallin M, Bledsoe J, et al. Utility of the emergency department observation unit in ensuring stress testing in low-risk chest pain patients. Crit Pathw Cardiol. 2009;8(3):122–4. https://doi.org/10.1097/hpc.0b013e3181b00782.
68. Mensah GA, Wei GS, Sorlie PD, et al. Decline in cardiovascular mortality. Circ Res. 2017;120(2):366–80. https://doi.org/10.1161/circresaha.116.309115.

# Reimbursement Considerations: Chest Pain Observation


**Michael A. Granovsky**


## 1 Chest Pain Observation: Professional Reimbursement Considerations

Physician documentation, coding requirements, and reimbursement realities for chest pain observation units have been an area of great confusion in the past. This section will attempt to provide clarity and simplification of the seemingly complex reimbursement process. At a high level, chest pain observation unit patients receive physician's services during their stay including evaluation and management services as well as diagnostic services.

## 2 General Physician Documentation Requirements

The Centers for Medicare and Medicaid Services (CMS) defines observation care as "A well-defined set of specific, clinically appropriate services, which include ongoing short term treatment, assessment, and reassessment, that are furnished while a decision is being made regarding whether patients will require further treatment as hospital inpatients or if they are able to be discharged from the hospital" [1].

Observation is an outpatient service and, using Medicare as an example, falls under Medicare part B. AMA CPT codes are used to describe cognitive and diagnostic services provided to chest pain observation services. CMS states, "In only rare and exceptional cases do reasonable and necessary outpatient observation services span more than 48 h. In the majority of cases, the decision whether to


M. A. Granovsky (✉)
LogixHealth, Bedford, MA, USA
e-mail: mgranovsky@logixhealth.com



M. Pena et al. (eds.), *Short Stay Management of Chest Pain*, Contemporary
Cardiology, https://doi.org/10.1007/978-3-031-05520-1_3

discharge a patient from the hospital following resolution of the reason for the observation care or to admit the patient as an inpatient can be made in less than 48 h, usually in less than 24 h" [1]. Over a period of 24–48 h, patients may receive services that take place over three or more calendar days. The current procedural terminology (CPT) code sets include the ability to report multiple calendar day stays.

Additionally, with respect to the physician billing requirements, Medicare provides the following instruction: "For a physician to bill observation care codes, there must be a medical observation record for the patient which contains dated and timed physician's orders regarding the observation services the patient is to receive, nursing notes, and progress notes prepared by the physician while the patient received observation services" [1].

The CMS and CPT requirements are summarized below and include:

- A dated and timed order to place the patient in observation.
- The medical record should also contain a risk stratification statement and brief plan that demonstrates the medical necessity for the observation stay.

***Example*** *A 39-year-old female presents with vague chest pain. Will place in chest pain unit for ACS evaluation protocol including serial cardiac enzymes and stress test in the morning.*

- Progress notes demonstrating periodic assessments. Of note, there is currently not a minimum number of required progress notes. The progress note entries should reflect the variability in the patient's clinical course. A straight forward rule out ACS patient would have fewer progress notes than a patient who had a more complicated course.

***Example*** *A 57-year-old male placed in chest pain unit to rule out ACS:*

*9:00: No chest pain, first troponin normal, resting comfortably. RR 20 O2 saturation 97%.*

*12:00: Called to see patient for headache. BP noted 194/110. No chest pain. EKG normal. Patient had missed his BP meds this morning prior to coming to the hospital. Daily medications updated and provided.*

*17:00: Headache resolved. BP 160/78. Second troponin normal.*


## 3  Calendar Day Coding Scenarios

One of the more confusing aspects related to observation services is the seemingly myriad of coding scenarios relating to the timing of a patient's observation care (Table 1). This discussion will attempt to simplify the scenarios using the following two broad constructs:

1. All the care takes place on one calendar day.
2. The care spans more than one calendar day.

**Table 1** Examples of coding single and multiple calendar day stays in chest pain observation unit

| Observation complexity | Care all on the same day | Care covers 2 days | Care covers 3 days |
| --- | --- | --- | --- |
| Low | 99234 | 99218 + 99217 | 99218 + 99224 + 99217 |
| Moderate | 99235 | 99219 + 99217 | 99219 + 99225 + 99217 |
| High | 99236 | 99220 + 99217 | 99220 + 99226 + 99217 |

## 4  Chest Pain Observation: Admitted and Discharged on the Same Day

For example, the patient is placed in observation at 8 AM and discharged home at 8 PM the same day. There are three codes for reporting when the patient is admitted and discharged from observation on the same day.

- 99234: Low complexity
- 99235: Moderate complexity
- 99236: High complexity

The following relative value update committee (RUC) vignette is particularly relevant for chest pain observation units and provides a sense of the complexity of chest pain unit patients.

*RUC Vignette*  99236—A 52-year-old patient comes to the ED because of chest pain. The patient is admitted for observation and discharged later on the same day.

## 5  Medicare Time Requirements for 99234–99236

Importantly, Medicare requires 8 h of care to report the same day observation code set 99234–99236. "When a patient receives observation care for less than 8 h on the same calendar date, the Initial Observation Care, from CPT code range 99218–99220, shall be reported by the physician. The Observation Care Discharge Service, CPT code 99217, shall not be reported for this scenario" [1].

## 6  Chest Pain Observation: Admitted and Discharged on Different Calendar Days

For example, the patient is placed in observation at 8 PM on Monday and discharged home at 9 AM on Wednesday.

## 6.1 Day 1: The First Day

There are three codes for reporting the first day of observation for stays greater than 1 day:

- 99218: Low complexity
- 99219: Moderate complexity
- 99220: High complexity

## 6.2 The Middle Day(s)

There are three codes for reporting the middle days of observation for observation stays greater than 2 days:

- 99224: Low complexity
- 99225: Moderate complexity
- 99226: High complexity

Utilize 99224–99226 for observation care services provided on dates other than the initial or discharge date. These codes include reviewing the medical record and reviewing the results of diagnostic studies and changes in the patient's status since the last assessment by the physician.

## 6.3 The Discharge Day

There is one code for reporting the last day of observation for stays greater than 1 day:

- 99217: Observation care discharge
- 99217 Observation discharge management is reported for all services on the date of observation discharge and includes the following: a final examination, discussion of the observation stay, follow-up instructions, and documentation.
- 99217 (Observation discharge) is used for the management of care on the final day and is used in conjunction with CPT codes 99218–99220 and, if applicable, the middle day codes 99224–99226.

## 7 Evaluation and Management Service Documentation Requirements

Currently, chest pain observation unit documentation requirements are governed by the CMS and CPT rules which are in flux. For 2021 dates of service, the office visit codes 99201–99215 (not previously discussed) documentation requirements are governed by a collaborative effort between the AMA and CMS. Those updated office visit guidelines in future years may be applied to the observation codes.

However, currently, the 1995 CMS documentation guidelines as amended in 1997, along with CPT principles, typically determine the documentation requirements for chest pain observation patients.

Observation cases are scored primarily based on the key elements of the history, physical exam, and medical decision-making (Tables 2 and 3). With the exception of the lowest level of service, involving low complexity medical decision-making, observation services typically require a comprehensive history and physical examination.

## 8 Documentation Requirements 99218/99234 (Low Complexity Medical Decision-Making)

99218 and 99234 require a detailed history and examination which are further described in a more numeric fashion below:

- History of Present Illness: 4 elements
- Past, Family or Social History: 1 element
- Review of Systems: 2 systems
- Physical Exam 2-7 organ systems/body areas

## 9 Documentation Requirements 99219/99220/99235/99236 (Moderate and High Complexity MDM)

99219–99220 and 99235–99236 require a comprehensive and exam which are further described in a more numeric fashion below:

- History of present illness: 4 elements
- Past, family or social history: All 3 elements
- Review of systems: 10 systems
- Physical exam: 8 organ systems

**Table 2** Documentation requirements 99218–99220 and 99234–99236

| Level | HPI | ROS | PFSHx | PE | MDM |
| --- | --- | --- | --- | --- | --- |
| 99218/99234 | 4 | 2 | 1 | 2 | Low |
| 99219/99235 | 4 | 10 | 3 | 8 | Moderate |
| 99220/99236 | 4 | 10 | 3 | 8 | High |

Requires all three key components: history, exam, and medical decision-making

**Table 3** Documentation requirements summary 99224–99226

| Level | HPI | ROS | PFSHx | PE | MDM |
| --- | --- | --- | --- | --- | --- |
| 99224 | 1 | 0 | N/A | 1 | Low |
| 99225 | 1 | 1 | N/A | 2 | Moderate |
| 99226 | 4 | 2 | N/A | 2 | High |

Requires two of three key components: interval history, exam, and medical decision-making

## 10   Observation Services CPT Typical Times

CPT publishes typical times associated with observation services (Table 4). As part of the documentation guideline evolution mentioned earlier the office visit codes may be scored based on specifically time. It is possible that observation code assignment could also be based on a time component in the future and as such the published typical time values for the codes utilized in chest pain observation units are included below.

## 11   Chest Pain Observation Unit Reimbursement

Each CPT code is typically valued by the Relative Value Update Committee (RUC). Following an extensive survey and analysis process, the RUC assigns a number of relative value units (RVUs) to that specific code/service. CMS then applies certain technical adjustments, and each year publishes the RVUs assigned to each code. Using Medicare as an example, the RVU value is then multiplied by a published annual conversion factor (Medicare payment per RVU) to determine the final payment amount (Table 5).

**Table 4** Summary of CPT typical times associated with observation services

| CPT code | Typical CPT times (min) |
| --- | --- |
| 99218 | 30 |
| 99219 | 50 |
| 99220 | 70 |
| 99224 | 15 |
| 99225 | 25 |
| 99226 | 35 |
| 99234 | 40 |
| 99235 | 50 |
| 99236 | 55 |

**Table 5** RVUs and payment chest pain observation evaluation and management services

| Code | Total RVUs | Estimated payment ($) |
| --- | --- | --- |
| 99234 | 3.77 | 140 |
| 99235 | 4.77 | 175 |
| 99236 | 6.14 | 225 |
| 99224 | 1.12 | 40 |
| 99225 | 2.05 | 75 |
| 99226 | 2.95 | 110 |
| 99218 | 2.82 | 105 |
| 99219 | 3.83 | 140 |
| 99220 | 5.22 | 190 |
| 99217 | 2.05 | 75 |

In the scenario where a patient is admitted to observation on one day and discharged on the following day, the 99218–99220 codes will typically be assigned with the discharge code 99217. If the patient has a 3-day stay, the RVUs for day 1 (99218–99220), the middle day (99224–99226), and 99217 are added together to determine the final payment amount for the totality of the visit (Table 6).

## 12 Additional Diagnostic Services

Chest pain observation patients receive diagnostic testing in addition to the cognitive work reported using the observation evaluation management codes discussed above including EKGs, echocardiograms, chest X-rays (Table 7). The professional component of these services are also typically reported.

Chest pain observation services involve cognitive work represented by the CPT Evaluation and Management Codes. The specific codes chosen are dependent on the number of calendar days the patient spend in the chest pain unit, the history and physical examination documentation, and the complexity of Medical Decision-Making. Diagnostic studies, such as EKGs, are also reported. Each reported service has an assigned RVU value and corresponding payment amount. Attention to the professional side reimbursement detail is critical to ensuring the financial success of your unit.

**Table 6** Combined RVUs for chest pain observation multi day stays

| 2-Day stay: initial observation code + discharge code | RVUs | Combined RVUs |
|---|---|---|
| 99218 + 99217 | 2.82 + 2.05 | 4.87 |
| 99219 + 99217 | 3.83 + 2.05 | 5.88 |
| 99220 + 99217 | 5.22 + 2.05 | 7.27 |
| 3-Day stay initial observation code + middle day code + discharge code | RVUs | Combined RVUs |
| 99218 + 99224 + 99217 | 2.82 + 1.12 + 2.05 | 5.99 |
| 99219 + 99225+ 99217 | 3.83 + 2.05+ 2.05 | 7.93 |
| 99220 + 99226+ 99217 | 5.22 + 2.95+ 2.05 | 10.22 |

**Table 7** Example of professional diagnostic services performed in chest pain observation nits

| Description | CPT | Professional component RVUs | Approximate payment ($) |
|---|---|---|---|
| EKG | 93010 | 0.24 | 9 |
| Limited echocardiogram | 93308 | 0.73 | 26 |
| Central line | 36556 | 2.46 | 90 |
| Elective cardioversion | 92960 | 3.12 | 115 |

# Reference

1.  CMS Medicare Claims Processing Manual IOM Pub 100-04 30.6.8 A. Accessed July 13, 2020.

# Why Have Chest Pain Patients in a Short Stay Unit?

**Kushal Nandam and Michael Ross**

## 1  Background

Cardiovascular disease in the United States is one of the highest causes of mortality. The estimated prevalence of coronary heart disease is around 18 million Americans with a rate of about 6.7% of all adults [1]. The estimated direct and indirect cost of heart disease between 2014 and 2015 was $218.7 billion. Myocardial infarction (MI) and coronary heart disease (CHD) were two of the most expensive conditions treated in hospitals in 2013, roughly $12.1 and $9 billion, respectively [1]. In 2016, the number of inpatient hospital discharges was about 1.045 million unique hospitalizations for ACS. There were also 10 million visits every year in the ED with a chief complaint of chest pain [2]. From a glance at gross statistics, it is obvious that CHD has a profound impact on the health of patients, hospital resources utilized, and total financial cost on the healthcare system.

Chest pain is one of the most important chief complaints of a patient who presents to the Emergency Department (ED). It also involves some of the highest risk and highest acuity patients who present to the ED. Specifically, chest pain that involves coronary heart disease (CHD) is a complex decision-making process that can be a particularly difficult task to give a quick disposition. Emergency physicians (EPs) are the primary healthcare providers who sift, diagnose, and deliver appropriate care to the undifferentiated chest pain. Despite a number of tools, immediate diagnostic certainty can be elusive. It has been found that up to 8% of myocardial infarction patients can have a completely normal EKG, and less than half of AMI patients had positive diagnostic cardiac markers on arrival [3]. Chest pain also happens to be one of the highest legal risk of chief complaints to the emergency

K. Nandam · M. Ross (✉)
Emory University, Atlanta, GA, USA
e-mail: MAROSS@emory.edu



M. Pena et al. (eds.), *Short Stay Management of Chest Pain*, Contemporary
Cardiology, https://doi.org/10.1007/978-3-031-05520-1_4

department. Emergency physicians carried a 7.5% risk of litigation, annually [4]. In a 2010 study reviewing litigation in emergency departments, acute MI was found to be the top diagnosis of ED claims, with about 5% of the total claims and chest pain (unspecified) being 4%. For AMI, the average indemnity was roughly $245,000, and near the top of the list. Given the stakes, not only for patient outcomes, but also for protecting one's practice, it is clear that missed MI is a cause of high concern.

Coronary heart disease (CHD) constitutes the range from asymptomatic coronary artery disease (CAD) or CAD with stable angina to ACS, which includes unstable angina (UA) and acute MI (NSTEMI and STEMI). Coronary heart disease (CHD) manifesting as ACS, and in particular UA, is one of the most difficult chest pain diagnosis to select out for proper care. The diagnostic challenges has led to dramatic changes and testing in practices over the decades. The EKG was one of the first tools in the arsenal and is the standard initial evaluation for chest pain patients concerning for ACS. Laboratory diagnosis of ACS had advanced the field with cardiac biomarkers from CKMB to troponin and even high-sensitivity (hs) troponin. The options for noninvasive diagnostic testing started with the treadmill stress EKG and now have seen advances to stress echocardiography, nuclear medicine cardiac stress testing, sestamibi cardiac myocardial perfusion studies, and more recently coronary CT. Despite the advances in care, there are still a number of patients in whom it is difficult to create a quick snapshot diagnosis of ruling in or out ACS in the emergency department. This leads to further care and work-up beyond the ED, whether that is admitting the patient to the hospital or a short stay unit.

## 2   What Is a Short Stay Unit?

Observation medicine is a branch of medicine that takes care of patients who are too sick to go home but not sick enough to be admitted, or to determine their need for inpatient admission. CMS defines observation *services* as "outpatient care ordered by a physician and provided in a hospital bed" with a "well defined set of specific, clinically appropriate services, which includes ongoing short-term treatment, assessment and reassessment before a decision can be made regarding whether the patient will require further treatment as a hospital inpatient or if they are able to be discharged from the hospital" [5]. For the vast majority of patients, the decision to admit can be made within 48 hours and a large portion within 24 h [5].

Most observation patients enter the hospital through the emergency department [5]. The average emergency department length of stay of patients admitted to the hospital is 5 h. Subsequently, the average hospital inpatient length of stay is roughly 5 days. Hospital inpatient admissions with a length of stay less than 24 h are generally denied payment by health insurers as an "unnecessary inpatient admission." This creates a "6–24 h" orphan population of patients whose hospital needs are greater than 6 h, but less than 24 h. These "6–24 h patients" are generally managed using outpatient observation services. However, there is much variation in the hospital *settings* in which observation care is provided. The nomenclature used to

**Table 1** Hospital settings in which observation services are provided [6]

| Setting | Description | Characteristics |
| --- | --- | --- |
| Type 1 | Protocol driven, observation unit | Highest level of evidence for favorable outcomes<br>Care typically directed by ED |
| Type 2 | Discretionary care, observation unit | Care directed by a variety of specialists<br>Unit typically based in ED |
| Type 3 | Protocol driven, bed in any location | Often called a "virtual observation unit" |
| Type 4 | Discretionary care, bed in any location | Most common practice<br>Unstructured care<br>Poor alignment of resources with patients' needs |

describe these settings uses two variables: the use of a dedicated observation unit and the use of observation protocols. They are defined as type 1–4 settings (see Table 1). This chapter will focus on chest pain patients in a type 1 setting.

The type 1 setting is a protocol-driven observation unit, most commonly run by the emergency department [7]. These are typically the most efficient systems in delivering observation care because there are focused patient care goals, the staffing is aware of time constraints and urgency to having a quick disposition, and protocols are easily streamlined for specific chest pain complaints. The American College of Emergency Physicians' policy on the management of ED observation units states that this setting is a "best practice" for observation patients. It is one that requires a commitment of staff and resources. A number of terms are used by hospitals to describe these units that include Observation Unit (OU), Emergency Department Observation Unit (EDOU), Clinical Decision Unit (CDU), Short Stay Unit (SSU), and Chest Pain Observation Unit (CPOU). The majority of observation services are delivered by either internists or emergency medicine departments.

Type 2 setting is Discretionary Observation Unit, typically in the ED, where specialists direct care. Type 3 a virtual observation unit where patients can be placed anywhere in the hospital among admitted patients, but have protocol-derived care. Type 4 setting of observation care is for patients who obtain unstructured care in any hospital bed and is discretionary to the physician who takes care of them.

## 3  Why Have Short Stay Units?

Short Stay Units have been becoming more prevalent and established as essential cogs in the healthcare system. These units have allowed physicians to decrease diagnostic uncertainty when evaluating patients for ACS. They allow hospitals to efficiently care for patients with rapid diagnostic testing and turnaround times, with safe discharges. In terms of efficient care, structured-protocol-based OUs (type 1) have reportedly shown a cost savings of 27–42% relative to traditional inpatient care [6]. The length-of-stay in type 1 units is half that of inpatient settings [6]. It has been estimated that type 1 OUs could save the US health system between $5.5 billion and 8.5 billion annually [6]. The growth of Observation Medicine accelerated treatment protocols has been proven effective for other conditions, including asthma, syncope, TIA, and atrial fibrillation, and congestive heart failure [7]. Baugh et al. estimated that with general expansion of observation units, "the average cost savings per patient would be $1572, annual hospital savings would be $4.6 million, ad national cost savings would be $3.1 billion" [8]. By having a carefully selected group of patients treated in EDOUs, patients can avoid an inpatient admission. This allows the medical system to have shorter length of stay, improved resource utilization, and decreased patient costs without sacrificing outcomes.

## 4   Which Chest Pain Patients Should Go to SSU?

Patients should be appropriately selected to go to the SSU. First, all adult patients evaluated in the ED with undifferentiated chest pain with a concern of ACS should have essential diagnostic information. This includes an EKG, medical history and family medical history, appropriate physical examination, as well as laboratory tests which include cardiac marker (troponin). Once this information has been gathered, patients can be risk stratified based on a number of scoring systems as well as tri-aged into a protocol. Patients identified as low risk can be discharged from the ED. The patients that have clearly demonstrated signs of ACS such as STEMI and NSTEMI or very high risk of UA should be admitted to the hospital for further extensive management. It is this last group of undifferentiated patients that are in the middle that would most benefit admission to an SSU. They are higher risk based on scoring factors from history, but do not have clear concrete evidence of ACS on EKG and troponin, but would necessitate further testing.

In appropriately choosing the patients for a chest pain protocol for SSUs, one must first appropriately screen out low-risk patients who can be discharged from the ED. Over the past few decades, several risk stratification tools have been developed to achieve this and include the ADAPT, EDACS, and HEART scores. The HEART score has become one of the more commonly used tools [9]. ACEP Chest Pain Policy committee suggests that a missed diagnosis rate of $\leq 1\%$ for 30-day MACE is acceptable. Using the HEART score, patients with a score 3 or less has been stud-ied to have a MACE of 0.9–1.7% [2]. Scores are taken one step further in what is called "pathways." For example, the "HEART Pathway" involves combining a HEART score with repeat troponins over time. The HEART Pathway is a validated decision tool established to identify which low-risk patients can be discharged from the ED with low MACE [10]. It combines the HEART score and a 0 and 3 h tropo-nin lab testing to risk stratify patients. It has been shown to provide better sensitivity and negative predicted value than the HEART score alone. Other scoring pathways include the ADAPT and EDACS decision tools. A 2016 study showed that they both had high sensitivity for MACE, but HEART pathway was able to stratify a higher portion of percent of patients as low risk and safe for early discharge [11, 12]. A 2019 study of the HEART Pathway in the ED beyond just discharged patients and did show reduced inpatient and stress testing, thus conserving resources without worsening 30 days MACE [13].

When these low-risk patients are discharged, evidence also suggests that there is no benefit of early stress testing within 72 h [14]. Original ACC recommendations have recommended patients discharged with ED with need of stress testing (ordered by ED) have it done within 3 days. One study showed patients discharged with a recommendation for outpatient testing, only 30% completed it within 3 days, and 10% did not complete it within 30 days. MACE over these 30 days in this study was low with AMI at 0.7% and revascularization at 0.3% with no deaths.

The most obvious patients that should be admitted to the hospital and not go to an SSU, are high risk patients diagnosed with Acute MI (STEMI and NSTEMI) patients. Patients with EKG findings of ST elevation MI generally need immediate reperfusion with PCI (or tPA depending on circumstances). Their severity of illness and intensity of service needs exceed what is appropriate for a SSU setting. Beyond immediate intervention, these patients often will have further evaluation with echocardiograms, medication titration, and cardiac rehab therapy that requires greater than the two midnights of observation. Management of ACS in NSTEMI patients often requires patients on 48 hours of anticoagulation, trending cardiac markers, and continual assessment for the need for PCI which also would not fit criteria of being within the time period of observation care.

This leaves a group of patients who fall between "very low risk" and "high risk" of ACS. These are hemodynamically stable patients with no acute ischemic EKG changes and negative troponins. They have a concerning story for ACS and commonly fall into a HEART score of 4–6. In this range, a validation of the HEART score showed a MACE of 16.6% at 30 days [15], which would be a higher number than most EPs would feel comfortable discharging, without reliable follow-up short-term follow-up or clear shared decision-making. Patients in this group bound for an SSU could even have a HEART score of 7 with negative troponins, but with nonspecific EKG changes that could increase MACE to 50–65% (captured by any HEART score greater than 7). Some would argue that an EP could place these patients in the SSU for continued monitoring, provided they no longer had chest pain. These patients may benefit with a cardiology consultation in conjunction with their SSU placement in the direction of decision of which imaging modality to consider. The HEART Pathway broadly defined patients as high risk if they didn't fall in the low-risk category, with a HEART score of greater than or equal to 4, and then differentiated patients based on troponin results [10]. Those patients were placed in the SSU or inpatient unit for further imaging/testing.

## 5 Why Chest Pain Patients Should Be in Short Stay Unit

A patient presentation of chest pain is a notoriously high-risk medical concern and risk that providers routinely face in the emergency department. For patients, chest pain represents the fear of a heart attack. Acute coronary syndrome, in particular, is the diagnosis that one would like to ideally rule in or out completely. However, despite many advances in diagnostics, research, and technology, it is difficult to make an immediate diagnosis. The ultimate goals of selecting the right chest pain patients for an SSU would be to decrease risk of MACE in discharged patients, increase efficiency from a length of stay and resource utilization, and appropriately admit ACS patients.

When creating an SSU with chest pain protocols, there needs to be essential components to be a part of the pathway. First is the right patient selection. As stated before, those patients who have intermediate risk of ACS have not been definitely ruled out, with an initial evaluation of higher than 2% risk of MACE at 30 days from the ED visit. Having an SSU does not meet all chest pain patients should be placed in there. Low-risk patients should be discharged because they are too low risk that any extra care would likely not lead to any benefits and potential harm.

The essential components of an SSU chest pain protocol include appropriate patient selection, serial troponin and EKG testing, cardiac telemetry, and cardiac imaging. The final disposition of these patients during their observation period will be determined by the results of these tests. The CHEER study established a baseline for SSU protocols including minimum of 6 hours stay, serial cardiac enzymes, administration of aspirin, and advanced cardiac testing. If patients had negative testing, they were discharged. If they had positive findings of positive biomarkers or concerning findings on advanced cardiac testing, they were admitted [16, 17].

The first diagnostic component of chest pain patients in an SSU is to have serial troponin and EKGs during the stay. Cardiac troponins should be drawn at 3- and 6-h intervals for patients with suspicion of ACS and beyond 6 h after onset of symptoms if EKG changes are noted with negative troponins on initially evaluation (ACC).

The second important diagnostic component for chest pain patients in the SSU is imaging or provocative testing. Per the ACC guidelines, the "goals of noninvasive testing in patients with low or intermediate" risk of CAD are "to detect ischemia and estimate prognosis" [18]. The timing for patients with UA would be those that are asymptomatic and clinically stable at 12–24 h [18]. In addition to this, there are contraindications of stress testing that EPs keep in mind when ordering testing such as AMI within 2 days, high-risk unstable angina, uncontrolled arrhythmia, symptomatic severe aortic stenosis, uncontrolled heart failure, acute PE, myocarditis, pericarditis, endocarditis, aortic dissection (acute), active concurring medical issue such as sepsis [19].

Historically the main modality of additional testing to rule out ACS has traditionally been the stress treadmill EKG because of "its simplicity, lower cost, and widespread familiarity with its performance and interpretation" [18]. During this test, patients are required to increase their metabolic rate by engaging in strenuous activity (i.e., treadmill) and observe serial EKGs to assess for dynamic or ischemic changes. To select this test, the patient must be able to exercise to a reasonable degree and the baseline EKG must be free of resting ST changes (baseline ST abnormalities, Left Bundle Branch Blocks, LV hypertrophy with ST-T changes, intraventricular conduction defect, paced rhythms, pre-excitation, and digoxin) [18]. These restrictions do limit the patient population and should undergo other testing if they do not fall in the above requirements. If patients are able to exercise, but have ST changes on resting EKG, stress testing a patient with additional component of imaging modality should be used (i.e., transthoracic echocardiogram) [18]. Exercise echocardiography, even in the absence of abnormal baseline EKG, can add prognostic information (compared to EKG) as well as has a higher specificity to testing, giving the test an advantage. One recent study in Europe compared exercise echo vs exercise EKG with suspected ACS in SSU. The results showed incremental prognostic information and higher net clinical benefits [20]. Regardless, a negative stress EKG had very favorable outcomes with one meta-analysis result showing "the annual risk of cardiac death or myocardial infarction with normal exercise echocardiography was 0.54%" [21].

Over the years, as patient population has become more sedentary and more complex pathology, there has been an increased need for further advanced imaging options. In patients who are unable to exercise, patients must be induced to achieve an adequate heart rate, typically by pharmacological methods to get adequate results. Stress agents include vasodilators (adenosine, dipyrimadole, and regadensone) and positive chronotropes (dobutamine). Stress agents are often combined with nuclear imaging modalities. This includes myocardial perfusion imaging (MPI) with Sestamibi (MIBI) isotopes using Single Photon Emission Computer Tomography (SPECT) cameras or Rubidium isotopes with Positron Emission Tomography (PET) imaging cameras.

As seen here, there are a number of cardiac imaging modalities to assess the risk for ACS. Generally, the absence of inducible ischemia on negative stress testing and imaging is associated with low risk of 30-day MACE. In patients with intermediate risk of ACS, a normal MPI with MIBI testing was found to have a MACE of 3% at 30 days in a 2002 trial [22]. One meta-analysis "reported that normal images by both techniques accurately identify low-risk patients: annualized risk of cardiac death or myocardial infarction by SPECT, 0.45%; and by echocardiography, 0.54%" [21]. Patients who are found to have normal MPI or stress testing can be comfortably discharged as risk of ACS has been better defined and MACE determined to be sufficiently low enough.

A newer imaging modality has been coronary CT angiogram (cCTA). CT coronary studies have allowed more rapid assessment and a high negative predictive value. Hoffman compared early CCTA vs standard of care for chest pain and showed that length of stay was reduced by 7.6 h relative to standard care. Patients were discharged at a rate of 47% vs 12% in standard of care [23]. They reported that about 50% of the patients in the CCTA group were discharged within 8.6 h of presentation. However, there was a significant increase in diagnostic testing with the CCTA group, and a nonsignificant increase in the rate of invasive coronary angiography in the intermediate risk patients with CCTA group (11%) versus non-CCTA group (7%). Follow-up studies also showed durable safety in the rule outs. CT coronary angiogram also provided significant prognostic value over time to rule out significant ACS over a year. In a later study, in patients that were at low and moderate risk with chest pain, they were randomized between traditional care and CT coronary and those that had a negative coronary CT result had a low rate of cardiac death, AMI, or revascularization and had no statistical difference compared to standard of care [24]. Another argument for opting to use CCTA could be long-term benefits of finding non-intervenable atherosclerosis for early medical treatment. In the recently published SCOT-HEART trial, the "use of CTA in addition to standard of care in patients with stable chest pain resulted in a significantly lower rate of death from CHD or nonfatal MI at 5 years than standard of care alone" without increase in coronary angiography or revascularization [25]. The rate was about 1.6% lower than standard therapy; however, all-cause mortality did not change. The researchers suggested that the potential difference in CHD-related mortality was most likely secondary to additional changes in preventative treatment for coronary artery disease.

## 6 Improved Outcomes

There are a number of benefits for having chest pain patients evaluated in an SSU. These include lower hospital length of stay, lower costs for all stakeholders, improved resource allocation, and improved satisfaction for both EPs and patients.

SSU for chest pain allows for streamlined, focused protocols that allow us to answer specific question: "Can we rule out AMI?" First of all, the safety and efficacy of chest pain units have been established. The CHEER study randomized patients with chest pain and an intermediate risk of cardiovascular events to a CPU vs admission (standard of care). In this study, Farkouh found the MACE rate of both populations was equal at 6 months, with reduced use of resources without increasing adverse outcomes [16]. A subsequent analysis of the population in the CHEER study also showed no difference in primary outcomes (MI, death, CHF, stroke, or out of hospital cardiac arrest) for patients 5 years out between those assessed in the CPU vs admission [16, 17].

Hospitals are one large stakeholder that can benefit from a number of metrics by creating protocols for chest pain patients in an SSU. These include decreased resource utilization (inpatient beds and length of stay). The CHEPER study specifically addressed the resource allocation benefits of chest pain patients in observation units [26]. This study compared observation units with chest pain evaluations to prior studies on chest pain evaluation without the use of observation. The findings showed that 76% of these chest pain patients in observation units were discharged home without admission. The results also had a lower proportion of missed MIs (0.4 vs 4.5%) and had a final hospital admission rate that was lower. Further analysis showed that a higher portion of the patients had a "rule out MI" evaluation, which meant advanced diagnostic testing, despite lower length of stay. Another randomized control trial by Roberts et al. [27] measured a number of metrics with an ED-based accelerated diagnostic protocols (ADPs)/chest pain observation units vs inpatient admission. First, the hospital admission rates for ADPs were 45.2% vs 100% for control patients. The total cost per patient using ADPs was about $1528 vs $2085 in the control group, saving $567 per patient. The LOS was also significantly decreased by 11.3 h [27]. The primary benefit of decreased resource utilization of the hospital is though decreased length of stay. These and other studies show that a protocol-driven SSU can provide streamlined care, with higher specificity and lower readmit rates. EPs are cognizant about the risks that chest pain patients have, as well as being acutely aware of the limitation of resources available. Results of having quick turnaround times with diagnostic certainty allow EPs to have higher diagnostic comfort level as well as a higher satisfaction of safely discharging patients that are known to be low risk for AMI.

There are also patient-centered outcomes associated with SSUs, specifically in regard to chest pain patients. Rydman reported patient satisfaction of a CPU versus inpatient observation and found that patients evaluated in a CPU had higher levels for all satisfaction for all metrics measured [28]. The data suggested "that overall satisfaction was more strongly correlated with fewer problems in areas of communication" and other examples such as patient education and discharge preparation. With chest pain patients in a protocol-driven CPU, it is reasonable to see that a streamlined approach allows clearer communication with EPs, as well as clear patient education and discharge preparation because there is a standard structure to the process. Another small study in a hospital which compared observation patients in a dedicated OU vs a general inpatient bed also showed higher patient satisfaction scores [29]. This study also re-demonstrated that there was an improvement in communication with EPs. It can be difficult to assess the direct cost burden on patients in SSU versus inpatient stays because of differing insurance policies. An additional benefit to patients can potentially be cost savings. Medicare beneficiaries have had some concern because observation services are billed as outpatient services, and patients generally see a 20% co-pay for this. Despite this limitation, patients may see cost savings in SSU evaluations. One study looked at Medicare beneficiaries, and it showed Medicare observation copayments were generally lower by an average of $324 and 94% of observation co-pays lower than for inpatient care [6].

## 7    Conclusion

Chest pain patients are among the highest risk patients that enter the EDs today in terms of morbidity, finance, and liability. ED evaluations of a large percentage of these patients may not be able to immediately determine safely the requirement of inpatient care or safe discharge. Creating an SSU with chest pain protocols has been an incredible tool at the disposal of hospitals and EPs to help evaluate these patients. The evidence has consistently shown good outcomes with decreasing MACE of discharged patients and admitting appropriate patients to the inpatient units of hospitals. This has allowed improved length of stay, resource allocation, improved costs, and improved satisfaction among patients.

It is well known that healthcare expenditures are the largest portion of the US national GDP over the years, and it is increasing. Finding ways to improve cost and resource allocation is key to keep healthcare system solvent while improving care. Observation Units have been extremely useful in assisting to avoid costly inpatient stays. Further deploying SSUs for chest pain patients can further help the goal of improving allocation of care in the US healthcare system.

# References


1. Virani SS, et al. Heart disease and stroke statistics-2020 update: a report from the American Heart Association. Circulation. 2020;141(9):e139.
2. Tomaszewski CA, et al. Clinical policy: critical issues in the evaluation and management of emergency department patients with suspected non-ST-elevation acute coronary syndromes. Ann Emerg Med. 2018;72(5):e65–e106.
3. Wilkinson K, Severance H. Identification of chest pain patients appropriate for an emergency department observation unit. Emerg Med Clin North Am. 2001;19(1):35–66.
4. Ferguson B, et al. Malpractice in emergency medicine-a review of risk and mitigation practices for the emergency medicine provider. J Emerg Med. 2018;55(5):659–65.
5. Medicare benefit policy manual - chapter 6 - Hospital services covered under part B. 2020, pp. 20–21.
6. Ross MA, et al. Protocol-driven emergency department observation units offer savings, shorter stays, and reduced admissions. Health Aff. 2013;32(12):2149–56.
7. Ross MA, Granovsky M. History, principles, and policies of observation medicine. Emerg Med Clin North Am. 2017;35(3):503–18.
8. Baugh CW, et al. Making greater use of dedicated hospital observation units for many short-stay patients could save $3.1 billion a year. Health Aff. 2012;31(10):2314–23.
9. Mahler SA, et al. Can the HEART score safely reduce stress testing and cardiac imaging in patients at low risk for major adverse cardiac events? Crit Pathw Cardiol. 2011;10(3):128–33.
10. Mahler SA, et al. The HEART pathway randomized trial: identifying emergency department patients with acute chest pain for early discharge. Circ Cardiovasc Qual Outcomes. 2015;8(2):195–203.
11. Stopyra JP, et al. Chest pain risk stratification: a comparison of the 2-hour accelerated diagnostic protocol (ADAPT) and the HEART pathway. Crit Pathw Cardiol. 2016;15(2):46–9.
12. Stopyra JP, et al. Performance of the EDACS-accelerated diagnostic pathway in a cohort of US patients with acute chest pain. Crit Pathw Cardiol. 2015;14(4):134–8.
13. Sharp AL, et al. Effect of a HEART care pathway on chest pain management within an integrated health system. Ann Emerg Med. 2019;74(2):171–80.
14. Natsui S, et al. Evaluation of outpatient cardiac stress testing after emergency department encounters for suspected acute coronary syndrome. Ann Emerg Med. 2019;74(2):216–23.
15. Backus BE, et al. A prospective validation of the HEART score for chest pain patients at the emergency department. Int J Cardiol. 2013;168(3):2153–8.
16. Farkouh ME, et al. A clinical trial of a chest-pain observation unit for patients with unstable angina. N Engl J Med. 1998;339(26):1882–8.
17. Cullen MW, et al. Outcomes in patients with chest pain evaluated in a chest pain unit: the chest pain evaluation in the emergency room study cohort. Am Heart J. 2011;161(5):871–7.
18. Amsterdam EA, et al. 2014 AHA/ACC guideline for the management of patients with non-ST-elevation acute coronary syndromes: executive summary: a report of the American College of Cardiology/American Heart Association Task Force on Practice Guidelines. Circulation. 2014;130(25):2354–94.
19. Borawski JB, Graff LG, Limkakeng AT. Care of the patient with chest pain in the observation unit. Emerg Med Clin North Am. 2017;35(3):535–47.

20. Bouzas-Mosquera A, et al. Incremental value of exercise echocardiography over exercise electrocardiography in a chest pain unit. Eur J Intern Med. 2015;26(9):720–5.
21. Miller TD, Askew JW, Anavekar NS. Noninvasive stress testing for coronary artery disease. Cardiol Clin. 2014;32(3):387–404.
22. Udelson JE, et al. Myocardial perfusion imaging for evaluation and triage of patients with suspected acute cardiac ischemia: a randomized controlled trial. JAMA. 2002;288(21):2693–700.
23. Hoffmann U, et al. Coronary CT angiography versus standard evaluation in acute chest pain. N Engl J Med. 2012;367(4):299–308.
24. Hollander JE, et al. Coronary computed tomography angiography versus traditional care: comparison of one-year outcomes and resource use. Ann Emerg Med. 2016;67(4):460–8.
25. Newby DE, et al. Coronary CT angiography and 5-year risk of myocardial infarction. N Engl J Med. 2018;379(10):924–33.
26. Graff LG, et al. Impact on the care of the emergency department chest pain patient from the chest pain evaluation registry (CHEPER) study. Am J Cardiol. 1997;80(5):563–8.
27. Roberts RR, et al. Costs of an emergency department-based accelerated diagnostic protocol vs hospitalization in patients with chest pain: a randomized controlled trial. JAMA. 1997;278(20):1670.
28. Rydman RJ, et al. Patient satisfaction with an emergency department chest pain observation unit. Ann Emerg Med. 1997;29(1):109–15.
29. Plamann JM, Zedreck-Gonzalez J, Fennimore L. Creation of an adult observation unit: improving outcomes. J Nurs Care Qual. 2018;33(1):72–8.

# Value of Accreditation for Chest Pain Centers

Natalie Bracewell and David E. Winchester

## Abbreviations

| | |
|---|---|
| ACS | Acute coronary syndrome |
| ED | Emergency department |
| EMS | Emergency medical services |
| MI | Myocardial infarction |
| PCI | Percutaneous coronary intervention |
| STEMI | ST-elevation myocardial infarction |

The concept of a chest pain center dates back decades to Dr. Raymond Bahr and St. Agnes hospital in Baltimore, MD. In broadest terms, a chest pain center refers to a facility that has made special preparations to care for patients with acute chest pain syndromes, rapidly identifying and treating those with a coronary etiology. That may mean dedicated bed spaces, a stand-alone ward, or even a virtual unit where a specific care protocol is followed for chest pain patients who are intermixed with other patients. Because patients with chest pain syndromes receive care from a variety of clinicians, a multidisciplinary approach tends to produce the best outcomes. Chest pain is one of the most common presenting symptoms, and as such, care can be provided more efficiently when the work is standardized.

Nevertheless, many facilities face challenges in providing high-quality care for patients with acute chest pain syndromes. One potential solution which can help

N. Bracewell
Division of Cardiovascular Medicine, University of Florida College of Medicine, Gainesville, FL, USA

D. E. Winchester (✉)
Cardiology Section, Malcom Randall VAMC, Gainesville, FL, USA
e-mail: david.winchester@medicine.ufl.edu


M. Pena et al. (eds.), *Short Stay Management of Chest Pain*, Contemporary Cardiology, https://doi.org/10.1007/978-3-031-05520-1_5

facilities to navigate standardization of care, multidisciplinary collaboration, and a myriad of potential design elements is accreditation. If done earnestly and with buy-in from frontline clinicians, accreditation can raise the bar on the timeliness and quality of care, simultaneously giving patients greater satisfaction with the care they receive. In this chapter, we will discuss important structural and process elements of a comprehensive chest pain center and the ways that accreditation may benefit a facility, a healthcare system, and its surrounding community.

## 1 Accreditation Options

Multiple organizations offer accreditation or certification for comprehensive cardiac care as well as individual elements such as the coronary angiography suite, acute chest pain, heart failure, and others. Accreditation products differ in their cost, business model, level of engagement between the accreditation staff and facility personnel. Facility leadership needs to carefully select accreditation products that are best aligned with their interests and patient/staff needs. Below we describe some of the elements of a comprehensive accreditation system that addresses the management of acute chest pain from pre-hospital care through the transition back to primary/specialty care follow-up.

## 2 Facility Leadership

Chest pain center accreditation is typically a facility-wide designation and not something that an individual unit or clinical service line can accomplish in isolation. As such, strong facility leadership is a necessary part of a successful accreditation. Depending on the state of a facility's infrastructure, capital costs may be incurred that again would not typically be borne by any one service line's budgeting. Directives from the executive suite may be necessary in order to adequately engage staff from multiple service lines and to facilitate cooperation between groups that may not traditionally collaborate directly, such as frontline clinicians and physical plant staff or laboratory technologists.

Engagement with staff at all steps of patient care helps ensure that valuable input is not overlooked; a core principle of process improvement. Armed with comprehensive feedback on how to improve care, individual leaders must accept responsibility for crafting plans and putting them into action. Identifying specific individual physicians who can serve as champions for the accreditation process works to minimize the risk that responsibility for the process is not diffused to the point of being ineffective. Physician champions from emergency medicine and cardiology should be identified, although it would also be reasonable to include other services such as hospital/inpatient medicine. As an example of how accreditation drives these best practices, any facility could easily identify champions for the management of chest pain processes, but only about half do so prior to seeking accreditation [1]. The same analysis showed that only about half of facilities seeking accreditation had engagement with frontline clinical personnel and laboratory staff.

# 3  Community Outreach

Recognizing the benefit of early medical activation for heart attack care, some accreditation products require evidence of engagement with the communities that the facility inhabits: internal, external, or both. Often this consists of some assessment of community cardiovascular risk, identifying the highest risk subpopulations, and developing educational activities to try and reduce risk. This many take the form of screenings and wellness programs both for employees and with community partnered organizations. One effective method for community education on symptoms of myocardial infarction (MI) includes using the Early Heart Attack Care program which promotes self-awareness of early signs of impending heat attacks and encourages timely medical assessment and care.

# 4  Pre-hospital Care

While door-to-balloon time often dominates discussions of acute MI care, it does not capture all of the time important to optimizing patients' outcomes. As such, care of patients before they reach the hospital should be another focus of chest pain care and accreditation. For example, administration of aspirin prior to hospital admission in an acute MI is associated with improved mortality compared to those who received aspirin after admission [2]. A close working relationship with surrounding area emergency medical services (EMS) helps to increase compliance with these measures to improve patient outcomes.

EMS are a crucial part of the multidisciplinary approach of establishing an accredited chest pain center. As with the aforementioned physician champions, an EMS champion should be identified and encouraged to participate with the chest pain center leadership to optimize pre-hospital care for patients with suspected acute coronary syndrome (ACS). Programs such as Early Heart Attack Care also offer additional education. EMS staff should receive reports on success with practice recommendations and patient-specific feedback for critical patients requiring timely care for continued feedback and improvement.

## 5   Early Stabilization

According to the 2017 National Hospital Ambulatory Medical Care Surgery, the second leading symptom for patients presenting to the emergency department (ED) was chest pain and related symptoms with an estimated 6.5 million encounters, surpassed only by stomach and abdominal pain, cramps, and spasms [3]. Due to the high volume of patients with chest pain presenting to the ED but the two times increased mortality in a missed MI, an efficient system must be established [4]. Despite these widely known facts, a minority of facilities seeking accreditation have an adequately documented, facility-specific plan of care for ST-elevation MI (STEMI), even fewer had an agreed process on which patients qualify as "low-risk" for decision-making about early discharge, observation services, and outpatient follow-up [1].

Some physicians notoriously bristle at the notion of care protocols, deriding them as "cookbook medicine." While every patient clearly has unique factors to consider in their evaluation, the use of a protocol for early stabilization of those with chest pain may yield substantial benefits. Even the most fiercely autonomous physician would doubt the value of an early electrocardiogram (ECG) in these patients. Over a third of facilities seeking accreditation fail to perform and interpret an ECG within 10 minutes of arrival for chest pain patients despite the professional society recommendations to do so [1, 5].

These substantial gaps in early chest pain care may be reduced through accreditation. Specifically, as noted above, having physician champions responsible for action can help facilitate standardization of processes. Some facilities may achieve significant improvements through teamwork with the ECG technologists. Having the right partner can also help through collaboration with accreditation staff who have the experience of seeing how hundreds of other facilities around the country have developed and adopted care protocols.

Use of programs that have a pathway for triaging and managing patients with chest pain to reduce time to initial assessment and guide the next steps has proven to reduce hospitalizations and increase detection of ACS. One example is having patients who present to the ED with chest pain evaluated using the HEART score (history, ECG, age, risk factors, and initial troponin). Implementation of this scoring system may reduce hospitalizations by 6% while maintaining <1% of patients with a missed MI [6]. Accreditation helps with adoption of workflow guidelines similar to this, and paired with continual feedback of the compliance, and patient outcomes will continue to sharpen the initial stabilization and care path for chest pain patients in the ED.

Another early stabilization care process option is to establish a stand-alone chest pain unit. These units are designed for patients who are considered low risk for ACS but still need a brief evaluation period to minimize the likelihood of acute MI. Depending on the facility resources, these patients may be monitored on telemetry, have serial enzyme testing obtained, and undergo a stress test without using an acute care bed or having a prolonged stay in the ED. These processes are encouraged by most chest pain center accreditation products because multiple benefits have been observed including less missed MI, reduced costs, reduced length of stay and unneeded admissions, improved use of hospital resources, and fewer patients leaving without being evaluated in the ED [7, 8].

## 6    Acute Care

One area of CV care that most would likely agree benefits from a process-driven approach is for patients with an established ACS, specifically STEMI. Timely care is crucial for these patients, something we have known for decades. In GUSTO-IIb, delayed time to reperfusion or fibrinolytics in acute MI correlated with increased mortality [9]. Collaboration between Cardiology and ED staff, as well as the cardiac catheterization lab is required for shortened door-to-balloon times. Set protocols and resources brought to the institution by the chest pain center accreditation process can assist with communication and continual feedback to constantly improve the system. Required annual education with the staff as well as drills can help to hone these skills to be ready when a critically ill patient arrives.

Both time to procedure and prompt administration of medications are important for improving outcomes for acute coronary syndrome (ACS) patients. Multiple medications carry a class I indication including dual antiplatelet therapy, high-intensity statin, oral beta blocker, nitroglycerin if there is ongoing chest pain or hypertension, and systemic anticoagulation for non-STEMI patients. Due to the sheer number of medications recommended and need for rapid medical decision-making, it is very possible that there could be delays to medication administration in the ED. Accreditation as a chest pain center typically includes adoption of system enhancements, such as medication order sets, that reduce reliance on providers and improve standardized care of ACS patients [5, 10].

Some chest pain accreditation processes may encourage relationships between hospital centers or care networks. This can facilitate rapid transfer of critically ill patients requiring urgent percutaneous coronary intervention (PCI) or critical care post-MI. For STEMI patients who transfer from one hospital to another with a PCI-capable center, prolonged time spent at the initial hospital and delayed door-to-balloon times results in increased in-hospital mortality for those with delayed transfer and care [11]. Establishing transfer protocols between centers for patients can significantly reduce their time to intervention and therefore outcomes.

## 7    Transitions of Care

Outpatient follow-up after ACS is equally important as important in-hospital management. As just one example, from the PLATO study, patients with ACS on dual antiplatelet therapy still had around 11% incidence of re-infarction at 1 year [12]. In a study from Taiwan, 30-day readmission rates for NSTEMI patient were significantly less for patients who had 7-day outpatient follow-up with physicians than those who did not have close follow-up [13]. Close follow-up with a cardiologist is crucial for post-ACS patients to ensure medication optimization and continued assessment of symptoms. In a comprehensive chest pain center, the focus on patient care is not isolated to just the hospital stay itself but extends to after the patient is discharged. There are expectations for timely clinical follow-up and cardiac rehabilitation referrals, which help to improve outcomes and reduce readmissions. Despite clear value of close outpatient follow-up, only about half of accreditation-seeking facilities routinely refer patients to cardiac rehabilitation or have adequate discharge instructions on dosing and duration of cardiac medications; only 13% have a clear process on how to schedule outpatient stress testing [1].

## 8  Clinical Quality

Ultimately, the hope is that through better processes and reducing variation in care, that patients will experience improvement in clinical outcomes. For a variety of reasons, high-quality data showing improved outcomes with accreditation is limited. This is especially true in countries such as the US that do not have a national health database and where accrediting bodies have limited access to patient data for linkage to accreditation status. Starting more broadly, adherence to guidelines from professional societies on the management of ACS and STEMI is associated with reduced mortality. This was shown in a 2005 analysis from the CRUSADE registry where patient mortality was worst for the quartile of facilities with the lowest adherence to guidelines (6.31%) compared to the highest adherence quartile (4.15%, $P <$ 0.001) [14]. Ross et al. used data from the Medicare and Medicaid and found that compliance with core measures for acute MI was better at accredited chest pain centers. The metrics evaluated included aspirin on arrival, beta blocker on arrival, PCI <120 min after arrival, fibrinolytics <30 min after arrival, aspirin at discharge, beta blocker at discharge, angiotensin-converting enzyme inhibitor or angiotensin II receptor blocker at discharge, and smoking cessation counseling [15]. Together, these data suggest accreditation is a promising strategy to improve outcomes.

Other countries have databases suitable for investigating the clinical benefits of accreditation and have begun to do so. In China, a study evaluated 7-day in-hospital outcomes of acute MI patients before and after the hospitals had gone through the chest pain center accreditation process. This study showed that after accreditation, both major cardiac events (8.0% versus 6.7%, $p = 0.0003$) and mortality (1.6% versus 1.1%, $p = 0.021$) were reduced. This effect persisted with proportional hazard modeling (cardiac event hazard ratio 0.78, 95% confidence interval 0.68–0.91; mortality hazard ratio 0.71, 95% confidence interval 0.51–0.99) [16].

# 9   Conclusions

Accreditation in a chest pain center helps encourage clinicians to engage in best practices for patient care. Improvements are achieved through adoption of process improvement strategies, adherence to clinical guidelines, reducing unwanted variation in care, adoption of best practices demonstrated by other facilities, multidisciplinary teamwork, and a holistic approach that begins with prevention and ends after care has been transitioned to a long-term care provider. Data have shown substantial improvements in process measures, and emerging data are demonstrating reductions in important outcome measures including adverse cardiac events and mortality.

# References


1. Winchester DE, Osborne A, Peacock WF, et al. Closing gaps in essential chest pain care through accreditation. J Am Coll Cardiol. 2020;75(19):2478–82.
2. Barbash I, Freimark D, Gottlieb S, et al. Outcome of myocardial infarction in patients treated with aspirin is enhanced by pre-hospital administration. Cardiology. 2002;98(3):141–7.
3. US Department of Health and Human Services. National Hospital Ambulatory Medical Care Survey: 2017 Emergency Department Summary Tables. Centers for Disease Control and Prevention. Available at https://www.cdc.gov/nchs/ahcd/index.htm.
4. Pope JH, Aufderheide TP, Ruthazer R, et al. Missed diagnoses of acute cardiac ischemia in the emergency department. N Engl J Med. 2000;342(16):1163–70.
5. Amsterdam EA, Wenger NK, Brindis RG, et al. 2014 AHA/ACC guideline for the management of patients with non-ST-elevation acute coronary syndromes: executive summary: a report of the American College of Cardiology/American Heart Association Task Force on Practice Guidelines. Circulation. 2014;130(25):2354–94.
6. Mahler SA, Lenoir KM, Wells BJ, et al. Safely identifying emergency department patients with acute chest pain for early discharge. Circulation. 2018;138(22):2456–68.
7. Winchester DE, Stomp D, Shifrin RY, Jois P. Design and implementation of a stand-alone chest pain evaluation center within an academic emergency department. Crit Pathw Cardiol. 2012;11(3):123–7.
8. Storrow AB, Gibler WB. Chest pain centers: diagnosis of acute coronary syndromes. Ann Emerg Med. 2000;35(5):449–61.
9. Berger PB, Ellis SG, Holmes DR Jr, et al. Relationship between delay in performing direct coronary angioplasty and early clinical outcome in patients with acute myocardial infarction: results from the global use of strategies to open occluded arteries in Acute Coronary Syndromes (GUSTO-IIb) trial. Circulation. 1999;100(1):14–20.
10. O'Gara PT, Kushner FG, Ascheim DD, et al. 2013 ACCF/AHA guideline for the management of ST-elevation myocardial infarction: executive summary: a report of the American College of Cardiology Foundation/American Heart Association Task Force on Practice Guidelines. J Am Coll Cardiol. 2013;61(4):485–510.
11. Wang TY, Nallamothu BK, Krumholz HM, et al. Association of door-in to door-out time with reperfusion delays and outcomes among patients transferred for primary percutaneous coronary intervention. JAMA. 2011;305(24):2540–7.

12. Wallentin L, Becker RC, Budaj A, et al. Ticagrelor versus clopidogrel in patients with acute coronary syndromes. N Engl J Med. 2009;361(11):1045–57.
13. Tung YC, Chang GM, Chang HY, Yu TH. Relationship between early physician follow-up and 30-day readmission after acute myocardial infarction and heart failure. PLoS One. 2017;12(1):e0170061.
14. Peterson ED, Roe MT, Mulgund J, et al. Association between hospital process performance and outcomes among patients with acute coronary syndromes. JAMA. 2006;295(16):1912–20.
15. Ross MA, Amsterdam E, Peacock WF, et al. Chest pain center accreditation is associated with better performance of centers for Medicare and Medicaid services core measures for acute myocardial infarction. Am J Cardiol. 2008;102(2):120–4.
16. Fan F, Li Y, Zhang Y, et al. Chest pain center accreditation is associated with improved in-hospital outcomes of acute myocardial infarction patients in China: findings from the CCC-ACS Project. J Am Heart Assoc. 2019;8(21):e013384.

# Pathophysiology and Definition
# of the Acute Coronary Syndromes

Mani M. Alavi and Deborah B. Diercks

Understanding the pathophysiology of acute coronary syndromes (ACS) is essential to understand the diagnosis, risk stratification, and management strategies [1]. Patients with ACS are a high-risk group, and the contemporary classification, based on the related but distinctive pathophysiology of the syndromes, has provided a useful framework and rational therapeutic targets upon which to base the broad range of current management. Also, with the advent of high-sensitivity troponins, it is important to differentiate myocardial injury from myocardial infarction (MI). To that extent, the understanding of the condition of myocardial infarction with nonobstructive coronary syndrome (MINOCA) is relevant in any discussion of ACS.

## 1 Spectrum of the Acute Coronary Syndromes

ACS are viewed as a continuum of increasing severity, from unstable angina (UA) to non-ST-segment elevation myocardial infarction (NSTEMI) and ST-segment elevation MI (STEMI) [1, 2]. UA and NSTEMI comprise the NSTE ACS. The continuity of the syndromes is traditionally differentiated by electrocardiographic changes and increasingly sensitive serum markers of cardiac injury such as the troponins, which have blurred the distinction between UA and NSTEMI [2].

ACS are typically characterized by episodes of chest pain compatible with myocardial ischemia/infarction, although patients may occasionally present with

---

Update of original chapter by Ezra Amsterdam and Doug Kirk.

---

M. M. Alavi · D. B. Diercks (✉)
Department of Emergency Medicine, University of Texas, Southwestern Medical Center, Dallas, TX, USA
e-mail: Deborah.Diercks@utsouthwestern.edu

© The Author(s), under exclusive license to Springer Nature Switzerland AG 2022
M. Pena et al. (eds.), *Short Stay Management of Chest Pain*, Contemporary Cardiology, https://doi.org/10.1007/978-3-031-05520-1_6

complaints such as dyspnea, epigastric pain, or fatigue. Definitive diagnosis of each form of ACS is based on the accompanying electrocardiogram (ECG) and serum markers of cardiac injury, with troponin being the current gold standard [3]. STEMI is defined by ST-segment elevation indicative of acute injury; NSTEMI syndromes are typically associated with ischemic ST-segment and/or T wave abnormalities; however, there may also be no ECG alterations in NSTEMI.

Characteristic ECG alterations of injury in ACS have been categorized as transmural (ST elevation) and subendocardial (ST segment depression and T wave inversion). Both STEMI and NSTEMI are defined by increases in cardiac injury markers denoting myocardial necrosis. The most sensitive and specific cardiac injury markers are the cardiac troponins. The term acute myocardial infarction may be used when there is acute myocardial injury with clinical evidence of acute myocardial ischemia and with the detection of a rise and/or fall of cardiac troponin values with at least one value above the 99th percentile URL. In addition, patients must have symptoms suggestive of myocardial ischemic, or new ECG changes, based on the current universal definition of myocardial infarction [3]. NSTEMI and UA account for a large majority of ACS, a proportion that is likely to rise even further with the increasing sensitivity of diagnostic methods for cardiac necrosis.

## 2 Myocardial Injury Vs. Myocardial Infarction (MI)

With the recent wide adoptions of high-sensitivity troponins, the determination of myocardial injury has become both easier and prevalent [3]. Therefore, it is important to differentiate myocardial injury from MI. In fact high-sensitivity cardiac markers have made it necessary to re-evaluate the definition of MI and a distinction be made of myocardial injury in the absence of MI. It is true that myocardial injury is a requirement for the diagnosis of MI. However, myocardial injury is by itself a condition that needs to be understood. Myocardial injury is defined as evidence of elevated cardiac troponin value with a value above the 99th percentile [3, 4]. Further, this can be defined as an acute myocardial injury if change in the value of the cardiac biomarker exists.

Serial measurement of cardiac troponins can be used to determine ACS in order to determine changes in time [4]. In 2016, high-sensitivity troponins were approved for use in the United States. Troponins can be utilized to help make the diagnosis of ACS. Troponin levels rise after injury to cardiac muscle and detect elevations as early as 2–4 h after initial injury [5]. Of note cardiac markers including troponins are specific for myocardial injury. It is safe to say that high-sensitivity troponins have made it easier to detect myocardial injury, and this makes understanding the entity of myocardial injury more relevant. In general, high-sensitivity troponin helps decrease the time needed between testing but have also made detection of myocardial injury more prevalent [6]. The relevance of differentiating myocardial injury from MI is more important as more centers adopt high-sensitivity troponins.

As discussed, the diagnosis of MI requires biomarker evidence along with additional features. It is evident that myocardial injury can arise from both cardiac and non-cardiac conditions. It therefore makes it important to distinguish myocardia injury from different MI subtypes. In other words, when there is not an evidence of MI, a diagnosis of myocardia injury should be considered. Certainly, this diagnosis can be altered or changed if further diagnosis provides evidence of criteria meeting the definition of MI [3]. Studies have made it clear that myocardia injury which is defined as elevated cardiac troponin is encountered clinically and can have an adverse prognosis [4]. It is important to note that myocardial injury is not a benign entity and can be associated with high mortality and morbidity. In fact patients with myocardial injury (acute) had a significant rate of cardiovascular injury when compared to other types of MI. However, the prognosis and treatment of non-ischemic myocardia injury depends ultimately on the underlying cause. Consequently, for patients with elevated troponins, it is important to differentiate whether patients experienced myocardial injury versus one MI and if no evidence of myocardial ischemia a diagnosis of myocardial injury can be made [3].

# 3  Vulnerable Plaque and Plaque Rupture

## 3.1  Inflammation and Morphology

The central pathophysiologic event in the great majority of ACS is rupture of a vulnerable or unstable atherosclerotic plaque that induces coronary thrombosis and occlusion which results in myocardial ischemia and/or injury [7–9]. According to current concepts, the plaque that ulcerates and sets in motion the cascade of thrombogenesis and coronary occlusion possesses a thin fibrous cap and a large lipid pool [10]. The site of multiple mediators of inflammation such as macrophages, foam cells, and T lymphocytes releases matrix metalloproteinases and collagenases that promote erosion, ulceration, and rupture of the fibrous cap [8, 9, 11]. By contrast, the presence of smooth muscle cells, which promote plaque stability by secreting collagen, an essential component of the fibrous cap, is diminished at the site of atherosclerotic inflammation [12]. The size of the lipid pool is also an important determinant of plaque stability. In this regard, it has been reported that the threshold for rupture conferred by this lesion is a lipid pool comprising 50% of plaque volume [10, 13].

The foregoing pathoanatomic factors establish a plaque characterized by a large lipid pool, an inflammatory milieu, and a thin fibrous cap, all of which render it prone to rupture. Rupture typically occurs at the margins of the plaque where it is thinnest, inflammatory cells are densely concentrated and sheer stress is highest [7,

10, 14]. Because of its susceptibility to disruption and rupture, it is referred to as a *vulnerable* plaque in contrast to a stable plaque. The latter is characterized by a relatively thick fibrous cap, smaller lipid pool, and little evidence of inflammatory activity and is, thus, less subject to rupture and consequent coronary thrombosis. Using optical coherence tomography, investigators have shown that the lack of a lipid-rich plaque underneath an intact fibrinous cap in patients with an ACS is associated with reduced risk of major cardiac events [10]. It should be noted that plaque structure is not static and may shift between the more stable and the relatively vulnerable during the course of a patient's disease, in relation to the influence of risk factors, therapy, and hemodynamic alterations.

## 3.2  Coronary Thrombosis

Plaque rupture, which can be catastrophic, initiates thrombosis by exposure of circulating platelets to tissue factor within the subendothelial collagen matrix of the plaque [8]. Tissue factor is derived from endothelial cells and macrophages within the plaque and is highly thrombogenic. It activates the coagulation cascade and induces surface aggregation of platelets and fibrin deposition resulting in thrombogenesis at the site of plaque ulceration. Activated platelets intensely express the IIB/IIA receptor and release factors such as thromboxane A2 and serotonin that provoke vasospasm and augment platelet activity promoting further aggregation, hemostasis, and thrombogenesis [15]. ACS result when these pathogenic mechanisms overwhelm endogenous cardioprotective vasodilator and antithrombotic factors, whose production by abnormal endothelium of atherosclerotic arteries is deficient [16].

Thrombus forms on the surface of the plaque or can be initiated within the plaque after loss of integrity of the fibrous cap, which is followed by progression and protrusion of thrombus into the coronary lumen [8]. Thrombogenesis progresses in stages from partial to complete occlusion as platelets aggregate and finally are bound within a secondary fibrin network. Prior to complete occlusion, platelet aggregates from the thrombus in the path of circulating blood can embolize downstream to occlude the distal coronary vascular bed and increase the extent of jeopardized myocardium.

Appreciation of the pathogenesis of ACS provides the foundation for treatment directed at the underlying physiologic derangements. The basis of thrombolytic therapy for STEMI is susceptibility of the fibrin component of thrombus to dissolution by fibrinolytic agents. By contrast, the platelet core, which is the basis of NSTEMI ACS, is not responsive to fibrinolytic therapy and requires specific antiplatelet agents for inhibition of its genesis. Of course, antiplatelet therapy also has an important role in STEMI treatment. Therapeutic targets include preventive therapy to reduce atherosclerosis and favorable modification of the adverse characteristics of unstable atherosclerotic plaques by decreasing inflammation, strengthening the fibrous cap, and reducing the lipid pool [7].

## *3.3   Degree of Coronary Stenosis*

The vulnerable plaque is typically noncritical in its quiescent state in terms of degree of obstruction of coronary lumen diameter, which is usually less than 50% stenosis. Indeed, it has been established that the majority of myocardial infarctions are associated with coronary stenoses of less than 50% prior to the advent of thrombotic obstruction [17]. Symptoms of myocardial ischemia are unusual with this degree of stenosis, which does not significantly impair coronary blood flow at rest or ability to augment flow with increased myocardial oxygen demand. Reduction of coronary blood flow reserve is associated with stenosis greater than 70%, while impairment of resting coronary flow occurs when lumen diameter is reduced by more than 90% [18, 19]. It however should be noted that the risk of future cardiac events increases based on the degree of stenosis, and those patients with <50% stenosis are still at increased risk compared to those with normal coronary arteries. Additional risk for ACS can be identified by the presence of a high-risk plaque which may be defined by plaque composition when using new technology such as coronary computed tomography even when stenosis is <50% [7].

# 4   Clinico-Pathologic Correlations

As previously noted, the degree of thrombotic coronary obstruction typically determines the form of ACS that ensues after plaque ulceration and coronary thrombosis. The extent of ECG changes and degree of elevation of cardiac injury markers generally correlate with the magnitude of myocardial damage and, thereby, morbidity and mortality [20–22]. Because NSTEMI usually involves less myocardial damage than STEMI, mortality and other serious complications, such as cardiogenic shock, congestive heart failure, and arrhythmias, are less frequent during the initial hospitalization in NSTEMI. However, in some cases, NSTEMI may result in extensive damage, and STEMI may be associated with lesser injury. Further, patients with NSTE ACS are commonly older and have more extensive CAD and more frequent recurrent events. In addition, posthospital mortality in the first year is higher than with STEMI [23]. The basis for the latter finding may be related to delayed diagnosis and less aggressive therapy of NSTE ACS patients compared to those with STEMI. In general, because there is little or no evidence of acute myocardial necrosis in UA, early complications and mortality are lowest with this form of ACS.

Extent of ischemia and infarct size are also related to additional factors, such as the specific "culprit" coronary artery, site of vessel occlusion, presence of collateral coronary arteries, and hemodynamic factors influencing myocardial oxygen demand and supply during evolution of ACS. Thus, because it usually supplies the largest extent of myocardium, occlusion of the left anterior descending coronary artery generally results in more extensive ischemia/injury and greater morbidity and higher mortality than occlusion of the right or left circumflex arteries. Proximal coronary occlusion is associated with greater ischemia/injury than distal occlusion; collateral coronaries can limit the extent of infarction as can factors favoring reduced myocardial oxygen demand (e.g., lower heart rate and blood pressure). Finally, the therapeutic background (beta blockers, antiplatelet agents, statins, and other cardioprotective drugs) at the onset of ACS can alter its evolution.

Myocardial infarction with non-obstructive coronary syndrome (MINOCA) is a condition that is defined as clinical evidence of MI with normal or near normal coronary arteries [24]. It is important to understand the basics of MINOCA since it is reported to be present in 5–25% of MI. The diagnosis of MINOCA is made after coronary angiography in a patient who presents with criteria of MI with non-obstructive coronary arteries. The first steps of diagnosing MINOCA include ECG, history, cardiac biomarkers, echocardiography, coronary angiography, and left ventricular angiography [24]. This approach may also help differentiate the causes of MINOCA, and the two main categories are epicardial causes vs. microvascular causes [25]. There are a variety of causes of MINOCA. Causes of epicardial pattern can include coronary artery spasm (as occurs in cocaine and methamphetamine use), coronary artery plague, and coronary dissection. Microvascular causes of MINOCA include coronary microvascular spasm (CMS), coronary embolism, myocarditis, and Takotsubo syndrome. It is important to note that patients with MINOCA are often younger, and plaque disruption is fairly common [24]. Management depends on the underlying condition, and a mainstay of treatment includes modifiable CAD risk factor including medical management with aspirin, beta blockers, clopidogrel, etc. The prognosis of MINOCA is varied depending on the etiology and comorbidities. The specifics of the prognosis depend on the etiology and cause of the MINOCA. In the current culture, cocaine and other drugs of abuse such as methamphetamines require consideration in all patients presenting with ACS but especially young individuals and those with no cardiovascular risk factors [26].

## 5 Conclusions

The acute coronary syndromes include a continuum of acute myocardial ischemia manifested by STEMI, NSETMI, and UA. The diagnosis of myocardial injury has become more prevalent with the recent advent of high-sensitivity troponins. This has made it relevant to differentiate myocardial injury from MI. The clinical classification of the syndromes, which is based primarily on electrocardiographic and cardiac injury marker data, correlates closely with the underlying pathoanatomy. The central event is rupture of a vulnerable coronary atherosclerotic plaque. An inflammatory milieu and multiple other destabilizing features characterize the vulnerable plaque. Plaque rupture induces thrombotic coronary occlusion which results in an acute coronary syndrome, the specific type of which is determined by the degree of coronary obstruction and associated anatomic and hemodynamic factors.

Understanding of the pathophysiology of the acute coronary syndromes has provided a rational basis for current therapy and investigational approaches targeted at these derangements.

# References


1. Amsterdam EA, Wenger NK, Brindis RG, et al. AHA/ACC guideline for the management of patients with non-ST-elevation acute coronary syndromes: a report of the American College of Cardiology/American Heart Association Task Force on Practice Guidelines. Circulation. 2014;130(25):e344–426.
2. Hedayati T, Yadav N, Khanagavi J. Non-ST-segment acute coronary syndromes. Cardiol Clin. 2018;36(1):37–52.
3. Thygesen K, Alpert JS, Jaffe AS, et al. Fourth universal definition of myocardial infarction. J Am Coll Cardiol. 2018;72(18):2231–64.
4. Tamis-Holland JE, Jneid H, Reynolds HR, et al. Contemporary diagnosis and management of patients with myocardial infarction in the absence of obstructive coronary artery disease: a scientific statement from the American Heart Association. Circulation. 2019;139(18):e891–908.
5. Shah ASV, Anand A, Strachan FE, et al. High-sensitivity troponin in the evaluation of patients with suspected acute coronary syndrome: a stepped-wedge, cluster-randomised controlled trial. Lancet. 2018;392(10151):919–28.
6. Chapman AR, Adamson PD, Shah ASV, et al. High-sensitivity cardiac troponin and the universal definition of myocardial infarction. Circulation. 2020;141(3):161–71.
7. Raber L, Koskinas KC, Yamaji K, et al. Changes in coronary plaque composition in patients with acute myocardial infarction treated with high-intensity statin therapy (IBIS-4): a serial optical coherence tomography study. JACC Cardiovasc Imaging. 2019;12(8):1518–28.
8. Badimon L, Vilahur G. Thrombosis formation on atherosclerotic lesions and plaque rupture. J Intern Med. 2014;276(6):618–32.
9. Libby P. Current concepts of the pathogenesis of the acute coronary syndromes. Circulation. 2001;104(3):365–72.
10. Hoshino M, Yonetsu T, Usui E, et al. Clinical significance of the presence or absence of lipid-rich plaque underneath intact fibrous cap plaque in acute coronary syndrome. J Am Heart Assoc. 2019;8(9):e011820.
11. Davies MJ. Coronary disease: the pathophysiology of acute coronary syndromes. Heart. 2000;83:361–6.
12. Bennett MR. Apoptosis of vascular smooth muscle cells in vascular remodelling and atherosclerotic plaque rupture. Cardiovasc Res. 1999;41(2):361–8.
13. Davies MJ, Richardson PD, Woolf N, Katz DR, Mann J. Risk of thrombosis in human atherosclerotic plaques: role of extracellular lipid, macrophage, and smooth muscle cell content. Br Heart J. 1993;69(5):377–81.
14. Davies MJ. Stability and instability: two faces of coronary atherosclerosis: The Paul Dudley White Lecture 1995. Circulation. 1996;94(8):2013–20.
15. Sibbing D, Angiolillo DJ, Huber K. Antithrombotic therapy for acute coronary syndrome: past, present and future. Thromb Haemost. 2017;117(7):1240–8.
16. Kinlay S, Libby P, Ganz P. Endothelial function and coronary artery disease. Curr Opin Lipidol. 2001;12(4):383–9.
17. Ledru F, Reiber JC, Tuinenburg JC, Koning G, Lesperance J. Coronary angiography and the culprit lesion in acute coronary syndromes. In: Theroux acute coronary syndromes. Philadelphia: Saunders; 2003. p. 226–49.
18. Gould KL, Lipscomb K. Effects of coronary stenoses on coronary flow reserve and resistance. Am J Cardiol. 1974;34(1):48–55.

19. Biasco L, Pedersen F, Lonborg J, et al. Angiographic characteristics of intermediate stenosis of the left anterior descending artery for determination of lesion significance as identified by fractional flow reserve. Am J Cardiol. 2015;115(11):1475–80.
20. Antman EM, Tanasijevic MJ, Thompson B, et al. Cardiac-specific troponin I levels to predict the risk of mortality in patients with acute coronary syndromes. N Engl J Med. 1996;335:1342–9.
21. Tiller C, Reindl M, Holzknecht M, et al. Biomarker assessment for early infarct size estimation in ST-elevation myocardial infarction. Eur J Intern Med. 2019;64:57–62.
22. Goodman SG, Fu Y, Langer A, et al. The prognostic value of the admission and predischarge electrocardiogram in acute coronary syndromes: the GUSTO-IIb ECG Core Laboratory experience. Am Heart J. 2006;152(2):277–84.
23. Savonitto S, Ardissino D, Granger CB, et al. Prognostic value of the admission electrocardiogram in acute coronary syndromes. JAMA. 1999;281(8):707–13.
24. Scalone G, Niccoli G, Crea F. Editor's choice-pathophysiology, diagnosis and management of MINOCA: an update. Eur Heart J Acute Cardiovasc Care. 2019;8(1):54–62.
25. Niccoli G, Scalone G, Crea F. Acute myocardial infarction with no obstructive coronary atherosclerosis: mechanisms and management. Eur Heart J. 2015;36(8):475–81.
26. McCord J, Jneid H, Hollander J. Management of cocaine-associated chest pain and myocardial infarction: a scientific statement from the American Heart Association Acute Cardiac Care Committee of the Council on Clinical Cardiology. Circulation. 2008;117:1897–907.

# Chest Pain Risk Stratification by History, Physical Examination, and ECG

**Maria Aini**

## 1 Introduction

Chest pain is the second most common presenting chief complaint to the Emergency Department (ED), and heart disease continues to be the leading cause of death in the USA [1]. Chest pain accounts for eight million annual visits to the ED [1]. It can result from multiple etiologies including diseases of heart, lung, esophagus, gastro-intestinal system, and aorta. Distinguishing an acute versus nonacute chest pain presentation is paramount to emergency medicine clinicians. Acute atraumatic etiologies of chest pain include acute coronary syndrome (ACS), aortic dissection, pulmonary embolism, pericardial tamponade, pneumothorax, pneumonia, mediastinitis, and esophageal perforation. The high prevalence of chest pain as a presenting chief complaint compounded by a broad differential diagnosis makes the evaluation and ultimate disposition of chest pain challenging for clinicians. On the one hand, it is important to rule out acute etiologies of chest pain, and on the other hand, it is also important to consider overutilization of resources for the work-up of nonacute chest pain or low-risk ACS etiologies.

ACS is a life-threatening and time-dependent condition. It is a spectrum of coronary artery disease (CAD) defined by myocardial ischemia and/or myocardial infarction. ACS is classically divided into ST-segment elevation myocardial infarction (STEMI), non-ST-segment elevation myocardial infarction (NSTEMI) as well as unstable angina [UA]. UA traditionally was a category based on high clinical suspicion for ACS in the absence of biomarker instability. However, due to the advancement of high-sensitivity biomarkers, UA accounts for a smaller, declining group of ACS [2].

M. Aini (✉)
Clinical Operations, Department of Emergency Medicine, Thomas Jefferson University Hospital, Philadelphia, PA, USA

© The Author(s), under exclusive license to Springer Nature Switzerland AG 2022
M. Pena et al. (eds.), *Short Stay Management of Chest Pain*, Contemporary Cardiology, https://doi.org/10.1007/978-3-031-05520-1_7

Of overall chest pain presentations, 10–20% are evaluated for suspicion of ACS, and approximately one quarter of those admitted are ultimately confirmed to have a diagnosis of ACS [3, 4]. Due to the high stakes of the timely and accurate diagnosis of ACS specifically acute myocardial infarction (AMI) or STEMI, chest pain also accounts for one of the most common malpractice claims [5]. The generally accepted lower limit of pretest probability for ACS is 1–2% [6]. Some three million patients with chest pain are discharged from the ED each year, and 40,000 of these will ultimately undergo ACS. This group unfortunately accounts for 20–39% of malpractice dollars awarded in emergency medicine [7–9]. Recent evidence shows that half of a percent of patients with low-risk chest pain had an AMI or major adverse cardiac event (MACE) within 30 days [10]. Particularly in adult patients with recurrent, low-risk chest pain, there is currently insufficient evidence to recommend hospitalization (either standard inpatient admission or observation stay) versus discharge as a strategy to mitigate major adverse cardiac events within 30 days [11]. In the ED chest pain patient, the presence of a clear-cut alternative noncardiac diagnosis reduces the likelihood of a composite outcome of death and cardiovascular events within 30 days. However, it does not reduce the event rate to an acceptable level to allow ED discharge of these patients [12].

Over the years, different predictive modeling tools have been developed for risk stratification of patients to low versus moderate to high risk for ACS. That said, the proper evaluation and diagnosis of ACS as well as other acute diagnoses that cause chest pain starts with a proper history, physical examination, and electrocardiogram (ECG). An ECG is performed as a part of EMS or ambulatory triage and often done prior to a history and physical examination.

## 2 History

History taking in a patient presenting with chest pain should include questions pertaining to the onset of pain, pain quality and location, radiation of pain, associated symptoms, personal, and family risk factors for CAD and prior work-ups for chest pain. Cardiac chest pain describes pain that is ischemic in etiology. Ischemic chest pain has some features that can help to differentiate it from nonischemic chest pain. Ischemic chest pain is typically gradual in onset, the quality is described as pressure and tightness more often than pain, it is exacerbated by activity due to increased oxygen demand [13] and relieved with rest, and importantly, radiation of discomfort to upper extremities is very suggestive of chest pain associated with ACS [14]. Ischemic chest pain can often be associated with dyspnea, diaphoresis, vomiting, and fatigue. The most common anginal equivalent symptom of ischemic chest pain associated with ACS is isolated new onset or worsening exertional dyspnea [15, 16].

Nonischemic chest pain is associated with pain that is pleuritic or sharp, pain location identifiable with one finger, reproducible with palpation, and pain that is constant over days. Patients with continuous chest pain for greater than 24 h are unlikely to have an AMI and chest pain lasting less than a minute does not exclude AMI [17].

Atypical symptoms are other non-chest pain symptoms that can also suggest ACS. These typically include dyspnea alone, generalized weakness, nausea/vomiting, epigastric pain, palpitations, and syncope. It is important to consider these as anginal equivalents especially in women, patients with diabetes, and older patients [18]. In fact, AMI can present with no chest pain a third of the time which correlates with an increase in-hospital mortality in comparison to AMI presenting with chest pain [19, 20]. It is also equally important to consider that in chest pain presentations that present atypically or deemed low-risk ACS are other life-threatening etiologies causing acute chest pain as described above.

As atherosclerosis is responsible for most cases of CAD, patient evaluation for ACS should also include personal and familial risk factors for CAD. Traditional cardiac risk factors (family history, tobacco use, hypertension, diabetes mellitus, and hypercholesterolemia) are designed for the prediction of CAD but are somewhat limited for the prediction of ACS during an acute presentation [21–23]. More than 90% of coronary heart disease patients have prior exposure to at least one of the following risk factors: high total cholesterol, current treatment with cholesterol or high blood pressure lowering drugs, hypertension, current cigarette use, and clinical report of diabetes [24]. According to a large international case–control study, nine easily modifiable risk factors account for over 90% of the risk of an initial AMI: cigarette smoking, abnormal blood lipid levels, hypertension, diabetes, abdominal obesity, lack of physical activity, low daily fruit and vegetable consumption, alcohol overconsumption, and psychosocial index [25]. Lastly, more than 90% of coronary heart disease events will occur in individuals with at least one risk factor and approximately 8% will occur in people with only borderline levels of multiple risk factors [26].

It is important to remember that assessment for ACS remains a composite of the patient's history as well as risk factors, physical examination, and ECG [27].

## 3 Physical Examination

The physical examination in the ED often happens after or in parallel to ECG completion and interpretation. In a patient presenting with ACS, physical examination findings can often be non-diagnostic and normal. That said, initial assessment by the clinician should always focus on hemodynamic stability. Rapid assessment of airway, breathing, circulation, responsiveness can guide immediate interventions needed. Patients can appear dyspneic and/or diaphoretic. Vital signs can be completely normal to abnormal given the degree of associated failure or shock and based on the particular cardiac artery or geographic location of ischemia/infarct involved. Bradycardic rhythms on cardiac monitoring can specifically indicate inferior wall ischemia.

Evidence of acute heart failure in ACS includes jugular venous distention, pulmonary rales, hypotension, tachycardia, new S3 gallop, or new mitral regurgitation murmur. Cardiogenic shock as a result of ACS is the result of systemic hypoperfusion presenting with hypotension, tachycardia, altered mental status, or cold/clammy skin. These conditions should be recognized and treated immediately. In the case of STEMI-related cardiogenic failure, shock, or arrest, this should be done in conjunction with catherization lab activation for percutaneous coronary intervention [PCI] [28].

## 4 ECG

The ECG is one of the most important diagnostic tools to rule-in ACS as in the case of STEMI. Although its sensitivity is for AMI is low, it is a modality that is inexpensive, noninvasive, and fast. ECG makes it possible for prehospital assessment for STEMI and therefore appropriate transfer to cardiac catheterization centers for PCI ideally within 2 h [28]. Per guidelines from the American College of Cardiology and American Heart Association (ACC/AHA), an ECG should be performed within 10 min of arrival to the ED for patients as standard of care [15]. The typical accepted criteria for an ECG in triage are: greater than or equal to 25 years of age with chest pain, greater than or equal to 50 years of age with chest pain or an anginal equivalent symptom, greater than or equal to 80 years of age with chest pain, anginal equivalent symptom including abdominal pain, nausea, vomiting, altered mental status. The exception to this is a prehospital ECG diagnostic for STEMI which should go directly to a cardiac catheterization lab.

Any ST-segment elevation, even subtle elevation of less than 1 mm, that occurs in two or more contiguous leads should prompt concern for ischemia. ST-segment elevation with anatomically reciprocal ST-segment depression improves the specificity of the ST-elevation for diagnosis of ACS. The temptation to interpret ST-segment elevation as benign early repolarization, especially in patients older than 30 years, should be resisted [29]. In addition, there are several conditions that can manifest themselves through ST-segment elevation, most commonly ventricular aneurysm, aortic dissection through coronary ostia, hyperkalemia, pericarditis, left ventricular hypertrophy, Wolff-Parkinson-White syndrome, and left bundle branch block (LBBB). The primary distinguishing factor between early repolarization and acute myocardial injury is the presence of chest pain and age greater than 30 years old which warrants more concern for ACS.

While ST-segment depression alone is not an indication for PCI or thrombolytic [30], ST-segment depression in leads V1-V4 may indicate a posterior wall MI due to the reciprocal electrical view of the infarct. This finding may be misinterpreted as anterior wall ischemia unless the diagnosis of a posterior MI is entertained. Anterior ST-segment depression should be considered a posterior wall infarct until proven otherwise, and the initial ECG displaying this finding can be followed by a posterior lead ECG.

Similarly, inferior ST-segment elevation should be evaluated with a right-sided ECG to look for right ventricle (RV) infarction. This is clinically important for management purposes, as patients with acute RV infarction are preload-dependent in order to maintain adequate cardiac output. Nitrates should be avoided in these patients, as they can lead to hypotension and shock with little warning.

T-wave inversion occurs in many conditions, but in the setting of chest pain may be an indication of cardiac ischemia. T-wave inversion may also represent reperfusion of a completed infarct. Wellens sign is a biphasic T wave with terminal T-wave inversion in the anterior leads V2-V4 [31, 32]. This finding has a high specificity for proximal to mid-LAD occlusion, and patients at high risk for reocclusion.

Pathologic Q waves, which are usually wider and deeper than the normal deflections that represent septal wall depolarization, often indicate ischemia or dead myocardium. Generally speaking, Q waves are considered significant if the amplitude is greater than one third of the amplitude of the corresponding QRS complex. Preexisting Q waves from a previous myocardial infarction should not be ignored in patients presenting with chest pain, as they demonstrate strong evidence of coronary artery disease. It is also possible to see Q waves appear in the setting of STEMI/NSTEMI as the infarct evolves into myocardial wall necrosis.

New LBBB is the presenting ECG finding in approximately 7% of patients with AMI [33, 34]. It should be considered a sign of ischemia or infarction and prompt an ischemic work-up, especially when seen in the setting of acute chest pain. A set of clinical criteria that allows for ECG diagnosis of AMI in the setting of LBBB have been published [35, 36]. These criteria are: (1) ST-segment elevation of 1 mm or more that is concordant with the QRS complex; (2) ST-segment depression of 1 mm or more in lead V1, V2, or V3; and (3) ST-segment elevation of 5 mm or more that is discordant with the QRS complex. Similar criteria were developed for the diagnosis of AMI in the setting of an internal pacemaker device, which produces an ECG pattern similar to that of an LBBB. In this setting, discordant ST-segment elevation greater than 5 mm was the most statistically significant criterion associated with AMI [37].

New rhythm disturbances in the setting of chest pain are disturbing and warrant investigation. Examples include second- or third-degree heart block, tachydysrhythmia, and bradyarrhythmia. Patients with chest pain due to ischemia or infarction may have disrupted intrinsic pacemaker function or conduction pathways; conversely, such arrhythmias may lead to poor diastolic coronary artery perfusion with further ischemia or infarct. These patients are high risk and should be considered for coronary angiography; patients with active chest pain and arrhythmia should not be stress tested.

The challenge is that most initial ECGs in patients with ACS are non-diagnostic for ischemia or infarction [38]. It is important to analyze an ECG in the context of clinical evaluation including history, physical examination, biomarker testing, and overall risk stratification. A review of prior ECGs is important for determining whether abnormalities are new versus old increasing the sensitivity of a lone ECG. Patients with normal or nonspecific ECGs still have a 1–5% incidence of AMI and a 4–23% incidence of unstable angina [39]. A repeat ECG should be performed if the initial ECG is non-diagnostic, but the patient remains symptomatic, and there remains high clinical suspicion for AMI.

## References


1. National Center for Health Statistics. National hospital ambulatory medical care survey: 2017 emergency department summary tables. Hyattsville, MD: National Center for Health Statistics; 2020. https://www.cdc.gov/nchs/data/nhamcs/web_tables/2017_ed_web_tables-508.pdf. Accessed 2 Jun 2020.
2. Amsterdam EA, Wenger NK, Brindis RG, Casey DE Jr, Ganiats TG, Holmes DR Jr, Jaffe AS, Jneid H, Kelly RF, Kontos MC, Levine GN, Liebson PR, Mukherjee D, Peterson ED, Sabatine MS, Smalling RW, Zieman SJ, ACC/AHA Task Force Members. 2014 AHA/ACC guideline for the management of patients with non-ST-elevation acute coronary syndromes: a report of the American College of Cardiology/American Heart Association Task Force on Practice Guidelines. Circulation. 2014;130(25):e344–426. https://doi.org/10.1161/CIR.0000000000000134. Erratum in: Circulation. 2014;130(25): e433-4. Dosage error in article text. PMID: 25249585.
3. Möckel M, Searle J, Muller R, et al. Chief complaints in medical emergencies: do they relate to underlying disease and outcome? The Charité Emergency Medicine Study (CHARITEM). Eur J Emerg Med. 2013;20:103–8.
4. Ekelund U, Akbarzadeh M, Khoshnood A, et al. Likelihood of acute coronary syndrome in emergency department chest pain patients varies with time of presentation. BMC Res Notes. 2012;5:420.
5. Ferguson B, Geralds J, Petrey J, Huecker M. Malpractice in emergency medicine-a review of risk and mitigation practices for the emergency medicine provider. J Emerg Med. 2018;55(5):659–65.
6. Kline JA, Johnson CL, Pollack CV Jr, Diercks DB, Hollander JE, Newgard CD, Garvey JL. Pretest probability assessment derived from attribute matching. BMC Med Inform Decis Mak. 2005;5:26.
7. Braunwald E, Jones RH, Mark DB, et al. Diagnosing and managing unstable angina. Agency for Health Care Policy and Research. Circulation. 1994;90(1):613–22.
8. McCarthy BD, Beshansky JR, D'Agostino RB, Selker HP. Missed diagnoses of acute myocardial infarction in the emergency department: results from a multicenter study. Ann Emerg Med. 1993;22(3):579–82.
9. Rosamond W, Flegal K, Furie K, et al. Heart disease and stroke statistics--2008 update: a report from the American Heart Association Statistics Committee and Stroke Statistics Subcommittee. Circulation. 2008;117(4):e25–146.
10. Lindsell CJ, Anantharaman V, Diercks D, Han JH, Hoekstra JW, Hollander JE, Kirk JD, Lim SH, Peacock WF, Tiffany B, Wilke EK, Gibler WB, Pollack CV Jr, EMCREG-International i*trACS Investigators. The Internet Tracking Registry of Acute Coronary Syndromes (i*trACS): a multicenter registry of patients with suspicion of acute coronary syndromes reported using the standardized reporting guidelines for emergency department chest pain studies. Ann Emerg Med. 2006;48(6):666.
11. Musey PI, Bellolio F, Upadhye S, et al. Guidelines for reasonable and appropriate care in the emergency department (GRACE): recurrent, low-risk chest pain in the emergency department. Acad Emerg Med. 2021;28:718–44. https://doi.org/10.1111/acem.14296.
12. Hollander JE, Robey JL, Chase MR, et al. Relationship between a clear-cut alternative noncardiac diagnosis and 30-day outcome in emergency department patients with chest pain. Acad Emerg Med. 2007;14:210.

13. Goodacre S, Locker T, Morris F, Campbell S. How useful are clinical features in the diagnosis of acute, undifferentiated chest pain? Acad Emerg Med. 2002;9(3):203–8. https://doi.org/10.1111/j.1553-2712.2002.tb00245.x. PMID: 11874776.

14. Panju AA, Hemmelgarn BR, Guyatt GH, Simel DL. The rational clinical examination. Is this patient having a myocardial infarction? JAMA. 1998;280(14):1256–63. https://doi.org/10.1001/jama.280.14.1256. PMID: 9786377.

15. Anderson JL, Adams CD, Antman EM, et al. ACC/AHA 2007 guidelines for the management of patients with unstable angina/non ST-elevation myocardial infarction: a report of the American College of Cardiology/American Heart Association Task Force on Practice Guidelines (Writing Committee to Revise the 2002 Guidelines for the Management of Patients With Unstable Angina/Non ST-Elevation Myocardial Infarction): developed in collaboration with the American College of Emergency Physicians, the Society for Cardiovascular Angiography and Interventions, and the Society of Thoracic Surgeons: endorsed by the American Association of Cardiovascular and Pulmonary Rehabilitation and the Society for Academic Emergency Medicine. Circulation. 2007;116(7):e148–304.

16. Brogan GX. Risk stratification for patients with non-ST-segment elevation acute coronary syndromes in the emergency department. Cincinnati, OH: Emergency Medicine Cardiac Research and Education Group; 2007. p. 1–10.

17. Zitek T, Chen E, Gonzalez-Ibarra A, Wire J. The association of chest pain duration and other historical features with major adverse cardiac events. Am J Emerg Med. 2020;38(7):1377–83. https://doi.org/10.1016/j.ajem.2019.11.020. PMID: 31843326.

18. Pope JH, Aufderheide TP, Ruthazer R, Woolard RH, Feldman JA, Beshansky JR, Griffith JL, Selker HP. Missed diagnoses of acute cardiac ischemia in the emergency department. N Engl J Med. 2000;342(16):1163–70. https://doi.org/10.1056/NEJM200004203421603. PMID: 10770981.

19. Gupta M, Tabas JA, Kohn MA. Presenting complaint among patients with myocardial infarction who present to an urban, public hospital emergency department. Ann Emerg Med. 2002;40(2):180–6. https://doi.org/10.1067/mem.2002.126396. PMID: 12140497.

20. Canto JG, Shlipak MG, Rogers WJ, Malmgren JA, Frederick PD, Lambrew CT, Ornato JP, Barron HV, Kiefe CI. Prevalence, clinical characteristics, and mortality among patients with myocardial infarction presenting without chest pain. JAMA. 2000;283(24):3223–9. https://doi.org/10.1001/jama.283.24.3223. PMID: 10866870.

21. Jayes RL Jr, Beshansky JR, D'Agostino RB, Selker HP. Do patients' coronary risk factor reports predict acute cardiac ischemia in the emergency department? A multicenter study. J Clin Epidemiol. 1992;45(6):621–6.

22. Selker HP, Griffith JL, D'Agostino RB. A time-insensitive predictive instrument for acute myocardial infarction mortality: a multicenter study. Med Care. 1991;29(12):1196–211.

23. Selker HP, Griffith JL, D'Agostino RB. A tool for judging coronary care unit admission appropriateness, valid for both real-time and retrospective use. A time-insensitive predictive instrument (TIPI) for acute cardiac ischemia: a multicenter study. Med Care. 1991;29(7):610–27.

24. Greenland P, Knoll MD, Stamler J, et al. Major risk factors as antecedents of fatal and nonfatal coronary heart disease events. JAMA. 2003;290(7):891–7.

25. Yusuf S, Hawken S, Ounpuu S, et al. Effect of potentially modifiable risk factors associated with myocardial infarction in 52 countries (the INTERHEART study): case-control study. Lancet. 2004;364(9438):937–52.

26. Vasan RS, Sullivan LM, Wilson PW, et al. Relative importance of borderline and elevated levels of coronary heart disease risk factors. Ann Intern Med. 2005;142(6):393–402.

27. Lee TH, Cook EF, Weisberg M, Sargent RK, Wilson C, Goldman L. Acute chest pain in the emergency room. Identification and examination of low-risk patients. Arch Intern Med. 1985;145(1):65–9. PMID: 3970650.

28. Ibanez B, James S, Agewall S, et al. 2017 ESC Guidelines for the management of acute myocardial infarction in patients presenting with ST-segment elevation: the Task Force for the

Management of Acute Myocardial Infarction in Patients Presenting with ST-segment Elevation of the European Society of Cardiology (ESC). Eur Heart J. 2018;39:119–77.
29. Patton KK, Ellinor PT, Ezekowitz M, Kowey P, Lubitz SA, Perez M, Piccini J, Turakhia M, Wang P, Viskin S. American Heart Association Electrocardiography and Arrhythmias Committee of the Council on Clinical Cardiology and Council on Functional Genomics and Translational Biology. Electrocardiographic early repolarization: a scientific statement from the American Heart Association. Circulation. 2016;133(15):1520–9. https://doi.org/10.1161/CIR.0000000000000388. PMID: 27067089.
30. Savonitto S, Ardissino D, Granger CB, et al. Prognostic value of the admission electrocardiogram in acute coronary syndromes. JAMA. 1999;281(8):707–13.
31. de Zwaan C, Bar FW, Janssen JH, et al. Angiographic and clinical characteristics of patients with unstable angina showing an ECG pattern indicating critical narrowing of the proximal LAD coronary artery. Am Heart J. 1989;117(3):657–65.
32. Wellens HJ. Bishop lecture. The electrocardiogram 80 years after Einthoven. J Am Coll Cardiol. 1986;7(3):484–91.
33. Wong CK, White HD. The HERO-2 ECG sub-studies in patients with ST elevation myocardial infarction: implications for clinical practice. Int J Cardiol. 2013;170(1):17–23. https://doi.org/10.1016/j.ijcard.2013.10.008. PMID: 24182674.
34. Shlipak MG, Go AS, Frederick PD, Malmgren J, Barron HV, Canto JG. Treatment and outcomes of left bundle-branch block patients with myocardial infarction who present without chest pain. National Registry of Myocardial Infarction 2 Investigators. J Am Coll Cardiol. 2000;36(3):706–12. https://doi.org/10.1016/s0735-1097(00)00789-0. PMID: 10987588.
35. Sgarbossa EB. Recent advances in the electrocardiographic diagnosis of myocardial infarction: left bundle branch block and pacing. Pacing Clin Electrophysiol. 1996;19(9):1370–9.
36. Sgarbossa EB, Pinski SL, Barbagelata A, et al. Electrocardiographic diagnosis of evolving acute myocardial infarction in the presence of left bundle-branch block. GUSTO-1 (Global Utilization of Streptokinase and Tissue Plasminogen Activator for Occluded Coronary Arteries) Investigators. N Engl J Med. 1996;334(8):481–7.
37. Sgarbossa EB, Pinski SL, Gates KB, Wagner GS. Early electrocardiographic diagnosis of acute myocardial infarction in the presence of ventricular paced rhythm. GUSTO-I investigators. Am J Cardiol. 1996;77(5):423–4.
38. Gibler WB, Lewis LM, Erb RE, et al. Early detection of acute myocardial infarction in patients presenting with chest pain and nondiagnostic ECGs: serial CK-MB sampling in the emergency department. Ann Emerg Med. 1990;19(12):1359–66.
39. Hathaway WR, Peterson ED, Wagner GS, Granger CB, Zabel KM, Pieper KS, Clark KA, Woodlief LH, Califf RM. Prognostic significance of the initial electrocardiogram in patients with acute myocardial infarction. GUSTO-I Investigators. Global utilization of streptokinase and t-PA for Occluded Coronary Arteries. JAMA. 1998;279(5):387–91. https://doi.org/10.1001/jama.279.5.387. PMID: 9459474.

# The Role of Biomarkers in Chest Pain Evaluation

**Robert Christianson and Quinten Meadors**

## 1    Introduction

In the 1950s researchers discovered that the enzyme aspartate transaminase is released into circulation after cardiac injury was the first step in biomarkers becoming fundamental to diagnosis, risk stratification, and management of patients presenting with signs and symptoms of the acute coronary syndromes. The evolution of cardiac biomarkers continued through the 1970s with the routine measurement of lactate dehydrogenase and its LD1 to LD5 isoenzymes, and later with the emergence of total creatine kinase (CK) activity and its CK-MB isoenzyme. In the 1980s, vastly improved CK-MB "mass" immunoassays became available that do not rely on enzymatic activity. In the 1990s, the "era of troponin" occurred with the development of cardiac troponin T (cTnT) and cardiac troponin I (cTnI) testing. Along with clinical features and the electrocardiogram (ECG), cardiac cTnI and cTnT measurements have become fundamental in the assessment of the suspected acute coronary syndrome patient. In fact, in 2007 the National Academy of Clinical Biochemistry (NACB) issued the following Class I recommendation: "Biomarkers of myocardial necrosis should be measured in all patients who present with symptoms consistent with acute coronary syndromes." [1] The evidence base for biomarkers, i.e. cardiac troponin, is so compelling that the very diagnostic criteria for MI have been redefined based on cardiac troponin measurements [2]. Through recommendations set


R. Christianson
Clinical Chemistry Labs, University of Maryland, Baltimore, MD, USA
e-mail: rchristenson@umm.edu

Q. Meadors (✉)
Department of Emergency Medicine, Emory University School of Medicine,
Atlanta, GA, USA
e-mail: quinten.dashawn.meadors@emory.edu




M. Pena et al. (eds.), *Short Stay Management of Chest Pain*, Contemporary
Cardiology, https://doi.org/10.1007/978-3-031-05520-1_8

forth by the NACB guidelines, cardiac biomarkers have been utilized in conjunction with elements of the patient's clinical presentation (history, physical exam), and ECG to direct patient care and management in the workup of the acute coronary syndromes [1].

Incentives among diagnostic manufacturers have led to the development of increasingly precise and sensitive troponin assays and thus ushering in the "high-sensitivity troponin" era. The high-sensitivity cardiac troponin test (hs-cTnT) is among the latest generation of assays able to detect Troponin concentrations (cTn) concentrations in at least 50% of healthy individuals with high precision (coefficient of variation of $\leq$10%) at the 99th percentile; fivefold to 100-fold lower than the early conventional assays [3]. In comparison to conventional troponin assays, hs-cTn assays augments and accelerates a clinician's ability to rule-in or rule-out acute coronary syndromes, enables more rapid serial sampling, reduce costs, and identifies a larger number of patients at high risk for future cardiovascular events [4–7].

High-sensitivity cardiac troponin assays have drastically enhanced the clinical evaluation of acute coronary syndromes and are now used throughout the globe, routinely embedded within various algorithms for ruling in or out acute coronary syndromes [8]. However, the increased sensitivity of hs-cTn assays have unmasked many circumstances in which myocardial injury occurs in the absence of acute ischemic heart disease. Nonischemic myocardial injury may arise secondary to many cardiac conditions such as myocarditis or may be associated with noncardiac conditions such as renal failure [9]. Recently, through joint sponsorship from the American College of Cardiology, the American Heart Association, the European College of Cardiology, and the World Heart Federation, the fourth Universal Definition of Myocardial Infarction was released in 2018. The fourth universal definition reflects considerations in the clinical evaluation of patients using hs-cTn, while retaining the clinical definition of MI as the presence of acute myocardial injury detected by abnormal cardiac biomarkers in the setting of evidence of acute myocardial ischemia. For patients with increased cTn values, it is paramount that clinicians distinguish whether patients have suffered a nonischemic myocardial injury or one of the MI subtypes [10].

## 1.1  MI Subtypes

### 1.1.1  Type 1

Type 1 MI is due to acute coronary atherothrombotic myocardial injury with either plaque rupture or erosion and, often, associated thrombosis. Most patients with ST-segment elevation MI (STEMI) and many with non-ST-segment elevation MI (NSTEMI) fit into this category.

### 1.1.2 Type 2

Type 2 MI includes patients with evidence of acute myocardial ischemia who do not have acute coronary atherothrombotic injury but instead have oxygen supply–demand imbalance from other reasons. This occurs most often due to the presence of coronary artery disease, which limits increases in coronary perfusion in cases of severe anemia, significant arrhythmias, and other stressors. However, the presence of fixed coronary obstruction is not obligatory, including primary coronary causes such as vasospasm, coronary embolus, and coronary artery dissection. All of these can lead to a disparity between oxygen supply and demand in the myocardium. Most of these individuals do not have STEMI but more often have NSTEMI at presentation. Often, the distinction between type 1 and type 2 MIs can be made clinically based on the presentation; however, there are circumstances in which there is ambiguity, at which point imaging studies including angiography and, at times, more sophisticated coronary imaging may be helpful.

### 1.1.3 Type 3

Type 3 MI continues the concept that there may be an occasional patient who has characteristic symptoms of myocardial ischemia but whose cTn values have not become elevated because the patient succumbs before values are measured or who is stricken by sudden death with evidence of MI by autopsy.

### 1.1.4 Types 4 and 5

Types 4 and 5 MIs are related to coronary procedural events. However, it is emphasized that an isolated procedural elevation of cTn values is indicative of cardiac procedural myocardial injury that does not alone meet the criteria for percutaneous coronary intervention (PCI)-related type 4a MI or for coronary artery bypass grafting (CABG)-related type 5 MI. These MI categories that are applied within 48 h of the index procedure include an elevation of cTn values greater than 5 times the 99th percentile URL in the case of PCI and greater than 10 times the indicated URL in the case of CABG, along with evidence of new myocardial ischemia. Ischemia can be recognized by electrocardiogram changes, findings on imaging procedures, or as a result of a procedure-related complication that lead to reduced coronary blood flow. The selection of these biomarker cut-points rests on the assumption that the pre-procedural cTn values have a normal baseline. In patients with elevated pre-procedural values in whom the cTn level are stable ($\leq 20\%$ variation) or falling, the post-procedural values must rise by $>20\%$ but still must be more than 5 or 10 times the URL. The presence of procedure-related stent thrombosis (i.e., type 4b MI) and post-procedural restenosis (i.e., type 4c MI) are diagnosed applying the same criteria utilized for type 1 MI [10].

**Table 1** MI subtypes—Reference [10]

| MI Subtypes | Definition |
| --- | --- |
| Type 1 MI | MI due to acute coronary atherothrombotic injury with either plaque rupture or erosion and, often, associated thrombosis. |
| Type 2 MI | Acute myocardial ischemia secondary to oxygen supply-demand imbalance including coronary artery disease, vasospasm, coronary embolus, and coronary artery dissection. |
| Type 3 MI | Myocardial ischemia absent of increase in cTn elevation because the patient succumbs before increase in values are measured or is stricken by sudden death with evidence of MI by autopsy. |
| Type 4 MI | MI associated with stent thrombosis in the setting of myocardial ischemia in combination with a change in cardiac biomarkers with at least one value above the 99th percentile URL. |
| Type 4A MI | MI $\leq$48 h following coronary artery bypass grafting, defined by an elevation of cTn values >5 times the 99th percentile URL. |
| Type 5 MI | MI $\leq$48 h following coronary artery bypass grafting, defined by an elevation of cTn values >10 times the 99th percentile URL. |

In summary, there are many ways in which there can be necrosis of myocardium and release of troponin. These conditions are not limited to atherosclerosis and are listed in Table 1.

Cardiac Necrosis Markers

The troponin complex is comprised of three structural proteins termed troponin T, troponin C, and troponin I. The troponin complex is fundamental for the contraction of all striated muscle, both skeletal and cardiac. Because of the unique physiological demands on myocardium, cardiac specific isoforms of the troponin T and troponin I proteins evolved. The cardiac isoforms of TnT and TnI have amino sequences that are different from their skeletal muscle counterparts, and are virtually exclusive for myocardial tissue. Thus assays for cTnT and cTnI have exquisite cardiac specificity, and is one important reason why cTnT and cTnI have become the preferred marker for assessment of the acute coronary syndromes [1, 2].

While CKMB was once an important test previously for diagnosis of MI, it is no longer recommended by guidelines and may only add cost to the evaluation [11]. Similarly, myoglobin and LDH, once thought to be integral to diagnosis of MI are now of very limited clinical value in this this process [12].

For purposes of this discussion, the terms "Contemporary" and "Sensitive" will be used interchangeably. The "highly sensitive" and "high-sensitivity" assays will be discussed together.

## 1.2   Contemporary Troponin

Cardiac troponin is the preferred marker for the diagnosis of MI in patients suspected of having an acute coronary syndrome be it contemporary or high-sensitive [1, 2]. One must keep in mind that troponin is a structural protein such that some hours are frequently required for release and detection in circulation. Thus a critically important point when utilizing cardiac troponin is timing of blood sample collection. In general, blood should be obtained at hospital presentation, followed by serial sampling based on the clinical circumstances. With serial sampling in the presence of a clinical history suggestive of acute coronary syndrome, guidance is that a cardiac troponin value on at least one occasion during the first 24 h after the acute event above the maximal concentration exceeding the 99th percentile of values for reference control group is indicative of myocardial necrosis consistent with MI [1, 2]. The timing of the serial testing has varied somewhat. Contemporary troponin values were often regarded as needing 6–9 h after onset of pain to detect a rise which is physiologically true, but very few patients can present to the emergency department at the exact time of onset of pain. However, in the fourth definition of MI, the timing has been reduced for contemporary troponin to 3–6 h. Observation of a rise over the 99th percentile of the assay in use would be diagnostic if either the first (time 0) or second value has this feature.

Use of the 99th percentile of a reference control (normal) population as a cutpoint for cTnT or cTnI can be a source of confusion and some variability. This is because manufacturers of cardiac troponin assays have not used a common set of samples for establishing the characteristics of control populations. Currently, the best approach is for clinicians and laboratory medicine staff to jointly decide what the 99th percentile cutpoint concentration should be using information provided by the manufacturers, characteristics of the local population, their own studies and experience with the specific cardiac troponin assay.

## 1.3   Highly Sensitive Troponin Assays

The technical characteristics of cardiac troponin assays are an important consideration for both clinicians and laboratorians particularly in the age of marketing "sensitive," "ultrasensitive," "highly sensitive" assays. The previous generations of cTn assays usually reported the presence of troponin in terms of mcg/ml. The newer high-sensitivity assays (hs-cTnT) report results using ng/ml or ng/L and an assay is regarded as highly sensitive when it can detect troponin in 50% of normal individuals [13]. As there are few studies directly comparing contemporary to highly sensitive troponin assays with patient outcomes, there may be a disconnect in the actual

**Table 2** Highly Sensitive Diagnostic Troponin Assays [15]

| Assay name | Manufacturer | Troponin type | Limit of detection | 99th Percentile |
| --- | --- | --- | --- | --- |
| Elecsys 2010 | Roche Diagnostics | hs-cTnT | <5 ng/L | 19 ng/L |
| ARCHITECT i2000SR | Abbott Diagnostics | hs-cTnI | 1.7 ng/L | 28 ng/L |
| HsVista | Siemens Diagnostics | hs-cTnI | <2 ng/L | 58.9 ng/L |

clinical utility of detecting troponin at levels this low [14]. However, the Fourth Universal Definition of MI recommends the use of high-sensitivity assays. Finally, troponin and other biomarker assays must be characterized with respect to potential interferences that may cause either false positive or false negative results. Potential interferences include rheumatoid factor(s), human anti-mouse antibodies, heterophile antibodies, and other related proteins that can interfere with immunoassays [1]. Preanalytical assay characteristics that should be established include acceptable specimen type and stability of the measurements over time and across temperature ranges. Identification of antibody/epitope/recognition sites for each biomarker is also important; assays should target certain epitopes on the troponin molecule, such as the stable 41–49 amino acid region of troponin I that is less susceptible to interferences. Currently, there are three assays for hs-cTnT approved for use in the US by the Food and Drug Administration listed in Table 2 [15]. Clinicians should work with laboratory medicine staff to assure that performance of their cardiac troponin assay remains stable over time. One strategy for helping to assure stability is performing routine quality control in the relevant measurement concentrations range; this includes routine quality control at low troponin concentrations where clinical decisions are made.

## 1.4  Early Risk Stratification and Diagnosis of MI

A troponin level, be it contemporary, highly sensitive is the preferred marker for risk stratification and should be measured in all patients with suspected acute coronary syndrome [1]. The troponin concentration that confers increased risk of death and recurrent ischemic risk among patients with a compelling clinical history suggesting acute coronary syndromes was determined to be very low, near the upper limit of the normal or detectable range [16–19]. These data, in part, provided strong justification for setting the MI cutpoint at the 99th percentile of the reference control population. Values above the 99th percentile with an appropriate history of chest pain should prompt the start of treatment for NSTEMI. In terms of high-sensitivity troponin, the course of action may not be as straightforward.

## 1.5   Rapid Rule-Out Pathways

Development of a more efficient and expeditious method of ruling out acute coronary syndromes is the primary goal of cTn based chest pain risk stratification protocols. Rapid rule-out of hs-cTn allows for efficient identification and discharge of low-risk patients from the ED without need for excessive resource utilization. Such allocation of resources leads to improved outcomes through the application of more aggressive, evidence-based therapies for high-risk ACS patients. When combined with multidisciplinary care pathways based upon objective risk stratification using hs-cTn, implementation of a treatment strategy that is clinically efficacious and cost effective may be achievable. These considerations may drastically improve patient care and reduce ED transit time [20].

A number of diagnostic algorithms have been created that utilize the performance of hs-cTn assays in conjunction with various risk stratification tools and clinician judgment. Previous to the advent of these assays, the standard of practice using cTn equated to 3- to 6-h rule-outs, allowing for an adequate duration of time to elapse in ensuring the accurate detection of troponins, as well as allowing for serial sampling. Through exploitation of the increased sensitivity of the new assays, however, rapid rule-out pathways have created that permit shorter intervals between repeat cTn measurements for patients presenting for chest pain in as little as 1-h post-ED arrival. Furthermore, these assays have found little value in further testing beyond 3 h, and little value in serial testing for patients presenting with symptom onset >6 h, as rule-out based on a single negative hs-cTn has found to be reasonable [20].

While many emergency departments have already begun to incorporate rapid rule-out pathways for acute coronary syndromes into their workflow practices, some have not, particularly in the USA. Currently, there exists a plethora of data evaluating high-sensitivity troponin testing in patients with suspected acute coronary syndrome, including two prospective, randomized controlled trials, demonstrating very low rates of future ACS or death as far as 1 year after index presentation [21]. Incorporating rapid rule-out pathways into bedside ED practice allows for the implementation of a more rapid and safe disposition of patients who present with chest pain. Further incorporation of such protocols seek to decrease hospital overcrowding, hospital admission, and the need for additional cardiac testing [22].

## 1.6   Rule-Out at Presentation

In a meta-analysis study involving 22,457 patients from 19 studies, 49.1% of patients had a hs-cTnI <5 ng/L, and the 30-day major adverse cardiac event (MACE) rate was 0.5% [23]. Another multicenter randomized study of 31,492 patients compared a rapid rule-out strategy at presentation with hs-cTnI <5 ng/L to serial hs-cTnI over 6–12 h after symptom onset and found no significant difference between 30-day MACE between the strategies 0.3% in the rapid rule-out strategy and 0.4% in the standard strategy [24].

### 1.7  Rule-Out by 0/1-h Algorithm

A retrospective study with 1282 patients using the hs-cTnT assay applied the HEART score to distinguish between very low-risk and higher-risk patients. Those with a HEART score ≤3 had a 30-day MACE rate of only 0.2%; those with a HEART score ≥4 had a MACE rate of 2.3% using the 0/1 h algorithm. In another prospective study involving two centers (2296 patients) and no prospective risk score, it was found that 71% of patients who met the criteria for 0/1 h rule-out were discharged for outpatient management. At 30 days, the MACE rate was 0.2% among those discharged using the 0/1-h algorithm [25, 26].

### 1.8  Rule-Out by 0/3-h Algorithm

Patients with hs-cTn values who cannot be ruled out at presentation or by the 0/1-h algorithm require at least a 3-h value ≤99th percentile in evaluation of ACS. In a prospective implementation study utilizing the HEART score to stratify 4761 patients, 30.7% were deemed low risk and considered for discharge if their HEART score was ≤3 and serial hs-cTn was <99th percentile over 3 h. Among those discharged, the 30-day MACE rate was 0.4% [27, 28].

While there has yet to be an established "gold standard" clinical decision-making pathway, it remains clear that an early invasive management strategy has demonstrated benefit in patients who are cardiac troponin positive at presentation. Evidence showed a ~55% reduction in the odds of death or MI when a strategy of early angiography (within 4–48 h) and revascularization (when appropriate) was used in cardiac troponin positive acute coronary syndrome patients compared with a conservative management strategy [19]. Thus patient outcomes can be improved when an elevated concentration of troponin at presentation is used guide utilization of early angiography and revascularization if appropriate [1, 19].

## 2  Newer Ischemia Markers

Although hs-cTn assays allow for earlier detection of myocardial injury and a reduction in time to ACS diagnosis, cardiac troponins remain clinically employed as markers of necrosis, only indicative of an increased risk profile in patients for whom cardiac tissue has undergone irreversible injury [29]. It has previously been documented that patients with acute coronary syndromes who were contemporary troponin negative still had ~7% increased risk of adverse events in the 6 months after initial presentation [16, 30]. Markers of cardiac ischemia or other mechanisms are of potential value because about 40–60% of the acute coronary syndrome continuum do not have necrosis, so other indicators of increased risk may add information to cardiac troponin and the ECG. Markers of cardiac ischemia or other mechanisms remain an area of intense investigation and a litany of biochemical markers have been suggested as ischemia markers and risk stratification tools. Various candidate markers have been reviewed and a few will be specifically discussed here [31, 32].

## 2.1 Ischemia Modified Albumin

Oxidative stress and other physiological processes that occur during myocardial ischemia reportedly cause modifications in circulating albumin; the resulting modified albumin form has been coined "ischemia modified albumin" (IMA) and has diminished capacity for binding cobalt and other metals. This observation led to development of an albumin cobalt binding test for measurement of IMA and therefore the presence (or absence) of myocardial ischemia. The albumin cobalt binding test for IMA was FDA cleared as a serum biomarker of cardiac ischemia and risk stratification tool in suspected acute coronary syndrome patients.

A meta-analysis was conducted that included all studies evaluating the sensitivity and negative predictive value (NPV) of IMA in suspected acute coronary syndromes patients evaluated in an ED (25). This analysis showed that using three indicators together—an ECG that is nondiagnostic for ischemia, a negative cardiac troponin and a negative IMA test—yielded a sensitivity of 94.4%, and a NPV of 97.1% for diagnosis of acute coronary syndrome. The respective sensitivity and NPV for longer-term outcomes were 89.2% and 94.5% [33].

Although the clinical evidence for IMA indicates promise for use in ruling-out acute coronary syndromes and early risk stratification in the ED, the high-sensitivity assays for troponin have been better studied. One analysis by Mehta et al. suggests that there is a possible synergistic role for the IMA test when used with hs-cTnI [34].

## 2.2 Myeloperoxidase

Myeloperoxidase (MPO) is an enzyme which catalyzes the in vivo production of hypochlorite (bleach) from chloride and hydrogen peroxide; MPO is stored in abundant quantities in the azurophilic granules of polymorphonuclear neutrophils and macrophages. MPO may be an active player in destabilizing coronary plaque by degrading collagen, which is particularly troublesome when it occurs at the vulnerable plaque shoulder. This degradation can lead to plaque erosion and increased susceptibility for rupture, an important root cause of acute coronary syndromes. However, the full extent of all mechanisms generating this negative effect are not fully established [35].

Several studies have demonstrated that acute coronary syndrome patients having increased MPO in their blood are at increased risk [36]. One study conducted in the ED environment showed that the odds of major adverse events at 30 days and 6 months increased with each quartile increase in MPO blood concentration. Importantly, this increase in risk was 4.4-fold higher in patients who had elevated MPO but were persistently negative for cardiac troponin [37].

## 2.3  High-Sensitivity C-Reactive Protein

As atherosclerosis has been established as an inflammatory process, and the most well-described inflammatory marker is C-Reactive Protein (CRP), the studies seeking to evaluate this as a marker for CAD survival are plentiful, yet not specific [38, 39].

CRP has been shown to rise in patients presenting with acute coronary syndrome as a consequence of the inflammatory response to myocardial necrosis [40]. However elevated levels of CRP are also frequent in a large proportion of ED patients without myocardial necrosis. Numerous studies have indicated that hs-CRP is an independent predictor of short- and/or long-term outcome among patients with acute coronary syndrome, but beyond the thrombotic events, there is less of a relationship between CRP levels and atherosclerotic burden [41]. In fact, a study from 2008 showed that persons who had genetically higher CRP values did not have the expected outcomes for severe coronary disease [42]. Specifically, measurement of hs-CRP appears to contribute additional prognostic value in patients who are cardiac troponin negative and helps differentiate these levels from persons who are not symptomatic for coronary disease [43, 44]. Of interest, studies indicate that the relationship between hs-CRP and outcome is most robust with respect to mortality with a weaker relationship to recurrent MI [44]. However, the benefits of therapy based on hs-CRP remain uncertain and guidance of management should not be based solely upon measurement of CRP [1].

## 2.4  B-type Natriuretic Peptide and N-terminal proBNP

BNP is a heart hormone which has powerful physiological effects including natriuresis, vasodilatation, and inhibition of the renin-angiotensin-aldosterone system [45]. Ischemia appears to be an important stimulus for B-type natriuretic peptide (BNP) synthesis and release. BNP and its inert co-metabolite Amino-terminal proBNP (NT-proBNP) are released from cardiac myocytes in response to hemodynamic stress and specifically increased wall stress in the ventricles of the heart [46].

Impairment of ventricular relaxation and resulting non-systolic ventricular dysfunction is one of the earliest consequences of myocardial ischemia, preceding angina, and ST-segment deviation. This pathophysiology and a strong association between BNP and NT-proBNP with mortality in patients with unstable angina supports the idea that cardiac ischemia can stimulate release of BNP in the absence of necrosis [47].

Furthermore, in community based studies, risk for adverse events can be demonstrated with levels of BNP lower than what has been used for heart failure diagnosis [48]. However, given the data available for other markers management guidelines for acute coronary syndromes should not be based solely upon BNP or NT-proBNP values [1].

## 2.5 *Future Development*

At this time, there exist significant differences among hs-cTn assays in stratifying samples of patients with intermediate likelihood of ACS, which may result in different management recommendations [15]. The continued introduction of hs-cTn immunoassays to clinical practice will ultimately depend upon the determination of more accurate, suitable cut-offs in addition to the optimization of timing for serial sampling [49].

## 3 Point of Care Testing for Cardiac Biomarkers

Point of care testing (POCT) involves measurement of cardiac biomarkers at or near the patient bedside. Implementation of POCT for any clinical application is always driven by a "need for speed" that exceeds a central laboratory's ability to deliver information in time to improve either clinical or economic outcomes. POCT testing is invariably more costly than central lab testing and is encumbered by regulatory requirements. POCT is typically considered an option of last resort because virtually all organizations would prefer to measure cardiac markers within the infrastructure of the central laboratory, rather than going through all the trouble and expense of implementing POCT. Although the need for a rapid turnaround time for cardiac troponin has not been linked to improved clinical outcomes [50]. Faster results have been shown to facilitate patient flow and expedite decision-making and may even decrease patient charges in the right setting [50, 51]. Current guidelines strongly recommend that cardiac marker results be available within 1 h and optimally within 30 min of collection for care of patients in the ED [52].

As the implementation of hs-cTn into hospitals around the world continues, the value within POC testing decreases. cTn POC testing still does have a clinical role, but it's role is now complimentary to hs-cTn laboratory measurements. CTn POC testing may be useful when timely access to laboratory facilities for decision-making is not possible [53]. Outside of such scope, however, POC cTn limitations including the potential for false negative results on admission and the need for serial testing, yield it largely inferior the overall efficiency provided by rapid rule-out protocols using hs-cTn [54].

# 4   Future Developments

In the context of cardiac necrosis and MI, few analytes in laboratory medicine have the clinical value and impact of cTnT and cTnI. After all, cardiac troponin was mainly responsible for the re-definition of MI. For this reason it is difficult to conceive of a marker to replace cardiac troponin for the diagnosis of MI.

Very high-sensitivity cardiac troponin assays that are capable of reliable tenfold to 100-fold lower detection compared to current assays appear to be the path forward. Demonstrating an acute rise in cardiac troponin that is significantly higher than the sum of biological and analytical variation has led to detection of very subtle cardiac injury. Current developments that seek to demonstrate and quantify the rise of these values in terms of outcomes are ongoing. Further research is required to maximize the medical and economic value of hs-cTnT to patients and institutions [55].

# References


1. Morrow DA, Cannon CP, Jesse RL, et al. National Academy of Clinical Biochemistry Laboratory Medicine Practice Guidelines: clinical characteristics and utilization of biochemical markers in acute coronary syndromes. Clin Chem. 2007;53(4):552–74. https://doi.org/10.1373/clinchem.2006.084194.
2. Thygesen K, Alpert JS, White HD, et al. Universal definition of myocardial infarction. Circulation. 2007;116(22):2634–53. https://doi.org/10.1161/CIRCULATIONAHA.107.187397.
3. Apple FS, Sandoval Y, Jaffe AS, Ordonez-Llanos J, IFCC Task Force on Clinical Applications of Cardiac Bio-Markers. Cardiac troponin assays: guide to understanding analytical characteristics and their impact on clinical care. Clin Chem. 2017;63(1):73–81. https://doi.org/10.1373/clinchem.2016.255109.
4. Ar C, Pd A, Asv S, et al. High-sensitivity cardiac troponin and the universal definition of myocardial infarction. Circulation. 2019;141(3):161–71. https://doi.org/10.1161/circulationaha.119.042960.
5. Keller T, Zeller T, Peetz D, et al. Sensitive troponin I assay in early diagnosis of acute myocardial infarction. N Engl J Med. 2009;361(9):868–77. https://doi.org/10.1056/NEJMoa0903515.
6. McCarthy CP, Januzzi JL. Increasingly sensitive troponin assays: is perfect the enemy of good? J Am Heart Assoc. 2020;9(23):e019678. https://doi.org/10.1161/JAHA.120.019678.
7. Twerenbold R, Jaffe A, Reichlin T, Reiter M, Mueller C. High-sensitive troponin T measurements: what do we gain and what are the challenges? Eur Heart J. 2012;33(5):579–86. https://doi.org/10.1093/eurheartj/ehr492.

8. Eggers KM, Jernberg T, Ljung L, Lindahl B. High-sensitivity cardiac troponin-based strategies for the assessment of chest pain patients-a review of validation and clinical implementation studies. Clin Chem. 2018;64(11):1572–85. https://doi.org/10.1373/clinchem.2018.287342.

9. Ooi DS, Isotalo PA, Veinot JP. Correlation of antemortem serum creatine kinase, creatine kinase-MB, troponin I, and troponin T with cardiac pathology. Clin Chem. 2000;46(3):338–44.

10. Thygesen K, Alpert JS, Jaffe AS, et al. Fourth universal definition of myocardial infarction (2018). Glob Heart. 2018;13(4):305–38. https://doi.org/10.1016/j.gheart.2018.08.004.

11. Saenger AK, Jaffe AS. Requiem for a heavyweight: the demise of creatine kinase-MB. Circulation. 2008;118(21):2200–6. https://doi.org/10.1161/CIRCULATIONAHA.108.773218.

12. Eggers KM, Oldgren J, Nordenskjöld A, Lindahl B. Diagnostic value of serial measurement of cardiac markers in patients with chest pain: limited value of adding myoglobin to troponin I for exclusion of myocardial infarction. Am Heart J. 2004;148(4):574–81. https://doi.org/10.1016/j.ahj.2004.04.030.

13. Apple FS. A new season for cardiac troponin assays: it's time to keep a scorecard. Clin Chem. 2009;55(7):1303–6. https://doi.org/10.1373/clinchem.2009.128363.

14. Wildi K, Gimenez MR, Twerenbold R, et al. Misdiagnosis of myocardial infarction related to limitations of the current regulatory approach to define clinical decision values for cardiac troponin. Circulation. 2015;131(23):2032–40. https://doi.org/10.1161/CIRCULATIONAHA.114.014129.

15. Karády J, Mayrhofer T, Ferencik M, et al. Discordance of high-sensitivity troponin assays in patients with suspected acute coronary syndromes. J Am Coll Cardiol. 2021;77(12):1487–99. https://doi.org/10.1016/j.jacc.2021.01.046.

16. Kaul P, Newby LK, Fu Y, et al. Troponin T and quantitative ST-segment depression offer complementary prognostic information in the risk stratification of acute coronary syndrome patients. J Am Coll Cardiol. 2003;41(3):371–80. https://doi.org/10.1016/s0735-1097(02)02824-3.

17. Lagerqvist B, Diderholm E, Lindahl B, et al. FRISC score for selection of patients for an early invasive treatment strategy in unstable coronary artery disease. Heart. 2005;91(8):1047–52. https://doi.org/10.1136/hrt.2003.031369.

18. Morrow DA, Antman EM, Tanasijevic M, et al. Cardiac troponin I for stratification of early outcomes and the efficacy of enoxaparin in unstable angina: a TIMI-11B substudy. J Am Coll Cardiol. 2000;36(6):1812–7. https://doi.org/10.1016/s0735-1097(00)00942-6.

19. Morrow DA, Cannon CP, Rifai N, et al. Ability of minor elevations of troponins I and T to predict benefit from an early invasive strategy in patients with unstable angina and non-ST elevation myocardial infarction: results from a randomized trial. JAMA. 2001;286(19):2405–12. https://doi.org/10.1001/jama.286.19.2405.

20. Twerenbold R, Jaeger C, Rubini Gimenez M, et al. Impact of high-sensitivity cardiac troponin on use of coronary angiography, cardiac stress testing, and time to discharge in suspected acute myocardial infarction. Eur Heart J. 2016;37(44):3324–32. https://doi.org/10.1093/eurheartj/ehw232.

21. Chapman AR, Mills NL. High-sensitivity cardiac troponin and the early rule out of myocardial infarction: time for action. Heart. 2020;106(13):955–7. https://doi.org/10.1136/heartjnl-2020-316811.

22. Backus BE, Body R, Weinstock MB. Troponin testing in the emergency department—when 2 become 1. JAMA Netw Open. 2021;4(2):e210329. https://doi.org/10.1001/jamanetworkopen.2021.0329.

23. Chapman AR, Lee KK, McAllister DA, et al. Association of high-sensitivity cardiac troponin I concentration with cardiac outcomes in patients with suspected acute coronary syndrome. JAMA. 2017;318(19):1913–24. https://doi.org/10.1001/jama.2017.17488.

24. Anand A, Lee KK, Chapman AR, et al. High-sensitivity cardiac troponin on presentation to rule out myocardial infarction. Circulation. 2021;143(23):2214–24. https://doi.org/10.1161/CIRCULATIONAHA.120.052380.

25. McCord J, Cabrera R, Lindahl B, et al. Prognostic utility of a modified HEART score in chest pain patients in the emergency department. Circ Cardiovasc Qual Outcomes. 2017;10(2):e003101. https://doi.org/10.1161/CIRCOUTCOMES.116.003101.
26. Twerenbold R, Costabel JP, Nestelberger T, et al. Outcome of applying the ESC 0/1-hour algorithm in patients with suspected myocardial infarction. J Am Coll Cardiol. 2019;74(4):483–94. https://doi.org/10.1016/j.jacc.2019.05.046.
27. American College of Cardiology. Latest in ED risk stratification of chest pain: hs-cTn and risk scores. Washington, DC: American College of Cardiology; 2021. https://www.acc.org/latest-in-cardiology/articles/2021/04/30/13/47/http%3a%2f%2fwww.acc.org%2flatest-in-cardiology%2farticles%2f2021%2f04%2f30%2f13%2f47%2flatest-in-ed-risk-stratification-of-chest-pain. Accessed 25 Aug 2021.
28. Mahler SA, Lenoir KM, Wells BJ, et al. Safely Identifying Emergency Department Patients With Acute Chest Pain for Early Discharge. Circulation. 2018;138(22):2456–68. https://doi.org/10.1161/CIRCULATIONAHA.118.036528.
29. DAIC. Advantages of high sensitivity troponin assays. Arlington Heights, IL: DAIC; 2019. https://www.dicardiology.com/article/advantages-high-sensitivity-troponin-assays. Accessed 25 Aug 2021.
30. Morrow DA, de Lemos JA, Sabatine MS, et al. Evaluation of B-type natriuretic peptide for risk assessment in unstable angina/non-ST-elevation myocardial infarction: B-type natriuretic peptide and prognosis in TACTICS-TIMI 18. J Am Coll Cardiol. 2003;41(8):1264–72. https://doi.org/10.1016/s0735-1097(03)00168-2.
31. Apple FS, Wu AHB, Mair J, et al. Future biomarkers for detection of ischemia and risk stratification in acute coronary syndrome. Clin Chem. 2005;51(5):810–24. https://doi.org/10.1373/clinchem.2004.046292.
32. Morrow DA, Rifai N, Tanasijevic MJ, Wybenga DR, de Lemos JA, Antman EM. Clinical efficacy of three assays for cardiac troponin I for risk stratification in acute coronary syndromes: a thrombolysis in myocardial infarction (TIMI) 11B substudy. Clin Chem. 2000;46(4):453–60.
33. Bar-Or D, Lau E, Winkler JV. A novel assay for cobalt-albumin binding and its potential as a marker for myocardial ischemia-a preliminary report. J Emerg Med. 2000;19(4):311–5. https://doi.org/10.1016/s0736-4679(00)00255-9.
34. Mehta MD, Marwah SA, Ghosh S, Shah HN, Trivedi AP, Haridas N. A synergistic role of ischemia modified albumin and high-sensitivity troponin T in the early diagnosis of acute coronary syndrome. J Fam Med Prim Care. 2015;4(4):570–5. https://doi.org/10.4103/2249-4863.174295.
35. Ramachandra CJA, Ja KPMM, Chua J, Cong S, Shim W, Hausenloy DJ. Myeloperoxidase as a multifaceted target for cardiovascular protection. Antioxid Redox Signal. 2020;32(15):1135–49. https://doi.org/10.1089/ars.2019.7971.
36. Ndrepepa G. Myeloperoxidase - a bridge linking inflammation and oxidative stress with cardiovascular disease. Clin Chim Acta. 2019;493:36–51. https://doi.org/10.1016/j.cca.2019.02.022.
37. Brennan M-L, Penn MS, Van Lente F, et al. Prognostic value of myeloperoxidase in patients with chest pain. N Engl J Med. 2003;349(17):1595–604. https://doi.org/10.1056/NEJMoa035003.
38. Liuzzo G, Biasucci LM, Gallimore JR, et al. The prognostic value of C-reactive protein and serum amyloid a protein in severe unstable angina. N Engl J Med. 1994;331(7):417–24. https://doi.org/10.1056/NEJM199408183310701.
39. Pearson TA, Mensah GA, Alexander RW, et al. Markers of inflammation and cardiovascular disease: application to clinical and public health practice: a statement for healthcare professionals from the Centers for Disease Control and Prevention and the American Heart Association. Circulation. 2003;107(3):499–511. https://doi.org/10.1161/01.cir.0000052939.59093.45.
40. Pietilä K, Hermens WT, Harmoinen A, Baardman T, Pasternack A, Topol EJ, Simoons ML. Comparison of peak serum C-reactive protein and hydroxybutyrate dehydrogenase levels in patients with acute myocardial infarction treated with alteplase and streptokinase. Am J Cardiol. 1997;80(8):1075–7.

41. Folsom AR, Pankow JS, Tracy RP, et al. Association of C-reactive protein with markers of prevalent atherosclerotic disease. Am J Cardiol. 2001;88(2):112–7. https://doi.org/10.1016/s0002-9149(01)01603-4.
42. Zacho J, Tybjaerg-Hansen A, Jensen JS, Grande P, Sillesen H, Nordestgaard BG. Genetically elevated C-reactive protein and ischemic vascular disease. N Engl J Med. 2008;359(18):1897–908. https://doi.org/10.1056/NEJMoa0707402.
43. Lindahl B, Toss H, Siegbahn A, Venge P, Wallentin L. Markers of myocardial damage and inflammation in relation to long-term mortality in unstable coronary artery disease. FRISC Study Group. Fragmin during Instability in Coronary Artery Disease. N Engl J Med. 2000;343(16):1139–47. https://doi.org/10.1056/NEJM200010193431602.
44. Morrow DA, Rifai N, Antman EM, et al. C-reactive protein is a potent predictor of mortality independently of and in combination with troponin T in acute coronary syndromes: a TIMI 11A substudy. Thrombolysis in Myocardial Infarction. J Am Coll Cardiol. 1998;31(7):1460–5. https://doi.org/10.1016/s0735-1097(98)00136-3.
45. Azzazy HME, Christenson RH. B-type natriuretic peptide: physiologic role and assay characteristics. Heart Fail Rev. 2003;8(4):315–20. https://doi.org/10.1023/a:1026182912461.
46. de Lemos JA, McGuire DK, Drazner MH. B-type natriuretic peptide in cardiovascular disease. Lancet. 2003;362(9380):316–22. https://doi.org/10.1016/S0140-6736(03)13976-1.
47. de Lemos JA, Morrow DA. Brain natriuretic peptide measurement in acute coronary syndromes: ready for clinical application? Circulation. 2002;106(23):2868–70. https://doi.org/10.1161/01.cir.0000042763.07757.c0.
48. Wang TJ, Larson MG, Levy D, et al. Plasma natriuretic peptide levels and the risk of cardiovascular events and death. N Engl J Med. 2004;350(7):655–63. https://doi.org/10.1056/NEJMoa031994.
49. Lippi G, Sanchis-Gomar F. "Ultra-sensitive" cardiac troponins: requirements for effective implementation in clinical practice. Biochem Med (Zagreb). 2018;28(3):030501. https://doi.org/10.11613/BM.2018.030501.
50. Lee-Lewandrowski E, Corboy D, Lewandrowski K, Sinclair J, McDermot S, Benzer TI. Implementation of a point-of-care satellite laboratory in the emergency department of an academic medical center. Impact on test turnaround time and patient emergency department length of stay. Arch Pathol Lab Med. 2003;127(4):456–60. https://doi.org/10.5858/2003-127-0456-IOAPSL.
51. Apple FS, Chung AY, Kogut ME, Bubany S, Murakami MM. Decreased patient charges following implementation of point-of-care cardiac troponin monitoring in acute coronary syndrome patients in a community hospital cardiology unit. Clin Chim Acta. 2006;370(1–2):191–5. https://doi.org/10.1016/j.cca.2006.02.011.
52. Nichols JH, Christenson RH, Clarke W, et al. Executive summary. The National Academy of Clinical Biochemistry Laboratory Medicine Practice Guideline: evidence-based practice for point-of-care testing. Clin Chim Acta. 2007;379(1–2):14–28; discussion 29–30. https://doi.org/10.1016/j.cca.2006.12.025.
53. Apple FS, Fantz CR, Collinson PO. Implementation of high-sensitivity and point-of-care cardiac troponin assays into practice: some different thoughts. Clin Chem. 2020;67:hvaa264. https://doi.org/10.1093/clinchem/hvaa264.
54. Venge P, Ohberg C, Flodin M, Lindahl B. Early and late outcome prediction of death in the emergency room setting by point-of-care and laboratory assays of cardiac troponin I. Am Heart J. 2010;160(5):835–41. https://doi.org/10.1016/j.ahj.2010.07.036.
55. Mueller C, Boeddinghaus J, Nestelberger T. Downstream consequences of implementing high-sensitivity cardiac troponin. J Am Coll Cardiol. 2021;77(25):3180–3. https://doi.org/10.1016/j.jacc.2021.04.063.

# Emergency Department Presentation of Chest Pain

Natasia Terry and Kristin Aromolaran

## 1 Arrival to ED

In the US, chest pain is the second most common reason, after abdominal pain, for presentation to the emergency department according to the CDC [1]. Patients with this complaint may arrive via emergency medical services or self-transportation, often dependent on access and community. For patients transported via EMS, pre-hospital ECG acquisition is an internationally recognized recommendation for care of the ACS patient [2]. A recent audit of the prehospital MI program in the UK found a survival advantage in patients who obtained an ECG prior to arrival in the ED. This adds to the body of literature that has previously shown that paramedics can obtain a high quality ECG and it decreases door-to-balloon time (D2B) [3–5].

Despite the guidelines, patients may often choose to transport themselves to the ED. This could often result in a shorter trip to the ED door, but given EMS transport often expedites medical professionals arriving at the patient's bedside, may in fact lead to a longer time to treatment for these self-transporting patients [6].

Although multiple groups recommend EMS transport for chest pain and is a centerpiece of the American College of Cardiology's communication program, a recent Danish study suggests that transport via EMS is likely low yield. In their more than 71,000 cases reviewed, one in six ambulance trips involved chest pain, but had a discharge rate from the ED of more than 50% [7, 8]. However, given that ischemic heart disease remains the leading cause of death of humans worldwide, the low yield of this process for the sake of earlier treatment is likely reasonable [9].

N. Terry (✉) · K. Aromolaran
Department of Emergency Medicine, Emory University School of Medicine, Atlanta, GA, USA
e-mail: nataisia.terry@EMORY.EDU



M. Pena et al. (eds.), *Short Stay Management of Chest Pain*, Contemporary Cardiology, https://doi.org/10.1007/978-3-031-05520-1_9

93

## 2   Presentations of Acute Coronary Syndrome

Adult patients who present to the emergency department with chest pain or shortness of breath should prompt the care team to consider acute coronary syndrome (ACS). Although simple and seemingly broad, this approach does not fully take into account the nuance of this clinical situation.

A 2004 review defined "Typical Angina" as "Substernal discomfort, precipitated by exertion, improved with rest or nitroglycerin in less than 10 min" and further concluded that overall, it had the highest overall likelihood ratio in diagnosis of coronary artery disease. In diagnosis of MI, these same authors found that the presence of "pressure-like" chest pain had the highest LR which was only 1.3 [10].

Another way to conceptualize who should be evaluated for ACS is to examine the characteristics of those who ultimately have the most serious outcome of ACS short of sudden cardiac death and should receive an ECG rapidly. Criteria for a triage ECG, initially put forth by Graff, are listed in Table 1 [11]. Glickman and colleagues further added malaise and nausea for persons over 80, but Osborne et al. found that the addition of this criteria provided little yield in another hospital [12, 13]. That said, these criteria can serve as guidelines only and should not usurp physician judgment.

As discussed elsewhere in this text, the diagnosis of the myocardial infarction acute coronary syndrome may prove to be straightforward as the crux of the diagnosis rests on the acquisition of either an ECG or laboratory biomarkers. The remaining two acute coronary syndrome diagnoses of stable and unstable angina can provide significant diagnostic challenges. Classically, these are described as diagnoses in persons not exhibiting myocardial necrosis evidenced by lack of biomarkers and ECG findings suggestive of acute cellular death [14]. Descriptions of chest pain with effort date back to the eighteenth century and its association with myocardial infarction are also well documented [15]. With the use of more high-sensitivity troponin assays, the patients who were once thought to have angina, now would be more appropriately categorized as having a myocardial infarction [16, 17]. As such, the overall incidence of persons who have (or had) angina is decreasing with the increasing ability to detect lower levels of troponin indicative of myocardial cell death.

Therefore, the utility of parsing out differences between unstable and stable angina is also decreasing and the most prudent evaluation is one where the presentation for AMI is considered alongside anginal conditions in the broader search for the presence of coronary artery disease.

## 3   Confounders and Atypical Presentations

In classical teaching, ACS presents as crushing, substernal chest pain that radiates to the arm or jaw and is associated with nausea, weakness, and diaphoresis, many patients present with atypical symptoms. It may be more accurate to say is that "the typical presentation of acute coronary syndrome is atypical." Pain perception and descriptions vary widely among patients and are influenced by numerous factors including older age, diabetes mellitus, female gender, and non-white race [18]. Atypical presentations of patients with ACS include dyspnea, nausea, diaphoresis, syncope, or pain in the arms, epigastrium, shoulder, or neck. When these symptoms present without chest pain they are known as "anginal equivalents." Others may have no symptoms at all of myocardial infarction. A 2002 review suggested that approximately 50% of patients with AMI will not have chest pain as a chief complaint and researchers from a 2010 prospective study found that the classic "radiation to the left arm" component of the history was less predictive of MI than several of the more atypical complaints.

Unfortunately, patients with atypical presentations have continually been found to have poorer outcomes despite data published in 2000 showing worsening mortality [19]. These patients also are less likely to receive standard adjunct therapies shown to reduce mortality and are treated less aggressively even in the setting of an STEMI [20, 21].

Elderly patients are a population well known for their atypical presentations of ACS. In fact, findings from Bayer and colleagues suggest that a patient's age has a direct correlation with atypical presentations. In a review of over 700 patients with proven myocardial infarction (average age 76.0) chest pain was seen in only 66% of patients; 75% over the age of 70 and only 50% over the age of 80. Above age 85 years old, chest pain was present in only 38%, making a classic presentation in this age group an exception [22]. In many trials and database inquiries, the elderly have worse outcomes and less adherence to guideline recommended therapies despite the fact that no set of ACS guidlelines fractionates the adult treatment population [23]. In this population, other common symptoms include nausea and vomiting, dyspnea, palpitations, and diaphoresis. One study of 446 patients found that 39% presented with palpitations, 28% with fatigue, and 20% with nausea/vomiting. Furthermore, unlike the typical teaching, these symptoms are less likely to be induced by physical exertion in the elderly and instead by other stressors such as infection or dehydration [24, 25].

Unsurprisingly, CAD is the leading cause of death in women just like men and there are important gender differences to note in their presentations of coronary ischemia. On average, women are almost a decade older than men at the time of their MI with greater than 55% of their AMIs at 70 years or older [26]. Patients and physicians may not have a high enough suspicion that symptoms at a younger age of presentation could be from coronary ischemia as women are often given lower risk categories by their primary care physicians which, according to a 2005 survey, may be the driver of them receiving fewer preventative recommendations [27]. Some of the most recent studies show a that outcomes from CAD may be similar for women and men after controlling for risk factors, but disparities arise when examining Hispanic or African-American Women [28–30].

When women do present with symptoms, they are more likely to have more atypical presentation than men, however, both groups still present most commonly with chest pain. One meta-analysis found that both men and women present most often with chest pain (pooled prevalence, men 79%; 95% CI, 72–85, pooled prevalence, women 74%; 95% CI, 72–85), although men more than women. This same meta-analysis which included 27 studies also found that when compared to men, women had higher odds of presenting with several atypical symptoms. Specifically, pain between the shoulder blades (OR 2.15; 95% CI, 1.95–2.37), nausea or vomiting (OR 1.64; 95% CI, 1.48–1.82), and shortness of breath (OR 1.34; 95% CI, 1.21–1.48) [31]. This higher odds of atypical symptoms could be the underlying cause of data from the Framingham study which indicates that the percentage of unrecognized infarcts was highest in women and older men [18].

Non-white patients represent another population with disturbingly higher rates of missed ACS. From a multicenter prospective trial, Pope and colleagues showed that non-white patients were less likely to be hospitalized if they presented with either acute cardiac ischemia, but the findings of triage acuity may have diminished in more recent studies [32, 33]. One recent study looked at ACS symptom presentation among white, Chinese and South Asian patients. It found that midsternal pain was the most common presenting symptoms regardless of ethnicity. Furthermore, 33% of white participants, 19% of South Asian, and 20% of Chinese participants reported atypical symptoms ($p < 0.006$) [34]. While it may not be entirely clear why these disparities exist in presentation, another study interviewed patients of different ethnicities and found that that delayed presentation for minority groups was due to cost, language barriers, thinking their symptoms are "non-urgent" and concern about the disruptive effect that going to the hospital could have on their home and family [34]. Despite this initial qualitative data, there is a lack of in-depth analysis into the underlying reason for healthcare disparities among non-white patients. Further research must be done in order to truly understand why patients of non-white race have higher rates of missed ACS and poorer outcomes.

Diabetes has long been understood as an independent risk factor for coronary artery disease and has been demonstrated in meta-analysis [35]. Coronary atherosclerosis does not only appear to be more prevalent, but also more extensive in diabetic than nondiabetic patients [36, 37]. In fact, with a two- to fourfold increase in cardiovascular events compared to nondiabetics, the main cause of death for diabetics is cardiovascular morbidity [38].

In addition to the increased incidence and mortality of coronary heart disease in diabetics, their higher incidence of atypical presentations requires the emergency physician to be ever more vigilant in evaluating the diabetic with possible ACS. Their atypical presentations are most commonly believed to be due to their blunted appreciation for ischemic pain. Histologic and physiologic evidence of damage to cardiac afferent nerve fibers has been shown in diabetic patients, suggesting that neuropathy, as well as prolongation of the anginal perceptual threshold and an abnormality in metaiodobenzylguanidine uptake, may play a role in blunting the perception of ischemic pain [39, 40]. This may lead to symptoms that are mild, atypical, or truly silent and therefore accurate diagnosis of ACS based upon the history may be more difficult. The prevalence of silent MI in low-risk diabetic patients ranges from 6% to 23% in various studies and has been found to be as high as 60% in high-risk diabetic patients [41]. In the Framingham study, 12% of MIs were believed to be truly asymptomatic. It was more common in diabetic patients (39%) compared with their nondiabetic counterparts (22%) [18].

When symptoms do exist, several studies have found that diabetes is an independent risk factor for an atypical presentation of ACS [38]. Atypical symptoms such as confusion, dyspnea, fatigue or nausea, and vomiting may be the presenting complaint in 32–42% of diabetic patients with MI compared with 6–15% of nondiabetic patients, but other studies do not show much difference in the presentations [42, 43]. On balance, it does appear fair to conclude that atypical chest pain in diabetic patients leads to worse clinical outcomes most recently evidenced by an analysis of patients with DM presenting with atypical chest pain had the highest risk of all-cause death (HR 2.23, 95% CI 1.80–2.76) and any MI (HR 2.34, 95% CI 1.51–3.64) [44].

# 4 Differential Diagnosis

The emergency physician should use a thorough history and physical exam to not only help determine the risk of possible ACS, but also to recognize and distinguish anginal chest pain from other serious and life-threatening conditions. While the differential diagnosis for both "typical" and "atypical" anginal symptoms is broad, the most important alternative diagnoses include aortic dissection, pulmonary embolism, esophageal perforation (Boerhaave's syndrome), and spontaneous pneumothorax.

## *4.1 Aortic Dissection*

Patients with aortic dissection classically have risk factors that may include known atherosclerosis, uncontrolled hypertension, coarctation of the aorta, bicuspid aortic valves, aortic stenosis, Marfan syndrome or Ehlers-Danlos syndrome [45]. They complain of a ripping, searing or tearing chest pain that radiates to the intrascapular area of the back. It is typically maximal at onset and may be felt both above and below the diaphragm. Their physical exam may reveal a diastolic murmur from aortic insufficiency and unequal blood pressures in their upper extremities. The chest radiograph may show numerous nonspecific findings, the most helpful being a widened mediastinum. In a meta-analysis involving 21 studies with 1848 patients, the pooled sensitivity of a widened mediastinum was 83% in patients with proven dissection [46]. However, another study found that more than 20% of patients with confirmed aortic dissection lacked any abnormalities in the mediastinum or aortic contour, particularly in patients with a nondilated by dissected aorta [47]. Even though things like the Aortic Dissection Detection risk score shows promise for ruling out disease, specific imaging with CT, MRI or echocardiography may ultimately be necessary [48].

## *4.2   Pulmonary Embolism*

Pulmonary embolism (PE) is an often insidious and potentially lethal diagnosis. While the mortality of PE is traditionally estimated as high as 30%, it falls to 8% with timely diagnosis and treatment. Patients may present with any combination of chest pain, dyspnea, syncope, shock or hypoxia but, like ACS, may also present with atypical symptoms. Classic risk factors that promote a state of thrombosis include but are not limited to malignancy, lower extremity trauma, prolonged inactivity (bed rest, hospitalization) and thrombophilic disease states (e.g., protein C deficiency). If chest pain is present, it is classically described as sharp and pleuritic. The physical exam may be asymptomatic or include leg pain and swelling, tachypnea, tachycardia, hypoxia, or hypotension. Numerous studies have been performed to help risk stratify patients. A systematic review by Stein et al. showed that an ELISA D-dimer has a sensitivity of 0.95 (CL, 0.85–1.00), and negative likelihood ratio, 0.13 (CL, 0.03–0.58) [49]. Used with a low pre-test probability as determined by a clinical decision aid (such as the Wells criteria or Charlotte Rule), a rule with high negative predictive value can be achieved. Although d-dimer testing may be adequate in low-risk patients, those considered high risk require either a CT angiogram or *V/Q* scan to more accurately exclude the diagnosis.

## *4.3   Esophageal Rupture*

Esophageal rupture (Boerhaave's syndrome) is a rare but deadly cause of chest pain and must be considered by the evaluating physician, especially given mortality rates of up to 40% [50]. Most cases occur after endoscopy, or less commonly, after forceful vomiting. The patient classically describes a history of substernal, sharp chest pain with onset suddenly after emesis. They are usually ill-appearing, dyspneic, and diaphoretic. While the exam may be normal, it may reveal a pneumothorax or subcutaneous air. In a review at Rhode Island Hospital, 44 cases were identified (30 cases were after endoscopic procedures) [43]. Of those that did not undergo endoscopy, presenting signs and symptoms in this cohort included vomiting (50%), chest pain (43%), tachycardia (71%), decreased breath sounds (36%). All but one of these 14 patients had an abnormal chest X-ray and the correct diagnosis was made in only three cases. Once again, the "classic" presentation is more "classic" than common. Swallow studies (barium or gastrografin) are typically the initial study of choice but may be normal in 25% of cases and should not be used alone to exclude the diagnosis.

## *4.4   Spontaneous Pneumothorax*

Spontaneous pneumothorax is due to a sudden change in the barometric pressure in the lungs, most often in patients with obstructive lung disease (asthmatics and COPD). It is most typically described as a sharp, sudden pleuritic chest pain that is associated with dyspnea. Patients may be ill-appearing, dyspneic, and diaphoretic. The physical exam may be normal or reveal decreased breath sounds and hyperexpansion on the affected side. An upright inspiratory chest radiograph will usually reveal the diagnosis, with the increasing accessibility of ultrasound in emergency departments across the country, ultrasound has become a viable means of diagnosing a pneumothorax. One study looking at posttraumatic pneumothoraxes found that ultrasound had a sensitivity of 58.9% with a positive likelihood ratio of 69.7 and a specificity of 99.1% when compared to the composite standard. Furthermore, when compared to CXR, using CT scan as the gold standard, ultrasound had a higher sensitivity than CXR, 48.8% and 20.9%, respectively, and a similar specificity of 99.6% and 98.7%, respectively [51].

# 5  Electrocardiogram Analysis

The ECG is the single most important diagnostic test in the evaluation of patients with chest pain as it is so readily available and fast. The American College of Cardiology and the American Heart Association guidelines for ECG acquisition within the first 10 min upon the presentation of a patient with chest discomfort or symptoms consistent with ACS [52]. Time to ECG acquisition has also been identified as one of the key components of the National Heart Attack Alert Program's initiative to shorten time to interventional therapy (time to ECG acquisition). Diercks et al. found in a population of over 60,000 patients with NSTEMI, female gender was the most significant predictor of delayed ECG acquisition. This is significant because Diercks et al. also found that a delay in ECG acquisition led to an increase in clinical outcomes for STEMI patients at 30 days (odds ratio, 3.95; 95% confidence interval, 1.06–14.72; $p = 0.04$) [53].

Best practices put forth by the National Heart Attack Alert Program and AHA, beyond deciding to obtain an ECG, performing the ECG, and presenting the ECG to the treating physician for interpretation, suggests a prehospital ECG to decrease the time to diagnosis [54, 55]. They suggest that a protocol be in place to allow nurses to obtain a 12 lead EKG without a physician's order, and to do so with criteria liberal enough to include patients with atypical symptoms. The ECG still remains a challenge for many programs as a recent study described the missed case rate of several emergency departments varied widely despite the years of guidelines available preceding this evaluation [56].

Designing a program for this process should be intentional and simple criteria should be in place to capture the STEMI population within 10 min. Graff et al. developed criteria listed in Table 1 and this was later verified by Osborne et al. [11, 13]. Glickman and colleagues added nausea and malaise to an elderly group of patients, but ultimately, these criteria should be considered as a starting point for development of a pathway tailored to fit an ED's population [12]. Furthermore, one ECG is only a portion of a dynamic disease process. The ACC/AHA guidelines support obtaining serial 12-lead ECGs in the ED to improve sensitivity for detecting ACS if the initial ECG is nondiagnostic [57]

**Table 1** Graff criteria for triage (rapid) ECG

| Patients with age >30 with |
| --- |
| • Chest pain |
| Patients with age >50 with (any) |
| • Palpitations |
| • Weakness |
| • Syncope |
| • Dyspnea |

# References


1. CDC. National Hospital Ambulatory Medical Care Survey: 2018 Emergency Department summary tables. Atlanta, GA: CDC; 2018. p. 39.
2. O'Gara PT, Kushner FG, Ascheim DD, et al. 2013 ACCF/AHA guideline for the management of ST-elevation myocardial infarction: executive summary: a report of the American College of Cardiology Foundation/American Heart Association Task Force on Practice Guidelines. J Am Coll Cardiol. 2013;61(4):485–510. https://doi.org/10.1016/j.jacc.2012.11.018.
3. Aufderheide TP, Hendley GE, Thakur RK, et al. The diagnostic impact of prehospital 12-lead electrocardiography. Ann Emerg Med. 1990;19(11):1280–7. https://doi.org/10.1016/s0196-0644(05)82288-7.
4. Canto JG, Rogers WJ, Bowlby LJ, French WJ, Pearce DJ, Weaver WD. The prehospital electrocardiogram in acute myocardial infarction: is its full potential being realized? National Registry of Myocardial Infarction 2 Investigators. J Am Coll Cardiol. 1997;29(3):498–505. https://doi.org/10.1016/s0735-1097(96)00532-3.
5. Quinn T, Johnsen S, Gale CP, et al. Effects of prehospital 12-lead ECG on processes of care and mortality in acute coronary syndrome: a linked cohort study from the Myocardial Ischaemia National Audit Project. Heart. 2014;100(12):944–50. https://doi.org/10.1136/heartjnl-2013-304599.
6. Hutchings CB, Mann NC, Daya M, et al. Patients with chest pain calling 9-1-1 or self-transporting to reach definitive care: which mode is quicker? Am Heart J. 2004;147(1):35–41. https://doi.org/10.1016/s0002-8703(03)00510-6.
7. ACC Accreditation Services. Community education and EHAC. Washington, DC: ACC Accreditation Services; n.d.. https://cvquality.acc.org/accreditation/advocacy/Community-Education. Accessed 19 Jun 2021.
8. Pedersen C, Stengaard C, Friesgaard K, et al. Chest pain in the ambulance; prevalence, causes and outcome - a retrospective cohort study. Scand J Trauma Resusc Emerg Med. 2019;27:84. https://doi.org/10.1186/s13049-019-0659-6.
9. WHO. The top 10 causes of death. Geneva: WHO; 2020. https://www.who.int/news-room/fact-sheets/detail/the-top-10-causes-of-death. Accessed 19 Jun 2021.
10. Akita Chun A, McGee SR. Bedside diagnosis of coronary artery disease: a systematic review. Am J Med. 2004;117(5):334–43. https://doi.org/10.1016/j.amjmed.2004.03.021.
11. Graff L, Palmer AC, Lamonica P, Wolf S. Triage of patients for a rapid (5-minute) electrocardiogram: a rule based on presenting chief complaints. Ann Emerg Med. 2000;36(6):554–60. https://doi.org/10.1067/mem.2000.111057.
12. Glickman SW, Shofer FS, Wu MC, et al. Development and validation of a prioritization rule for obtaining an immediate 12-lead electrocardiogram in the emergency department to identify ST-elevation myocardial infarction. Am Heart J. 2012;163(3):372–82. https://doi.org/10.1016/j.ahj.2011.10.021.
13. Osborne A, Ali K, Lowery-North D, et al. Ability of triage decision rules for rapid electrocardiogram to identify patients with suspected ST-elevation myocardial infarction. Crit Pathw Cardiol. 2012;11:211–3. https://doi.org/10.1097/HPC.0b013e31826f4e8e.

14. Braunwald E, Antman EM, Beasley JW, et al. ACC/AHA guidelines for the management of patients with unstable angina and non-ST-segment elevation myocardial infarction: executive summary and recommendations. A report of the American College of Cardiology/American Heart Association task force on practice guidelines (committee on the management of patients with unstable angina). Circulation. 2000;102:1193–209.

15. Heberden W. Some account of disorder of the breast. Med Trans R Coll Phys (Lond). 1772;2:59–67.

16. Braunwald E, Morrow DA. Unstable angina. Circulation. 2013;127(24):2452–7. https://doi.org/10.1161/CIRCULATIONAHA.113.001258.

17. Mendis S, Thygesen K, Kuulasmaa K, et al. World Health Organization definition of myocardial infarction: 2008–09 revision. Int J Epidemiol. 2011;40(1):139–46. https://doi.org/10.1093/ije/dyq165.

18. Margolis JR, Kannel WS, Feinleib M, Dawber TR, McNamara PM. Clinical features of unrecognized myocardial infarction--silent and symptomatic. Eighteen year follow-up: the Framingham study. Am J Cardiol. 1973;32(1):1–7. https://doi.org/10.1016/s0002-9149(73)80079-7.

19. Canto JG, Shlipak MG, Rogers WJ, et al. Prevalence, clinical characteristics, and mortality among patients with myocardial infarction presenting without chest pain. JAMA. 2000;283:3223–9.

20. Hammer Y, Eisen A, Hasdai D, et al. Comparison of outcomes in patients with acute coronary syndrome presenting with typical versus atypical symptoms. Am J Cardiol. 2019;124(12):1851–6. https://doi.org/10.1016/j.amjcard.2019.09.007.

21. Zdzienicka J, Siudak Z, Zawiślak B, et al. Patients with non-ST-elevation myocardial infarction and without chest pain are treated less aggressively and experience higher in-hospital mortality. Kardiol Pol. 2007;65(7):769–75; discussion 776–7.

22. Bayer AJ, Chadha JS, Farag RR, Pathy MS. Changing presentation of myocardial infarction with increasing old age. J Am Geriatr Soc. 1986;34(4):263–6. https://doi.org/10.1111/j.1532-5415.1986.tb04221.x.

23. Carro A, Kaski JC. Myocardial infarction in the elderly. Aging Dis. 2010;2(2):116–37.

24. Engberding N, Wenger NK. Acute coronary syndromes in the elderly. F1000Research. 2017;6:1791. https://doi.org/10.12688/f1000research.11064.1.

25. Pour HA. Comparison of clinical presentation related on risk factors in older and younger patients with acute coronary syndrome. Int J Clin Cardiol. 2015;2:6. https://doi.org/10.23937/2378-2951/1410058.

26. Chandra NC, Ziegelstein RC, Rogers WJ, et al. Observations of the treatment of women in the United States with myocardial infarction: a report from the National Registry of Myocardial Infarction-I. Arch Intern Med. 1998;158(9):981–8. https://doi.org/10.1001/archinte.158.9.981.

27. Mosca L, Linfante AH, Benjamin EJ, et al. National study of physician awareness and adherence to cardiovascular disease prevention guidelines. Circulation. 2005;111(4):499–510. https://doi.org/10.1161/01.CIR.0000154568.43333.82.

28. Berger JS, Elliott L, Gallup D, et al. Sex differences in mortality following acute coronary syndromes. JAMA. 2009;302(8):874–82. https://doi.org/10.1001/jama.2009.1227.

29. Siabani S, Davidson PM, Babakhani M, et al. Gender-based difference in early mortality among patients with ST-segment elevation myocardial infarction: insights from Kermanshah STEMI Registry. J Cardiovasc Thorac Res. 2020;12(1):63–8. https://doi.org/10.34172/jcvtr.2020.10.

30. Williams RA. Cardiovascular disease in African American women: a health care disparities issue. J Natl Med Assoc. 2009;101(6):536–40. https://doi.org/10.1016/s0027-9684(15)30938-x.

31. van Oosterhout REM, de Boer AR, Maas AHEM, Rutten FH, Bots ML, Peters SAE. Sex differences in symptom presentation in acute coronary syndromes: a systematic review and meta-analysis. J Am Heart Assoc. 2020;9(9):e014733. https://doi.org/10.1161/JAHA.119.014733.

32. Mukhopadhyay A, D'Angelo R, Senser E, Whelan K, Wee CC, Mukamal KJ. Racial and insurance disparities among patients presenting with chest pain in the US: 2009-2015. Am J Emerg Med. 2020;38(7):1373–6. https://doi.org/10.1016/j.ajem.2019.11.018.

33. Pope JH, Aufderheide TP, Ruthazer R, et al. Missed diagnoses of acute cardiac ischemia in the emergency department. N Engl J Med. 2000;342(16):1163–70. https://doi.org/10.1056/NEJM200004203421603.

34. King-Shier K, Quan H, Kapral MK, et al. Acute coronary syndromes presentations and care outcomes in white, South Asian and Chinese patients: a cohort study. BMJ Open. 2019;9(3):e022479. https://doi.org/10.1136/bmjopen-2018-022479.

35. Selvin E, Marinopoulos S, Berkenblit G, et al. Meta-analysis: glycosylated hemoglobin and cardiovascular disease in diabetes mellitus. Ann Intern Med. 2004;141(6):421–31. https://doi.org/10.7326/0003-4819-141-6-200409210-00007.

36. Ravipati G, Aronow WS, Ahn C, Sujata K, Saulle LN, Weiss MB. Association of hemoglobin A(1c) level with the severity of coronary artery disease in patients with diabetes mellitus. Am J Cardiol. 2006;97(7):968–9. https://doi.org/10.1016/j.amjcard.2005.10.039.

37. Waller BF, Palumbo PJ, Lie JT, Roberts WC. Status of the coronary arteries at necropsy in diabetes mellitus with onset after age 30 years. Analysis of 229 diabetic patients with and without clinical evidence of coronary heart disease and comparison to 183 control subjects. Am J Med. 1980;69(4):498–506. https://doi.org/10.1016/s0149-2918(05)80002-5.

38. Khafaji HAH, Suwaidi JMA. Atypical presentation of acute and chronic coronary artery disease in diabetics. World J Cardiol. 2014;6(8):802–13. https://doi.org/10.4330/wjc.v6.i8.802.

39. Janand-Delenne B, Savin B, Habib G, Bory M, Vague P, Lassmann-Vague V. Silent myocardial ischemia in patients with diabetes: who to screen. Diabetes Care. 1999;22(9):1396–400. https://doi.org/10.2337/diacare.22.9.1396.

40. Scognamiglio R, Negut C, Ramondo A, Tiengo A, Avogaro A. Detection of coronary artery disease in asymptomatic patients with type 2 diabetes mellitus. J Am Coll Cardiol. 2006;47(1):65–71. https://doi.org/10.1016/j.jacc.2005.10.008.

41. Association AD. Consensus Development Conference on the Diagnosis of Coronary Heart Disease in People with Diabetes: 10–11 February 1998, Miami, Florida. Diabetes Care. 1998;21(9):1551–9. https://doi.org/10.2337/diacare.21.9.1551.

42. Nesto RW, Phillips RT. Asymptomatic myocardial ischemia in diabetic patients. Am J Med. 1986;80(4C):40–7. https://doi.org/10.1016/0002-9343(86)90451-1.

43. Richman PB, Brogan GX, Nashed AN, Thode HC. Clinical characteristics of diabetic vs nondiabetic patients who "rule-in" for acute myocardial infarction. Acad Emerg Med. 1999;6(7):719–23. https://doi.org/10.1111/j.1553-2712.1999.tb00441.x.

44. Lee J-W, Moon JS, Kang DR, et al. Clinical impact of atypical chest pain and diabetes mellitus in patients with acute myocardial infarction from prospective KAMIR-NIH registry. J Clin Med. 2020;9(2):505. https://doi.org/10.3390/jcm9020505.

45. Nienaber CA, Eagle KA. Aortic dissection: new frontiers in diagnosis and management: Part I: from etiology to diagnostic strategies. Circulation. 2003;108(5):628–35. https://doi.org/10.1161/01.CIR.0000087009.16755.E4.

46. Klompas M. Does this patient have an acute thoracic aortic dissection? JAMA. 2002;287(17):2262–72. https://doi.org/10.1001/jama.287.17.2262.

47. Evangelista A, Isselbacher EM, Bossone E, et al. Insights from the international registry of acute aortic dissection. Circulation. 2018;137(17):1846–60. https://doi.org/10.1161/CIRCULATIONAHA.117.031264.

48. Rogers AM, Hermann LK, Booher AM, et al. Sensitivity of the aortic dissection detection risk score, a novel guideline-based tool for identification of acute aortic dissection at initial presentation: results from the international registry of acute aortic dissection. Circulation. 2011;123(20):2213–8. https://doi.org/10.1161/CIRCULATIONAHA.110.988568.

49. Stein PD, Hull RD, Patel KC, et al. D-Dimer for the exclusion of acute venous thrombosis and pulmonary embolism. Ann Intern Med. 2004;140(8):589–602. https://doi.org/10.7326/0003-4819-140-8-200404200-00005.

50. Turner AR, Turner SD. Boerhaave syndrome. In: StatPearls. Treasure Island, FL: StatPearls Publishing; 2021. http://www.ncbi.nlm.nih.gov/books/NBK430808/. Accessed 1 Sep 2021.

51. Kirkpatrick AW, Sirois M, Laupland KB, et al. Hand-held thoracic sonography for detecting post-traumatic pneumothoraces: the Extended Focused Assessment with Sonography for Trauma (EFAST). J Trauma. 2004;57(2):288–95. https://doi.org/10.1097/01.ta.0000133565.88871.e4.
52. Amsterdam EA, Wenger NK, Brindis RG, et al. 2014 AHA/ACC guideline for the management of patients with non-ST-elevation acute coronary syndromes: executive summary: a report of the American College of Cardiology/American Heart Association Task Force on Practice Guidelines. Circulation. 2014;130(25):2354–94. https://doi.org/10.1161/CIR.0000000000000133.
53. Diercks DB, Peacock WF, Hiestand BC, et al. Frequency and consequences of recording an electrocardiogram >10 minutes after arrival in an emergency room in non-ST-segment elevation acute coronary syndromes (from the CRUSADE Initiative). Am J Cardiol. 2006;97(4):437–42. https://doi.org/10.1016/j.amjcard.2005.09.073.
54. Garvey JL, MacLeod BA, Sopko G, et al. Pre-hospital 12-lead electrocardiography programs: a call for implementation by emergency medical services systems providing advanced life support--National Heart Attack Alert Program (NHAAP) Coordinating Committee; National Heart, Lung, and Blood Institute (NHLBI); National Institutes of Health. J Am Coll Cardiol. 2006;47(3):485–91. https://doi.org/10.1016/j.jacc.2005.08.072.
55. Ting HH, Krumholz HM, Bradley EH, et al. Implementation and integration of prehospital ECGs into systems of care for acute coronary syndrome. Circulation. 2008;118(10):1066–79. https://doi.org/10.1161/CIRCULATIONAHA.108.190402.
56. Yiadom MYAB, Baugh CW, McWade CM, et al. Performance of emergency department screening criteria for an early ECG to identify ST-segment elevation myocardial infarction. J Am Heart Assoc. 2017;6(3):e003528. https://doi.org/10.1161/JAHA.116.003528.
57. Antman EM, Anbe DT, et al. ACC/AHA guidelines for the management of patients with ST-elevation myocardial infarction—executive summary. Circulation. 2004;110(5):588–636. https://doi.org/10.1161/01.CIR.0000134791.68010.FA.

# Risk Scoring Systems: Are They Necessary?

**Jaron Raper, Laura Goyack, and Matthew DeLaney**

## 1  Introduction

Chest pain is a common presentation to the emergency department. Various clinical scoring systems have been developed and implemented in effort to quantify a patient's risk of having a major adverse cardiac event (MACE) while simultaneously decreasing unnecessary testing and prevent unnecessary hospitalizations. Although there is no universal, agreed upon designation of what constitutes "High" versus "Low" risk outside of the rubrics of individual systems, the concept of a patient who has very low probability of having a MACE appears to stretch across the various scoring systems. Conversely, however, in the broader definitions of ACS, there may be some conflation of the designations of "high risk" for short-term mortality (i.e., currently having an MI) and "high risk" for MACE in the next 30–90 days which is more prudent for this this discussion.

These scoring systems often incorporate patient history, physical exam, ECG, and biomarkers. Early scoring systems, such as the thrombosis in myocardial infarction (TIMI) and GRACE, were derived to predict outcomes in patients with confirmed acute coronary syndrome (ACS). While not initially designed for use in the ED, these scores have been applied more broadly to patients presenting with undifferentiated chest pain. Recent novel scoring systems such as EDACS, ADAMT, and the HEART score have attempted to primarily evaluate risk in the undifferentiated cohort of patients who present to the ED with chest pain. They also serve to distinguish between patients who are safe for discharge and those who would benefit from admission.

---

The original version of this chapter has been revised. A correction to this chapter can be found at https://doi.org/10.1007/978-3-031-05520-1_20

---

J. Raper · L. Goyack · M. DeLaney (✉)
Department of Emergency Medicine, University of Alabama at Birmingham, Birmingham, AL, USA



M. Pena et al. (eds.), *Short Stay Management of Chest Pain*, Contemporary Cardiology, https://doi.org/10.1007/978-3-031-05520-1_10

## 2   TIMI

The thrombosis in myocardial infarction (TIMI) risk score was one of the first and most widely known chest pain rules comparing unfractionated heparin to enoxaparin in patients with confirmed ACS. The initial score, first published in 2000, was developed to prognosticate mortality, predict ischemic events, and help drive therapeutic decision making for patients presenting with unstable angina and non-ST segment elevation myocardial infarction (NSTEMI). The TIMI score uses the following seven elements, which are each assigned a potential value of one point: age >65 years, ≥3 classical risk factors for coronary artery disease (CAD), prior coronary stenosis if 50% or more, use of aspirin in the past 7 days, at least 2 anginal events in the past 24 h, elevated cardiac markers (troponin or CK-MB), and ST-deviation ≥0.5 mm on presentation. Each element is assigned either a score of 0 or 1 if present, resulting in a total TIMI Score between 0 and 7.

The initial TIMI publication found that event rates increased significantly as the TIMI risk score increased in the test cohort: 4.7% for a score 0/1; 8.3% for 2; 13.2% for 3; 19.9% for 4; 26.2% for 5; and 40.9% for 6/7 ($p < 0.001$ by ×2 for trend) [1].

Although, obviously not initially intended for ED use, several studies have proven that when applied to patients with chest pain in the ED, the TIMI risk score is useful in stratifying cardiovascular event risk and shows a linear relationship with the patient's overall incidence of cardiac events [2–5]. However, it does not perform well enough to reliably and safely guide patient disposition. In a meta-analysis including over 17,000 ED patients, Hess et al. found a 1.8% rate of MACE within 30 days when patients had a TIMI score of 0 (sensitivity 97.2%, specificity 25.0%) [6]. They concluded that the use of the TIMI risk score as the sole means of determining patient disposition was insufficient, and rather the score should be only used as an adjunct to clinical judgment.

A separate TIMI risk score for STEMI has also been developed, however, is not generally used in emergency medicine practice, as patients presenting with STEMI require revascularization regardless of the TIMI score. Therefore, the TIMI risk score for STEMI is more applicable and useful in the inpatient setting.

## 3   GRACE

The Global Registry of Acute Coronary Events (GRACE) risk score, first published in 2003, was developed from a multinational registry to estimate the in-hospital and 6-month mortality in patients with confirmed ACS. Unlike the TIMI score, GRACE included patients with ST-elevation myocardial infarction. Prior to the advent of this score, there was no validated risk model to predict mortality beyond 6 months.

The GRACE hospital post-discharge score contained eight independent risk factors derived after multivariate logistic regression analysis and accurately discriminated hospital survivors from death at 6 months, 1 year, 2 years, 3 years, and 4 years

**Table 1** Grace 2.0

| GRACE 2.0 | |
|---|---|
| Age | |
| Heart rate/pulse | |
| Systolic BP | |
| Creatinine | |
| Cardiac arrest at admission | |
| ST segment deviation on EKG | |
| Abnormal cardiac enzymes | |
| *Killip class* | |
| CHF | Rales and/or JVD |
| Pulmonary edema | Cardiogenic shock |

(Table 1). Each element has its own scoring, and it is possible to score from 1 to 372. The simplified model developed to be used for clinical practice found a *c* statistic of 0.83 to discriminate risk, nearly the same for the overall expanded model (0.84) [7].

The risk score was validated to work for all three subsets of ACS (STEMI, NSTEMI, unstable angina) [8]. Furthermore, it was externally validated to predict 6-month risk of death and myocardial infarction [9].

Utilizing the original GRACE risk score, patients were assigned a score and mortality risk was projected based on a range of risk scores. GRACE was then refined to the GRACE risk score 2.0 which not only allows for broader use due to eliminating some variables that might otherwise be unknown and allows for specific mortality calculations based on individual scores in comparison to the mortality ranges assigned by its predecessor. Studies have found that the updated GRACE risk score has better discrimination and is easier to use than the prior iteration based on linear associations [9].

Few studies have evaluated the use of the GRACE score in the emergency department in the role of risk stratifying patients to be able to discharge. The few that have, concluded that the GRACE score shows poor to moderate performance in stratifying ED chest pain patients in distinguishing MACE vs. non-MACE [10–12].

## 4  EDACS-ADP

The Emergency Department Assessment of Chest Pain Score (EDACS) (2014) was designed to predict short-term risk of MACE in patients presenting to the ED with chest pain (Table 2). The EDACS score was then combined with normal contemporary troponin results at 0 and 2 h, as well as an ECG without new ischemia to develop the EDACS-accelerated diagnostic protocol (EDACS-ADP). The purpose of this addition was to identify a subgroup of patients presenting to the ED with very low short-term risk of MACE who could be safely discharged with further cardiac evaluation in the outpatient study [13].

**Table 2** EDACS-ADP

| EDACS-ADP | |
| --- | --- |
| Age | |
| Sex (Male +6) | |
| Known CAD or 3 risk factors (+4) | |
| *Symptoms and signs* | |
| Diaphoresis (+3) | Pain radiates to shoulder, neck or jaw (+5) |
| Pain occurred or worsened with inspiration (−4) | Pain is reproduced by palpation (−6) |

The EDACS-ADP chest pain system can be reviewed in Table 2 below. The patient is considered to be low risk for MACE with an EDACS score of <16, an ECG without new ischemia, and both negative 0-h and 2-h troponin. A calculated score ≥16, or EKG shows new ischemia, or 0-h or 2-h troponin are positive, then the patient is not low risk and the patient should be further observed.

The EDACS-ADP was prospectively, internally validated, and classified more than 50% of patients as having low risk of MACE within 30 days of discharge. The risk score was determined to be >99% sensitive for correctly identifying patients at low risk of MACE [13].

External retrospective validation of the score has had differing results, however. Flaws et al. supported the safety of the score's use after they concluded that 41.6% of patients were classified as low risk by the EDACS-ADP rule, with 100% sensitivity for 30-day MACE [14]. Shin et al. classified 35.2% of patients as low risk by the EDACS-ADP score, however, five cases (1.1%) of MACE still arose [15]. As such, the authors concluded that the MACE rate among low risk patients is higher than considered acceptable to be discharged without further evaluation by most ED physicians.

## 5 HEART

The HEART score was specifically designed to stratify all chest pain patients in the ED, excluding those presenting with STEMI (Table 3). This scoring system differs from the previously discussed TIMI and GRACE scores, which were derived for high risk patients to determine the need for invasive therapy, rather than evaluating the undifferentiated chest pain patient.

The five elements of the score include the following: History, ECG, Age, Risk factors, and Troponin. Each can be scored with zero, one, or two points; with a max of 10 points. Refer to Table 3 below for scoring details. The score places patients into low, intermediate, or high risk groups for having a major adverse cardiac event(s) in the next 6 weeks. Patients identified as low risk are classified as having a 0.9–1.7% risk of adverse cardiac events in the next 6 weeks, and are typically discharged home, while those identified as intermediate (12–17%) and high risk

**Table 3** HEART score reinterpretation from Six, et al. [16]

| HEART score | | | |
|---|---|---|---|
| | Score 0 | Score 1 | Score 2 |
| History | Slightly suspicious | Moderately suspicious | Highly suspicious |
| ECG | Normal ECG | Nonspecific repolarization | Significant ST-depression |
| Age (years) | <45 | 45–65 | >65 |
| Risk factors | No risk factors | 1–2 risk factors | ≥3 risk factors or history of atherosclerotic disease |
| Troponin | ≤normal limit | 1–3 × normal limit | >3 × normal limit |

(50–65%) are usually admitted [17]. The HEART score has been externally validated in retrospective and prospective studies [10, 18, 19].

The initial HEART score originally incorporated a single troponin, and although the score has been validated in many trials, there was still hesitation with discharging the low risk patient. This led to the development of the HEART Pathway. Mahler et al. analyzed a cohort of around 1000 patients from ED observation units to evaluate the use of the HEART score with two troponin values, the latter obtained 3 h after patient arrival in the ED. For patients who were identified as low risk (HEART score of 0–3) and with a repeat 3 h troponin which was unremarkable, the rate of MACE was found to be 0.6%, down from 1.7% as reported in the original HEART study. If the HEART score with troponins at hours 0 and 3 had been applied to this patient cohort there would have been a 0.5% rate of missed MACE, with a ~0.001% rate of unexpected death. The authors noted that a combination of a HEART score >3 or elevated troponins obtained 4–6 h after arrival was 100% sensitive for MACE. In addition, in this patient cohort, there was the potential to reduce further cardiac testing by 82% [20].

In a follow-up study, Mahler et al. found that after enrolling over 5000 patients, the HEART Pathway decreased hospitalization for chest pain by 21%, reduced hospital length of stay by 12 h, and did not lead to any increase in adverse events or recurrent cardiac care. Based on their data, the authors concluded that the HEART pathway will shorten hospital LOS for patients with acute chest pain, resulting in significant cost savings and improvement of efficiency [21].

With the advent of high sensitivity troponin, the Heart Score continues to have high discrimination in differentiating the low risk patient. A prospective study found that the modified HEART scores were comparable among conventional troponin and high sensitivity troponin for 30 day MACE and were equally effective in risk stratifying chest pain patients for safe discharge [22]. Santi et al. also confirmed that it is possible to safely discharge emergency department chest pain patients with a low modified HEART score after an initial high-sensitive troponin [23]. In the Santi study, of the 512 (37.2%) patients with a low HEART score, none had an event within 180 days. They also found a statistically significant difference ($p < 0.0001$) between the cumulative incidents of events in the three HEART score groups using high sensitivity troponin.

## 6   ADAPT

The ADAPT pathway is similar to the HEART score and uses troponins collected at 0 and 2 h (Table 4). Initial derivation and subsequent validations reported sensitivities of 99.7% for MACE at 30 days [24]. When ADAPT was compared to the HEART pathway Stropoya et al. found that while both scores were 100% sensitive for MACE, the HEART pathway was able to categorize 47% as low risk compared to only 24% when using the ADAPT pathway [25].

## 7   NOTR

Various other chest pain decisions tools have been proposed to help identify a subset of patients who are low risk. The No Objective Testing Rule (NOTR) relies on objective criteria consisting of cardiac risk factors, history of myocardial infarction or coronary artery disease, age, serial troponin measures, and a nonischemic ECG (no ST-depression or T-wave inversion in >1 contiguous lead) (Table 5). In an initial derivation study Greenslade et al. reported that the NOTR was able to categorize 31.7% of patients as "low risk" with a reported sensitivity of 97.6% for ACS. In a subsequent study Stopyra et al. found that both the HEART Pathway and the NOTR were able to identify all cases of MACE at 30 days in a subset of low risk patients. Despite this diagnostic accuracy, the HEART pathway was able to identify a larger subset of patients who were suitable for early discharge [26].

**Table 4** ADAPT protocol

| ADAPT protocol |
| --- |
| Abnormal troponin at 0 or 2 h |
| Ischemic changes on EKG |
| Age ≥65 years |
| ≥3 CAD risk factors |
| Known CAD (stenosis ≥50%) |
| Aspirin use in past 7 days |
| Severe angina (≥2 episodes in 24 h or Persistent) |

**Table 5** NOTR

| NOTR |
| --- |
| Cardiac risk factors |
| History of MI/CAD |
| Age |
| Serial troponin measures |
| Nonischemic EKG |

**Table 6** Vancouver Chest Pain Rule

| Vancouver Chest Pain Rule |
| --- |
| **Step 1** |
| Abnormal initial EKG |
| Positive troponin at 2 h |
| Prior ACS or nitrate use |
| **Step 2** |
| Does palpation reproduce pain? |
| **Step 3** |
| Age 50 and above? |
| Does pain radiate to neck, jaw, or left arm? |

## 8  VCPR

Similarly the new Vancouver Chest Pain Rule (VCPR) uses objective criteria including electrocardiogram results, cardiac history, nitrate use, age, pain characteristics, and troponin results at 2 h after presentation (Table 6). While the initial derivation and validation studies reported sensitivities of −99.1%, further validations have found sensitivities as low as 78.1% [27–29]. Given this wide range of reported sensitivities future studies across a variety of patient populations are needed before the VCPR is used as a preferred diagnostic tool.

## 9  Clinical Impression

In a retrospective review of prospectively collected data, Greenslades et al. evaluated the performance of the m-ADAPT, EDACS, HEART, VCPR, and NOTR when used in conjunction with HST. While all of the pathways reported sensitivities ranging from 96.6% to 100% the pathways differed in terms of further risk stratification. When the VCPR and NOTER were used approximately $\frac{1}{3}$ of patients were able to be classified as low risk and discharged from the ED without further workup. Alternatively, the m-ADAPT, EDACS, and HEART pathways correctly identified almost half of the patients as being low risk and appropriate for outpatient management [30]. While the authors concluded that the VCPR and NOTR were safe and effective pathways, questions regarding the reproducibility and generalizability of these pathways remain. To date the HEART pathway has the largest body of literature supporting its use and seems to be the most robust tool available.

While the majority of patients who present to the ED do not have ACS, it is important to distinguish which patients are low risk for MACE (absence of known cardiovascular disease, a normal initial ECG, a normal initial troponin, and clinical stability) from those who are high risk. Over the last several decades, several scoring strategies have been developed in an effort to differentiate these patient populations.

Both the GRACE and TIMI scores were derived from patients with confirmed ACS and initially developed to predict in-hospital and 6-month mortality for patients presenting in the coronary care unit. The GRACE score risk stratifies patients presenting with STEMI, while TIMI predicts mortality for unstable angina and NSTEMI. The GRACE score also incorporated more variables, including Killip score, creatinine, and cardiac enzymes. Both are equally simple to calculate due to the advent of mobile phone based applications.

Studies have shown that the GRACE appears to outperform and have greater discriminative ability than the TIMI in predicting in-hospital and 6-month mortality when applied to NSTEMI patients [31–33]. However, few studies have assessed the performance of applying the GRACE score in the emergency department patients with potential ACS [31].

Reaney et al. prospectively compared the HEART, GRACE, and TIMI scores using a single troponin at admission and found that the HEART ($c$ −0.87) outperformed TIMI and GRACE ($c$ −0.78, 0.74, respectively) in overall discriminatory capacity for 30-day MACE [34].

In conclusion, these tools remain useful for some clinical decisions and communication to other providers about the patient's clinical condition. The TIMI and GRACE scores are well validated for predicting mortality and guiding therapeutics in the coronary care unit. The EDACS-ADP, ADAPT, NOTR, and VCPR show promise to assist with discharging the low risk chest pain patient in the emergency department, however, further studies are needed in order to further evaluate the performance of these scores across various patient populations. In the future, there will undoubtedly be a role for machine learning algorithms to aid in prediction of obstructive disease, but there remain computational limitations and the studies of this process are few [35]. However, currently the HEART score remains the most effective risk stratification tool for the undifferentiated chest pain patient presenting to the emergency department.

# References


1. Antman EM, Cohen M, Bernink PJ, et al. The TIMI risk score for unstable angina/non-ST elevation MI: a method for prognostication and therapeutic decision making. JAMA. 2000;284(7):835–42. https://doi.org/10.1001/jama.284.7.835.
2. Body R, Carley S, McDowell G, Ferguson J, Mackway-Jones K. Can a modified thrombolysis in myocardial infarction risk score outperform the original for risk stratifying emergency department patients with chest pain? Emerg Med J. 2009;26(2):95–9. https://doi.org/10.1136/emj.2008.058495.
3. García Almagro FJ, Gimeno JR, Villegas M, et al. Use of a coronary risk score (the TIMI Risk Score) in a non-selected patient population assessed for chest pain at an emergency department. Rev Esp Cardiol. 2005;58(7):775–81.
4. Hess EP, Perry JJ, Calder LA, et al. Prospective validation of a modified thrombolysis in myocardial infarction risk score in emergency department patients with chest pain and possible acute coronary syndrome. Acad Emerg Med. 2010;17(4):368–75. https://doi.org/10.1111/j.1553-2712.2010.00696.x.

5. Pollack CV, Sites FD, Shofer FS, Sease KL, Hollander JE. Application of the TIMI risk score for unstable angina and non-ST elevation acute coronary syndrome to an unselected emergency department chest pain population. Acad Emerg Med. 2006;13(1):13–8. https://doi.org/10.1197/j.aem.2005.06.031.

6. Hess EP, Agarwal D, Chandra S, et al. Diagnostic accuracy of the TIMI risk score in patients with chest pain in the emergency department: a meta-analysis. CMAJ. 2010;182(10):1039–44. https://doi.org/10.1503/cmaj.092119.

7. Granger CB, Goldberg RJ, Dabbous O, et al. Predictors of hospital mortality in the global registry of acute coronary events. Arch Intern Med. 2003;163(19):2345–53. https://doi.org/10.1001/archinte.163.19.2345.

8. Tang EW, Wong C-K, Herbison P. Global Registry of Acute Coronary Events (GRACE) hospital discharge risk score accurately predicts long-term mortality post acute coronary syndrome. Am Heart J. 2007;153(1):29–35. https://doi.org/10.1016/j.ahj.2006.10.004.

9. Fox KAA, Dabbous OH, Goldberg RJ, et al. Prediction of risk of death and myocardial infarction in the six months after presentation with acute coronary syndrome: prospective multinational observational study (GRACE). BMJ. 2006;333(7578):1091. https://doi.org/10.1136/bmj.38985.646481.55.

10. Backus BE, Six AJ, Kelder JC, et al. Chest pain in the emergency room: a multicenter validation of the HEART Score. Crit Pathw Cardiol. 2010;9(3):164–9. https://doi.org/10.1097/HPC.0b013e3181ec36d8.

11. Boubaker H, Beltaief K, Grissa MH, et al. Inaccuracy of Thrombolysis in Myocardial Infarction and Global Registry in Acute Coronary Events scores in predicting outcome in ED patients with potential ischemic chest pain. Am J Emerg Med. 2015;33(9):1209–12. https://doi.org/10.1016/j.ajem.2015.05.019.

12. Poldervaart JM, Langedijk M, Backus BE, et al. Comparison of the GRACE, HEART and TIMI score to predict major adverse cardiac events in chest pain patients at the emergency department. Int J Cardiol. 2017;227:656–61. https://doi.org/10.1016/j.ijcard.2016.10.080.

13. Than M, Flaws D, Sanders S, et al. Development and validation of the Emergency Department Assessment of Chest pain Score and 2 h accelerated diagnostic protocol. Emerg Med Australas. 2014;26(1):34–44. https://doi.org/10.1111/1742-6723.12164.

14. Flaws D, Than M, Scheuermeyer FX, et al. External validation of the emergency department assessment of chest pain score accelerated diagnostic pathway (EDACS-ADP). Emerg Med J. 2016;33(9):618–25. https://doi.org/10.1136/emermed-2015-205028.

15. Shin YS, Ahn S, Kim Y-J, Ryoo SM, Sohn CH, Kim WY. External validation of the emergency department assessment of chest pain score accelerated diagnostic pathway (EDACS-ADP). Am J Emerg Med. 2020;38(11):2264–70. https://doi.org/10.1016/j.ajem.2019.09.019.

16. Six AJ, Cullen L, Backus BE, et al. The HEART score for the assessment of patients with chest pain in the emergency department: a multinational validation study. Crit Pathw Cardiol. 2013;12(3):121–6. https://doi.org/10.1097/HPC.0b013e31828b327e.

17. Brady W, de Souza K. The HEART score: a guide to its application in the emergency department. Turk J Emerg Med. 2018;18(2):47–51. https://doi.org/10.1016/j.tjem.2018.04.004.

18. Patnaik S, Shah M, Alhamshari Y, et al. Clinical utility of the HEART score in patients admitted with chest pain to an inner-city hospital in the USA. Coron Artery Dis. 2017;28(4):336–41. https://doi.org/10.1097/MCA.0000000000000474.

19. Van Den Berg P, Body R. The HEART score for early rule out of acute coronary syndromes in the emergency department: a systematic review and meta-analysis. Eur Heart J Acute Cardiovasc Care. 2018;7(2):111–9. https://doi.org/10.1177/2048872617710788.

20. Mahler SA, Riley RF, Hiestand BC, et al. The HEART Pathway randomized trial: identifying emergency department patients with acute chest pain for early discharge. Circ Cardiovasc Qual Outcomes. 2015;8(2):195–203. https://doi.org/10.1161/CIRCOUTCOMES.114.001384.

21. Mahler SA, Burke GL, Duncan PW, et al. HEART pathway accelerated diagnostic protocol implementation: prospective pre-post interrupted time series design and methods. JMIR Res Protoc. 2016;5(1):e10. https://doi.org/10.2196/resprot.4802.

22. Tan JWC, Tan HJG, Sahlen AO, et al. Performance of cardiac troponins within the HEART score in predicting major adverse cardiac events at the emergency department. Am J Emerg Med. 2020;38(8):1560–7. https://doi.org/10.1016/j.ajem.2019.158420.
23. Santi L, Farina G, Gramenzi A, et al. The HEART score with high-sensitive troponin T at presentation: ruling out patients with chest pain in the emergency room. Intern Emerg Med. 2017;12(3):357–64. https://doi.org/10.1007/s11739-016-1461-3.
24. Than M, Cullen L, Aldous S, et al. 2-Hour accelerated diagnostic protocol to assess patients with chest pain symptoms using contemporary troponins as the only biomarker: the ADAPT trial. J Am Coll Cardiol. 2012;59(23):2091–8. https://doi.org/10.1016/j.jacc.2012.02.035.
25. Stopyra JP, Miller CD, Hiestand BC, et al. Chest pain risk stratification: a comparison of the 2-hour accelerated diagnostic protocol (ADAPT) and the HEART pathway. Crit Pathw Cardiol. 2016;15(2):46–9. https://doi.org/10.1097/HPC.0000000000000072.
26. Stopyra JP, Miller CD, Hiestand BC, et al. Validation of the no objective testing rule and comparison to the HEART pathway. Acad Emerg Med. 2017;24(9):1165–8. https://doi.org/10.1111/acem.13221.
27. Christenson J, Innes G, McKnight D, et al. A clinical prediction rule for early discharge of patients with chest pain. Ann Emerg Med. 2006;47(1):1–10. https://doi.org/10.1016/j.annemergmed.2005.08.007.
28. Cullen L, Greenslade JH, Than M, et al. The new Vancouver Chest Pain Rule using troponin as the only biomarker: an external validation study. Am J Emerg Med. 2014;32(2):129–34. https://doi.org/10.1016/j.ajem.2013.10.021.
29. Ong MEH, Hao Y, Yap S, et al. Validation of the new Vancouver Chest Pain Rule in Asian chest pain patients presenting at the emergency department. CJEM. 2017;19(1):18–25. https://doi.org/10.1017/cem.2016.336.
30. Greenslade JH, Parsonage W, Than M, et al. A clinical decision rule to identify emergency department patients at low risk for acute coronary syndrome who do not need objective coronary artery disease testing: the no objective testing rule. Ann Emerg Med. 2016;67(4):478–489.e2. https://doi.org/10.1016/j.annemergmed.2015.08.006.
31. Aragam KG, Tamhane UU, Kline-Rogers E, et al. Does simplicity compromise accuracy in ACS risk prediction? A retrospective analysis of the TIMI and GRACE risk scores. PLoS One. 2009;4(11):e7947. https://doi.org/10.1371/journal.pone.0007947.
32. Roy SS, Abu Azam STM, Khalequzzaman M, Ullah M, Arifur RM. GRACE and TIMI risk scores in predicting the angiographic severity of non-ST elevation acute coronary syndrome. Indian Heart J. 2018;70(Suppl 3):S250–3. https://doi.org/10.1016/j.ihj.2018.01.026.
33. Tun H. Diagnostic accuracy of TIMI versus GRACE score for prediction of death in patients presenting with Acute Non-ST Elevation Myocardial Infarction (NSTEMI). J Cardiol Cardiovasc Med. 2019;4:001–5. https://doi.org/10.29328/journal.jccm.1001032.
34. Reaney PDW, Elliott HI, Noman A, Cooper JG. Risk stratifying chest pain patients in the emergency department using HEART, GRACE and TIMI scores, with a single contemporary troponin result, to predict major adverse cardiac events. Emerg Med J. 2018;35(7):420–7. https://doi.org/10.1136/emermed-2017-207172.
35. Al'Aref SJ, Maliakal G, Singh G, et al. Machine learning of clinical variables and coronary artery calcium scoring for the prediction of obstructive coronary artery disease on coronary computed tomography angiography: analysis from the CONFIRM registry. Eur Heart J. 2020;41(3):359–67. https://doi.org/10.1093/eurheartj/ehz565.

# Emergency Department Disposition of Patients Presenting with Chest Pain

**Anwar Osborne and Svadharma Keerthi**

## 1 Introduction

The importance of identifying patients with life-threatening illness is the cornerstone of emergency care. In this lens, the most common chief complaint of "chest pain" focuses the diagnostic strategy in determining the presence of myocardial infarction. Symptoms of suspected myocardial infarction belong under the larger rubric of acute coronary syndromes (ACS). The end of the diagnostic pathway, previously contained ST elevation MI's, non-ST elevation MI's, and unstable angina. However, with the advent of higher sensitivity troponins that have functionally moved many patients from the diagnostic category of "unstable angina" to the diagnosis of NSTEMI, the acute diagnostic strategy rests largely on the identification of the myocardial infarction. This section discusses the possible disposition options for patients presenting to the ED with ACS with respect to ED use of modern modalities such as contemporary troponin and high sensitivity troponin. An overview of which is displayed in Fig. 1.

## 2 Risk Stratification

While there may be some semantic disagreement about an exact definition of the term "low risk," the American Heart Association defines it as a hemodynamically stable patient with a near normal ECG and negative initial biomarkers. However, in

A. Osborne · S. Keerthi (✉)
School of Medicine, Emory University, Decatur, GA, USA
e-mail: adosbor@emory.edu; svadharma.keerthi@emory.edu

© The Author(s), under exclusive license to Springer Nature Switzerland AG 2022

M. Pena et al. (eds.), *Short Stay Management of Chest Pain*, Contemporary Cardiology, https://doi.org/10.1007/978-3-031-05520-1_11

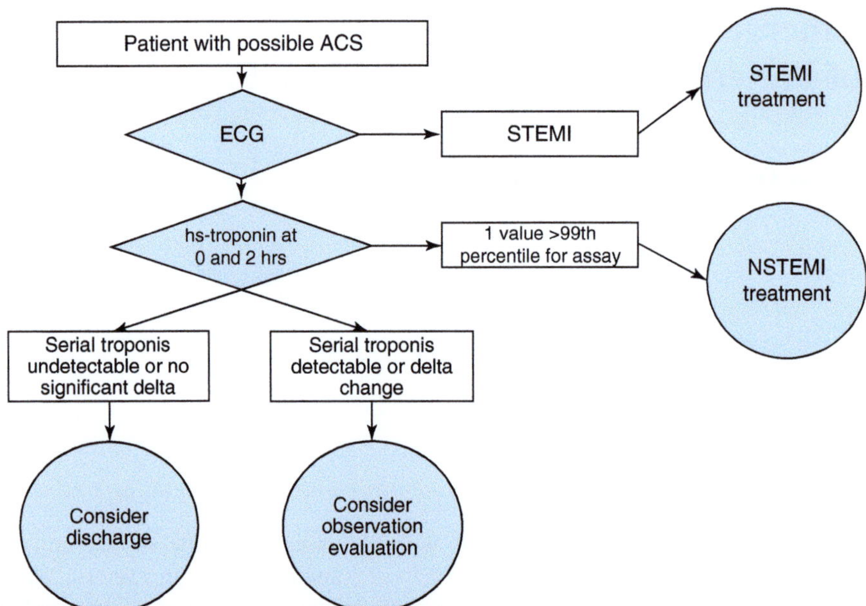


**Fig. 1** General approach to ED disposition w/ hs troponin. (Adapted from Sandoval Y, Jaffe AS. Using High-Sensitivity Cardiac Troponin T for Acute Cardiac Care. The American Journal of Medicine. 2017;130(12):1358–1365.e1. doi:https://doi.org/10.1016/j.amjmed.2017.07.033)

evaluation of the patient arriving to the emergency department with chest pain, several risk stratification tools have been proposed to help identify the patient that is high risk for a major adverse cardiac event (MACE) in the following 30 days, and have been good tools to aid the physician in the need for further work up. Prior popular risk scores such as the TIMI score are not as appropriate to use in the emergency department, as they focused on the need for patients who are already high risk who may need further invasive testing. Instead, the HEART score and the EDACS score have been widely used, as they help identify the patient with undifferentiated chest pain and their risk of MACE in the following 30 days. Having negative contemporary troponin and non-diagnostic ECG already confers a low 30 day event rate, but these scores were created to identify low risk patients who do not need further testing, they are great tools to help the emergency physician identify the patient that does not need any further testing and can be safely discharged [1]. With the addition of these scores to the work up of a patient arriving with chest pain, it can help identify the most appropriate patient who needs further testing to evaluate for ACS. In patients who are at moderate risk for MACE and who do not meet criteria for STEMI or NSTEMI in their initial work up are potential candidates for further testing in the observation unit. Details on the use and interpretation of the HEART and EDACS score are covered in detail elsewhere.

# 3 Inpatient Disposition

## 3.1 STEMI

According to the AHA/ACC guidelines for patients with chest pain, an initial screening ECG should be performed within 10 min of arrival to the ED or contact with the medical system. STEMI as defined by the Fourth Universal Definition of MI is an ECG showing ST-segment elevation greater than or equal to 1 mm (0.1 mV) in at least two contiguous leads. The exception of leads would be v2 and v3 which requires at least a 2 mm elevation in men over 40, at least 2.5 mm in men under 40, or 1.5 mm in women of any age. In previous guidelines from the AHA/ACC writing committee, the authors suggested "Door 2 Balloon" as a quality metric, but both the European guidelines and a 2013 update moved the metric to "First Medical Contact to reperfusion" with the healthcare system [2, 3]. This would indicate that ideally, a patient would have an ECG done and interpreted within 10 min whether or not they arrived to the walk-in area of the ED or were obtained from the scene and further, the intervention would take place within 90 min in either scenario. Other indications for acute reperfusion strategy are true posterior MIs or a new left bundle branch block.

## 3.2 NSTEMI

When an EKG is non-diagnostic for a STEMI, the subsequent step to evaluate a patient with chest pain is by using cardiac biomarkers. As discussed elsewhere in this text, most commonly used biomarker in modern medicine has been the troponin. In an NSTEMI, there is believed to be non-occlusive plaque rupture, which can lead to EKG changes suggestive of ischemia, and biomarker elevation. While it is standard practice to take a patient who meets criteria for a STEMI to PCI if available, this is not the case for NSTEMIs. Per the AHA guidelines, there is a Class 1A indication for urgent PCI in any patients having NSTEMIs with continued ischemic chest pain, arrhythmias, or hemodynamic instability. Other patients who must be considered for urgent PCI include patients with dynamic ST-T wave changes, significantly depressed LVEF <40%, ischemic chest pain with decompensated heart failure, patients with prior CABG, and patients who have received recent PCI within the last 6 months. In patients who are having the above, as immediate PCI is indicated, an urgent cardiology consult is indicated, with inpatient admission.

## 3.3 Delayed vs. Early PCI

Patients who are having NSTEMIs who do not meet the above criteria for urgent PCI often get delayed PCIs. There have been several randomized control trials that have compared urgent PCI to delayed PCIs in patients having NSTEMIs, however, the definition of early, delayed, and the medications each group received prior to PCI were largely varied across the trials, making it difficult to compare. A 2006 meta-analysis of early versus delayed PCI showed a significant mortality benefit for patients who received early PCI, and in 15 year follow-up of one of the studies, found a persistent decreased mortality benefit on average of 18 months for patient receiving early PCI. However, there is no specific guideline yet that recommends urgent PCI outside the indications mentioned previously, and without high risk features, patients having an NSTEMI often will receive delayed PCI. Suffice it to say that these patients should be admitted to an inpatient service soon after the diagnosis of NSTEMI is concerned.

## 4 Observation Unit Disposition

Appropriate selection of incoming patients is the cornerstone of the success of the ultimate safe disposition. In most cases, patients are placed in a short stay unit by a referring physician, typically from the ED, after some level of direct evaluation. Even though the leading cause of death of humans is cardiac disease, there are very few patients who present to the ED with chest pain that have an acute coronary syndrome [4, 5]. The details of this initial evaluation are discussed in detail elsewhere in this text, but as mentioned above the information obtained through this process should first identify patients with either a STEMI or NSTEMI. The contributing test to the STEMI diagnosis is the ECG and the key test for NSTEMI would be biomarkers. As with all patients placed in a protocol driven observation unit, there should be as few barriers to discharge as possible and as clear an endpoint feasible in this transfer process [6].

### *4.1 Appropriate Patients*

After determining which patients with possible ACS have either a STEMI or NSTEMI, this largest group of suspect patients should receive care in the acute setting to determine the presence of other possible life-threatening diagnoses such as aortic dissection, PE, pneumothorax, and esophageal rupture if possible. Then, the remaining group without these diagnoses, but also without so few risks as to make further testing valueless should be considered for the observation unit. With the advent of multiple scoring systems to categorize patients with ACS, there is a growing body of evidence around patients at very low risk for ACS. Placing patients in an observation unit will likely not yield a decrease in mortality in the low risk population. This is probably demonstrated best by a study in 2001 where patients received either an exercise stress test or a cardiac catheterization after being deemed low risk. Here, the exercise stress test performed worse than the coronary angiography for identifying coronary artery disease, but more importantly there were no significant differences in MACE at 1 year [7]. Furthermore, a review of insurance claims from over 900,000 patients similarly found that patients who were not immediately admitted for suspected MI who also underwent non-invasive testing and/or subsequent coronary angiography were as likely to be admitted for future MI as those who had no testing in 30 days [8]. Finally, the risk of placing a patient on a pathway that has limited value is a dubious proposition when there is a rate of false positive patients receiving a cardiac catheterization that may prove to be fatal that appears to be similar to the absolute risk reduction of the test at hand [9].

## 5  Outpatient Follow-Up Disposition [Discharge from the ED]

To be sure, observation stays are technically outpatient as defined by the Hospital Manual [10]. Thereby, arranging a follow-up evaluation by a primary care provider or cardiologist within the 10–12 h would be a reasonable strategy for this group, but most practicing physicians would agree that this arrangement would be an exception rather than a rule. Although the data would be regional and related to local factors, a study in California showed that very few providers had primary care appointments available within 10 days [11]. Therefore, the guideline recommended 72 h follow-up exists primarily as a construct to understand how soon suspected ACS patients may need to be evaluated again. Care pathways, or accelerated diagnostic pathways, have been discussed throughout this text, but in this discussion, they are framed for the purpose of leaving the ED for outpatient follow-up.

### 5.1  The HEART Pathway

Because of a myriad of factors, the HEART score is well studied for the purpose of discharging patients from the ED. Using contemporary troponin, Mahler et al. found no MACE at 30 days using 0 and 3 h measurements in patients with a HEART score 3 or less [12]. The findings of a study in the Netherlands found similarly low MACE rates without differences between usual care groups and treatment groups. Here, patients with HEART scores 0–3 were discharged home and many of the sites used hs troponin assay [13]. In a US study at eight sites, Mahler et al. used hs troponin assays and found that the HEART score was necessary to achieve low rates of MACE in the early discharge model [14].

### 5.2  European Society of Cardiology

Because of an abundance of data in European studies, the European Society of Cardiology recommends 0–1 and 0–2 h pathways with clinical criteria for early discharge if they have hs troponin available [15]. While the AHA and ACC have not updated their guidelines as of this publication to reflect rapid pathways with high sensitivity troponin, it stands to reason that there are a number of data driven ways to provide patients with the service of early discharge consistent with the types of troponin assays available at a given facility.

## 6 Special Considerations in Disposition

### *6.1 Known Coronary Artery Disease*

While it may be the place of the observation unit to determine coronary artery disease that has yet to be diagnosed in the chest pain patient, some patients arrive to the ED with known disease. Patients with appropriate history and the absence of cardiac biomarkers present on evaluation were determined to have "unstable angina." But with the advent of high sensitivity assays for troponin, these patients are rare [16]. Current guidelines recommend admission for patients with recurrent pain, but again, this would be rare in the setting of higher sensitivity assays. The treatment decision to place the patient in the hospital for pain control will likely be incongruent with disposition designed to decrease mortality. A 2014 meta-analysis including patients without acute MI found that there was no reduction in death in patients randomized to an invasive strategy for disease versus medical therapy alone [17]. These findings are further bolstered by the ISCHEMIA trial which found similarly, that the value of an initial invasive strategy did not extend to mortality benefit in patients with even moderate and severe disease [18]. This is not to suggest that there is no role for testing for possible prognosis for surgeries as from an office setting, but testing, be it invasive or non, has a very limited role in patients with known disease.

#### 6.1.1 Women

Women account for a significant proportion of UA/NSTEMI and cardiovascular disease is the leading cause of death worldwide for women, just like men [19]. However, their pathways to and around the disease may be different in that they tend to be older and have an increasing number of co-morbidities (hypertension, diabetes, and heart failure) [20]. Women are more likely to present with atypical symptoms and specifically, are less likely to have diaphoresis and complain of "chest pain" as their primary concern [21, 22]. Even though these presenting complaints require vigilance of the provider to determine the nature of the complaint, the most recent AHA guidelines do not distinguish treatment modalities between the sexes. With respect to disposition, the Fourth Definition of MI does change the requirement for ST elevation somewhat and several assays of hs troponin have sex based cut off values. Both of these factors would potentially change the disposition of a female patient in the proper setting.

## 6.2  Cocaine Induced Chest Pain

Even though cocaine associated chest pain is regarded as a reason for decrease suspicion for MI, it is the most common acute medical condition in users of this drug [23]. Also, as it may prove to be routine to check urine drug screens in these patients, obtaining one in a patient who already admits to use is redundant, but more importantly, cocaine is so rapidly metabolized in the blood that it would be rare that a laboratory would have a test on hand to determine its presence in acute intoxication. Benzoylecgonine is the most common metabolite tested for and it may be present in urine studies for 10 more days. In terms of disposition, the observation unit has been shown to be appropriate and feasible in these patients for repeating troponin evaluation serial ECGs.

# 7  Conclusions

Chest pain remains a common presenting symptom for ED visits. Generally, patients with STEMI and NSTEMI are admitted and have an invasive strategy implemented. The observation unit can aid in diagnosing new coronary disease and determining if patients with troponin values in an indeterminate range belong in the higher risk group. New risk strategies paired with high sensitivity troponin are allowing providers to discharge more patients safely than ever before.

# References


1. Wassie M, Lee M-S, Sun BC, et al. Single vs serial measurements of cardiac troponin level in the evaluation of patients in the emergency department with suspected acute myocardial infarction. JAMA Netw Open. 2021;4(2):e2037930. https://doi.org/10.1001/jamanetworkopen.2020.37930.
2. Ibanez B, James S, Agewall S, et al. 2017 ESC Guidelines for the management of acute myocardial infarction in patients presenting with ST-segment elevation: the Task Force for the management of acute myocardial infarction in patients presenting with ST-segment elevation of the European Society of Cardiology (ESC). Eur Heart J. 2018;39(2):119–77. https://doi.org/10.1093/eurheartj/ehx393.
3. O'Gara PT, Kushner FG, Ascheim DD, et al. 2013 ACCF/AHA guideline for the management of ST-elevation myocardial infarction: executive summary: a report of the American College of Cardiology Foundation/American Heart Association Task Force on Practice Guidelines. J Am Coll Cardiol. 2013;61(4):485–510. https://doi.org/10.1016/j.jacc.2012.11.018.
4. Goldman L, Cook EF, Johnson PA, Brand DA, Rouan GW, Lee TH. Prediction of the need for intensive care in patients who come to the emergency departments with acute chest pain. N Engl J Med. 1996;334:1498–504. https://doi.org/10.1056/NEJM199606063342303.
5. Mcdaniel M, Ross M, Rab T, et al. A comprehensive acute coronary syndrome algorithm for centers with percutaneous coronary intervention capability. Crit Pathw Cardiol. 2013;12:141–9. https://doi.org/10.1097/HPC.0b013e318292f168.

6. Ross MA, Aurora T, Graff L, et al. State of the art: emergency department observation units. Crit Pathw Cardiol. 2012;11:128–38. https://doi.org/10.1097/HPC.0b013e31825def28.

7. deFilippi CR, Rosanio S, Tocchi M, et al. Randomized comparison of a strategy of predischarge coronary angiography versus exercise testing in low-risk patients in a chest pain unit: in-hospital and long-term outcomes. J Am Coll Cardiol. 2001;37(8):2042–9. https://doi.org/10.1016/s0735-1097(01)01300-6.

8. Sandhu AT, Heidenreich PA, Bhattacharya J, Bundorf MK. Cardiovascular testing and clinical outcomes in emergency department patients with chest pain. JAMA Intern Med. 2017;177(8):1175–82. https://doi.org/10.1001/jamainternmed.2017.2432.

9. Arbab-Zadeh A. Stress testing and non-invasive coronary angiography in patients with suspected coronary artery disease: time for a new paradigm. Heart Int. 2012;7(1):e2. https://doi.org/10.4081/hi.2012.e2.

10. Inc H, CMS O. Medicare benefit policy manual. Baltimore, MD: CMS; 2021. p. 37.

11. Melnikow J, Evans E, Xing G, et al. Primary care access to new patient appointments for California Medicaid enrollees: a simulated patient study. Ann Fam Med. 2020;18(3):210–7. https://doi.org/10.1370/afm.2502.

12. Mahler SA, Burke GL, Duncan PW, et al. HEART Pathway accelerated diagnostic protocol implementation: prospective pre-post interrupted time series design and methods. JMIR Res Protoc. 2016;5(1):e10. https://doi.org/10.2196/resprot.4802.

13. Poldervaart JM, Reitsma JB, Backus BE, et al. Effect of using the HEART score in patients with chest pain in the emergency department: a stepped-wedge, cluster randomized trial. Ann Intern Med. 2017;166(10):689–97. https://doi.org/10.7326/M16-1600.

14. Allen BR, Christenson RH, Cohen SA, et al. Diagnostic performance of high-sensitivity cardiac troponin T strategies and clinical variables in a multisite US cohort. Circulation. 2021;143(17):1659–72. https://doi.org/10.1161/CIRCULATIONAHA.120.049298.

15. Collet J-P, Thiele H, Barbato E, et al. 2020 ESC Guidelines for the management of acute coronary syndromes in patients presenting without persistent ST-segment elevation. Eur Heart J. 2021;42(14):1289–367. https://doi.org/10.1093/eurheartj/ehaa575.

16. Braunwald E, Morrow DA. Unstable angina. Circulation. 2013;127(24):2452–7. https://doi.org/10.1161/CIRCULATIONAHA.113.001258.

17. Stergiopoulos K, Boden WE, Hartigan P, et al. Percutaneous coronary intervention outcomes in patients with stable obstructive coronary artery disease and myocardial ischemia: a collaborative meta-analysis of contemporary randomized clinical trials. JAMA Intern Med. 2014;174(2):232–40. https://doi.org/10.1001/jamainternmed.2013.12855.

18. Maron DJ, Hochman JS, Reynolds HR, et al. Initial invasive or conservative strategy for stable coronary disease. N Engl J Med. 2020;382(15):1395–407. https://doi.org/10.1056/NEJMoa1915922.

19. Woodward M. Cardiovascular disease and the female disadvantage. Int J Environ Res Public Health. 2019;16(7):1165. https://doi.org/10.3390/ijerph16071165.

20. Anderson JL, Adams CD, Antman EM, et al. ACC/AHA 2007 guidelines for the management of patients with unstable angina/non–ST-elevation myocardial infarction. J Am Coll Cardiol. 2007;50(7):e1–e157. https://doi.org/10.1016/j.jacc.2007.02.013.

21. Arslanian-Engoren C, Patel A, Fang J, et al. Symptoms of men and women presenting with acute coronary syndromes. Am J Cardiol. 2006;98(9):1177–81. https://doi.org/10.1016/j.amjcard.2006.05.049.

22. Patel H, Rosengren A, Ekman I. Symptoms in acute coronary syndromes: does sex make a difference? Am Heart J. 2004;148(1):27–33. https://doi.org/10.1016/j.ahj.2004.03.005.

23. Hollander JE, Hoffman RS. Cocaine-induced myocardial infarction: an analysis and review of the literature. J Emerg Med. 1992;10(2):169–77. https://doi.org/10.1016/0736-4679(92)90212-c.

# Short Stay Unit Requirements

**Matthew Wheatley**

## 1    Introduction and Short Stay Unit Concept

Short stay units (SSU) are dedicated areas within an acute care hospital where patients receive focused diagnostic tests and therapies. Typically, patients are treated as outpatients under observation status as they are undergoing treatment to determine the need for admission. This determination is expected to take less than two midnights. SSUs can go by many names: observation units, chest pain units, or clinical decision units. In this chapter, the term short stay unit (SSU) will be used to represent all of these dedicated patient care areas.

SSUs have been shown to be cost effective and efficient venues of care for patients who are being evaluated for acute coronary syndrome (ACS) [1, 2]. Their use is a level B recommendation by the ACC/AHA [3]. The greatest benefit terms of reducing patient length of stay and healthcare costs can be seen in SSUs that are dedicated units where patient care is protocol-driven (a type 1 unit) [4].

Greater than one-third of US hospitals have an SSU or are developing one [5, 6]. Most SSUs are closed units managed by the emergency department and run by emergency physicians, however, some are still run by internal medicine or cardiology.

M. Wheatley (✉)
Department of Emergency Medicine, Emory University School of Medicine,
Atlanta, GA, USA
e-mail: mwheatl@emory.edu


M. Pena et al. (eds.), *Short Stay Management of Chest Pain*, Contemporary
Cardiology, https://doi.org/10.1007/978-3-031-05520-1_12

## 2  Location

Many units that are administratively run by EM are co-located or adjacent to the ED and this can reduce logistical burdens [7]. However, in certain hospitals, the available space is on a different floor or geographically distant from the ED. These units may require different staffing and physician oversight.

## 3  Administration and Oversight

Strong physician and nursing leadership is essential for a successful SSU [8]. As mentioned above, leadership can be from EM, IM, or cardiology. The physician medical director is responsible for creating the patient care protocols and ensuring they are being followed appropriately. In addition, this person reviews unit utilization and throughput metrics to ensure patient care is efficient. The nursing manager for the SSU is responsible for ensuring adequate nursing staff and training the staff to carry out the patient care protocols.

These administrative officials should be in regular communication and conduct regular operations meetings that involve all stakeholders for the SSU. The purpose of the meeting is to review unit utilization and throughput data, discuss sentinel events and patient care barriers. With respect to a chest pain pathway, this meeting should include representatives from cardiology, radiology, and cardiac stress lab.

## 4  Staffing

Nurse staffing for an SSU that is caring for chest pain patients should be staffed similar to a cardiac telemetry floor. There should be a 1:4 or 1:5 nurse to patient ratio. This ratio is typically higher than regular nursing floor ratios of 1:8 but is necessary for the intensity of patient care. In several surveys, these ratios continue to appear as the standard for observation care. Larger units can employ patient care technicians to assist in patient care activities such as blood draws and transport. The SSU medical and nursing director are responsible for ensuring that the SSU has the appropriate level of other essential staff such as a unit clerk, environmental services, and security [9].

From a provider standpoint, an SSU should be staffed with a physician (DO or MD) working independently or in conjunction with an advanced practice provider (APP) [10]. SSUs that are contained within and operated by the ED may choose to have the responsible physician also seeing patients clinically in the ED. In these cases, APP coverage makes sense as it places a dedicated provider in the unit to primarily manage throughput and other patient care issues. Larger units have an APP present in the 24 h a day. However, it may make sense in smaller units to restrict staffing overnight when there are fewer new admissions. APP functions are to screen new admissions to the unit for appropriateness, ensure the patient care protocols are being followed, monitor essential testing and results, communicate with consultants, and ensure appropriate and timely disposition to and inpatients setting or home.

When patients with chest pain are being observed to rule out ACS, the APP ensures serial EKG and troponin testing happens as scheduled, interprets the results, and discusses them with the attending physician over the SSU. In addition, they must carry out the plan that was developed in the ED. Many times, this will involve provocative testing and/or cardiac imaging. Occasionally, formal cardiology consultation will be necessary to determine next steps such as coordinating these services for their patients.

## 5  Equipment and Supplies

Patient rooms in SSUs are outpatient spaces, so they need to meet those criteria in terms of size and function. Telemetry monitoring is necessary for an SSU that cares for chest pain patients. This should allow for continuous rhythm and ST segment analysis and should be centrally monitored. Patients are able to have telemetry monitoring discontinued once non-ST elevation myocardial infarction (NSTEMI) has been ruled out [11].

## 6  Conclusion

SSUs are essential in the work-up and care of patients with chest pain. While it is true that the type of care provided by these SSUs can conceptually be delivered in any bed within the hospital, these units serve as an option for certain low- and moderate-risk patients that avoids unnecessary use of these inpatient beds and can provide alternatives to patient discharge from the acute care setting.

## References


1. Graff LG, Dallara J, Ross MA, et al. Impact on the care of the emergency department chest pain patient from the Chest Pain Evaluation Registry (CHEPER) study. Am J Cardiol. 1997;80:563–8.
2. Gomez MA, Anderson JL, Karagounis LA, Muhlestein JB, Mooers FB. An emergency department-based protocol for rapidly ruling out myocardial ischemia reduces hospital time and expense: results of a randomized study (ROMIO). J Am Coll Cardiol. 1996;28:25–33.
3. Amsterdam EA, Wenger NK, Brindis RG, Casey DE, et al. 1014 ACC/AHA Guideline for the management of patients with non-ST-elevation acute coronary syndromes: executive summary. Circulation. 2014;130:2354–94.

 4. Ross MA, Hockenberry JM, Mutter R, et al. Protocol-driven emergency department observation units offer savings, shorter stays, and reduced admissions. Health Aff. 2013;32:2149–56.
 5. Wiler JL, Ginde AA. National study of emergency department observation services. Ann Emerg Med. 2010;56:S142.
 6. Ross MA, Aurora T, Graff L, et al. State of the art: emergency department observation units. Crit Pathw Cardiol. 2012;11(3):128–38.
 7. Baugh CW, Venkatesh AK, Bohan JS. Emergency department observation units: a clinical and financial benefit for hospitals. Health Care Manag Rev. 2011;36(1):28–37.
 8. Emergency department observation services. Ann Emerg Med. 2008;51:686.
 9. Baugh CW, Graff LG. Management – staffing. In: Graff LG, editor. Observation medicine: the healthcare system's tincture of time; 2009.
10. Conley J, Bohan JS, Baugh CW. The Establishment and Management of an Observation Unit. Emerg Med Clin North Am. 2017;35(3):519–33.
11. Sandau KE, Funk M, Auerbach A, et al. Update to practice standards for electrocardiographic monitoring in hospital settings: a scientific statement from the American Heart Association. Circulation. 2017;136:e273–344.

# Medical Therapy in Patients Managed in a Chest Pain Observation Unit

James McCord and Ahmed Kazem

## 1  Aspirin Therapy

The administration of aspirin (ASA) in the setting of ST-elevation myocardial infarction (STEMI) has been shown to dramatically decrease mortality, equaling that of fibrinolytic therapy [1]. In addition, ASA therapy decreases adverse cardiac events in the setting of unstable angina (UA) and non-ST segment elevation myocardial infarction (NSTEMI) [2–6]. ASA is inexpensive and has been shown to be safe and well tolerated in multiple randomized controlled trials [1, 2, 6–11]. The guidelines within the American Heart Association/American College of Cardiology as well as the European Society of Cardiology recommend the administration of ASA when the diagnosis of ACS is definite or suspected [12, 13]. In fact, one post hoc study demonstrated improved mortality rates with pre-hospital administration of ASA in patients with suspected ACS [14]. The International Consensus Conference on Cardiopulmonary Resuscitation Writing Group stated that it is reasonable for ASA to be administered in the pre-hospital setting, however, specifically in patients with suspected ACS [15].

Patients with undifferentiated chest pain managed in a CPU should have received ASA prior to transfer to the CPU, and even occasionally prior to presentation to the ED. For patients that did not receive ASA prior to transfer to the CPU, it is reasonable for ASA to be given to the patient in the CPU. For patients that cannot receive

J. McCord
Wayne State University, Detroit, MI, USA

Division of Cardiology, Henry Ford Heart and Vascular Institute, Detroit, MI, USA
e-mail: JMcCord1@hfhs.org

A. Kazem (✉)
Division of Internal Medicine, Henry Ford Hospital, Detroit, MI, USA
e-mail: akazem1@hfhs.org



M. Pena et al. (eds.), *Short Stay Management of Chest Pain*, Contemporary Cardiology, https://doi.org/10.1007/978-3-031-05520-1_13

ASA due to an allergy, other anti-platelet agents, such as clopidogrel, should probably not be administered until a diagnosis of ACS is made.


## 2   Anticoagulation

Unfractionated heparin (UFH) or low molecular weight heparin (LMWH) have been evaluated in six small randomized placebo-controlled studies that showed a 54% decrease in the combined endpoint of either death or MI in UA/NSTEMI [16–21]. There have been nine trials that have compared UFH to LMWH in UA/NSTEMI [9, 21–28]. In four of these trials, the LMWH enoxaparin had lower rates of death or MI when compared with UFH. LMWH can easily be administered in the ED as a subcutaneous injection. In addition, the other known anticoagulants bivalirudin [29] and fondaparinux [30] have been shown to decrease adverse cardiac events in the setting of UA/NSTEMI.

The most significant complication of anticoagulation use is bleeding. An analysis of four major trials with UFH and LWMH demonstrated a rate of major bleeding of 1–6.7%, and a transfusion rate of 0.6–12.2% [31]. In the international GRACE registry of over 24,000 ACS patients, the overall rate of major bleeding was 3.9%, however, in the US population, the major bleeding rate was significantly higher at 6.9%. In the ACTION registry (formerly known as CRUSADE), compromised of over 30,000 high-risk STEMI/NSTEMI US patients, the major bleeding rate was 11.5% [32]. The bleeding complications were in part attributed to excessive dosing of LMWH in 13.8% and with UFH in 32.8%. Major bleeding in patients anticoagulated for ACS is associated with higher mortality rates. In a combined analysis of the CURE and OASIS-2 trials, patients who suffered a major bleed had a 30-day mortality rate of 12.8% as compared to only 2.5% without [33]. Therefore, the administration of either UFH or LMWH should be in patients with definite ACS or in patients with high clinical suspicion for ACS due their significant risks [12]. These therapies can lead to significant bleeding complications and should not be used in patients with undifferentiated chest pain in a CPU.


## 3   Nitrates

Although an overview of several small studies of nitroglycerin (NTG) in MI in the pre-fibrinolytic era suggest a 35% reduction in mortality [34], two large randomized placebo-controlled studies (ISIS-4, GISSI-3) did not show any mortality benefit for use of NTG in acute MI [35, 36]. Most studies of NTG involved patients with STEMI, however the conclusions are applicable to patients with UA/

NSTEMI. Nonetheless, there are no randomized placebo-controlled studies that suggest symptom relief or reduction in cardiac events in UA/NSTEMI. Patients with known coronary artery disease are advised to use sublingual NTG at home in the setting of chest pain for symptom relief. In patients with electrocardiogram findings of ST segment elevation, NTG should be administered to evaluate for possible coronary vasospasm [12].

The use of sublingual NTG in the ED in patients with undifferentiated chest pain is commonly employed. However, the degree of relief of chest pain should not assist in the identification of a patient with ACS and should have no impact on the triage decision of these patients [37, 38]. NTG is commonly used to improve symptoms of esophageal spasm and is likely to have a significant placebo effect in this setting. Continuous administration of NTG, either in the form of nitropaste or intravenous infusion, should not be employed in the CPU.

# 4 Beta Blockers

The benefit of routine intravenous beta blocker in the setting of STEMI in the fibrinolytic era has been challenged by two large randomized trials [39, 40]. A meta-analysis of early beta blocker therapy in STEMI found no significant decrease in mortality [41]. More recently the large ACS COMMIT trial studied early intravenous therapy of beta blocker followed by oral administration in patients with MI (93% STEMI, 7% NSTEMI). Results demonstrated increased rates of cardiogenic shock and no improvement in mortality or adverse events at 8 days [42].

An overview of double-blind randomized trials of patients with UA or evolving MI suggest a 13% reduction in the risk of progression to MI [43]. However, it is important to note that these trials were conducted prior to the routine use of ASA, clopidogrel, GP IIb/IIIa inhibitors, and revascularization. Also, these trials lacked sufficient power to assess mortality in UA. Furthermore, pooled results from five trials in patients with ACS undergoing percutaneous intervention demonstrated a 6-month mortality rate of 1.7% in patients receiving beta blockers, and 3.7% in patients that did not [44].

There should be selective use of beta blockers in the CPU. Patients with atrial fibrillation may need beta blocker therapy for rate control, especially if they are taking it chronically. Patients that are taking a beta blocker at home may need this to be continued. It is important to note that patients who may be undergoing some form of stress testing may need to have the beta blocker withheld or the dose decreased to ensure an adequate heart rate response during testing. For the average patient in the CPU who has not already been on a beta blocker it should not be administered either intravenously or orally in the CPU.

# 5  Conclusion

The overwhelming majority of low-risk patients with undifferentiated chest pain that are evaluated and managed in a CPU are not diagnosed with an ACS. The only medical therapy that should be routinely administered to this patient population is ASA, as it is inexpensive, well-tolerated and highly effective across the spectrum of ACS. Anticoagulation with UFH or LMWH should not be administered routinely and should only be considered in the small fraction of patients that ultimately are diagnosed with ACS. NTG has never been shown to improve mortality or adverse cardiac events in ACS and cannot differentiate true ACS from non-ACS symptoms. Nonetheless, it may be given through its sublingual form as an attempt in symptom relief. Continuous administration of NTG in the form of nitropaste or intravenous infusion should not be employed in the CPU, but can be considered in patients diagnosed with ACS for control of symptoms. Finally, beta blockers are generally not recommended, however, they may be given to patients already taking them, or when other indications exist, such as rate control in patients with atrial fibrillation.

# References


1. Second International Study of Infarct Survival) Collaborative Group. Randomised trial of intravenous streptokinase, oral aspirin, both, or neither among 17,187 cases of suspected acute myocardial infarction: ISIS-2. ISIS-2 (Second International Study of Infarct Survival) Collaborative Group. Lancet. 1988;2:349–60.
2. Lewis HD Jr, Davis JW, Archibald DG, Steinke WE, Smitherman TC, Doherty JE III, et al. Protective effects of aspirin against acute myocardial infarction and death in men with unstable angina. Results of a Veterans Administration Cooperative Study. N Engl J Med. 1983;309:396–403.
3. Cairns JA, Gent M, Singer J, Finnie KJ, Froggatt GM, Holder DA, et al. Aspirin, sulfinpyrazone, or both in unstable angina. Results of a Canadian multicenter trial. N Engl J Med. 1985;313:1369–75.
4. Theroux P, Ouimet H, McCans J, Latour JG, Joly P, Levy G, et al. Aspirin, heparin, or both to treat acute unstable angina. N Engl J Med. 1988;319:1105–11.
5. The RISC Group. Risk of myocardial infarction and death during treatment with low dose aspirin and intravenous heparin in men with unstable coronary artery disease. Lancet. 1990;336:827–30.
6. Gaziano JM, Brotons C, Coppolecchia R, Cricelli C, Darius H, Gorelick PB, et al. Use of aspirin to reduce risk of initial vascular events in patients at moderate risk of cardiovascular disease (ARRIVE): a randomised, double-blind, placebo-controlled trial. Lancet. 2018;392:1036–46.
7. Steering Committee of the Physicians' Health Study Research Group. Final report on the aspirin component of the ongoing Physicians' Health Study. N Engl J Med. 1989;321:129–35.
8. Antithrombotic Trialists Collaboration. Collaborative meta-analysis of randomised trials of antiplatelet therapy for prevention of death, myocardial infarction, and stroke in high risk patients. BMJ. 2002;324:71–86.
9. Fragmin during Instability in Coronary Artery Disease (FRISC) study group. Low-molecular-weight heparin during instability in coronary artery disease. Lancet. 1996;347:561–8.
10. Hansson L, Zanchetti A, Carruthers SG, Dahlof B, Elmfeldt D, Julius S, et al. Effects of intensive blood-pressure lowering and low-dose aspirin in patients with hypertension: principal

results of the Hypertension Optimal Treatment (HOT) randomised trial. HOT Study Group. Lancet. 1998;351:1755–62.

11. Gurfinkel EP, Manos EJ, Mejail RI, Cerda MA, Duronto EA, Garcia CN, et al. Low molecular weight heparin versus regular heparin or aspirin in the treatment of unstable angina and silent ischemia. J Am Coll Cardiol. 1995;26:313–8.

12. Amsterdam EA, Wenger NK, Brindis RG, Casey DE Jr, Ganiats TG, Holmes DR Jr, et al. 2014 AHA/ACC guideline for the management of patients with non–ST-elevation acute coronary syndromes: a report of the American College of Cardiology/American Heart Association Task Force on Practice Guidelines. J Am Coll Cardiol. 2014;64:e139–228.

13. Knuuti J, Wijns W, Saraste A, Capodanno D, Barbato E, Funck-Brentano C, et al. 2019 ESC guidelines for the diagnosis and management of chronic coronary syndromes. Eur Heart J. 2020;41:407–77.

14. Barbash IM, Freimark D, Gottlieb S, Hod H, Hasin Y, Battler A, et al. Outcome of myocardial infarction in patients treated with aspirin is enhanced by pre-hospital administration. Cardiology. 2002;98:141–7.

15. Neumar RW, Shuster M, Callaway CW, Gent LM, Atkins DL, Bhanji F, et al. Part 1: Executive summary: 2015 American Heart Association guidelines update for cardiopulmonary resuscitation and emergency cardiovascular care. Circulation. 2015;132:S315–67.

16. Telford AM, Wilson C. Trial of heparin versus atenolol in prevention of myocardial infarction in intermediate coronary syndrome. Lancet. 1981;1:1225–8.

17. Williams DO, Kirby MG, McPherson K, Phear DN. Anticoagulant treatment of unstable angina. Br J Clin Pract. 1986;40(3):114–6.

18. Theroux P, Waters D, Qiu S, McCans J, de Guise P, Juneau M. Aspirin versus heparin to prevent myocardial infarction during the acute phase of unstable angina. Circulation. 1993;88:2045–8.

19. Neri Serneri GG, Gensini GF, Poggesi L, Trotta F, Modesti PA, Boddi M, et al. Effect of heparin, aspirin, or alteplase in reduction of myocardial ischaemia in refractory unstable angina. Lancet. 1990;335:615–8.

20. Holdright D, Patel D, Cunningham D, Thomas R, Hubbard W, Hendry G, et al. Comparison of the effect of heparin and aspirin versus aspirin alone on transient myocardial ischemia and in-hospital prognosis in patients with unstable angina. J Am Coll Cardiol. 1994;24:39–45.

21. Cohen M, Theroux P, Borzak S, Frey MJ, White HD, Van Mieghem W, et al. Randomized double-blind safety study of enoxaparin versus unfractionated heparin in patients with non-ST-segment elevation acute coronary syndromes treated with tirofiban and aspirin: the ACUTE II study. The Antithrombotic Combination Using Tirofiban and Enoxaparin. Am Heart J. 2002;144:470–7.

22. Cohen M, Demers C, Gurfinkel EP, Turpie AG, Fromell GJ, Goodman S, et al. A comparison of low-molecular-weight heparin with unfractionated heparin for unstable coronary artery disease. Efficacy and Safety of Subcutaneous Enoxaparin in Non-Q-Wave Coronary Events Study Group. N Engl J Med. 1997;337:447–52.

23. Klein W, Buchwald A, Hillis SE, Monrad S, Sanz G, Turpie AG, et al. Comparison of low-molecular-weight heparin with unfractionated heparin acutely and with placebo for 6 weeks in the management of unstable coronary artery disease. Fragmin in unstable coronary artery disease study (FRIC). Circulation. 1997;96:61–8.

24. The Frax.I.S. Study Group. Comparison of two treatment durations (6 days and 14 days) of a low molecular weight heparin with a 6-day treatment of unfractionated heparin in the initial management of unstable angina or non-Q wave myocardial infarction: FRAX.I.S. (FRAxiparine in Ischaemic Syndrome). Eur Heart J. 1999;20:1553–62.

25. Goodman SG, Fitchett D, Armstrong PW, Tan M, Langer A. Integrilin and Enoxaparin Randomized Assessment of Acute Coronary Syndrome Treatment (INTERACT) Trial Investigators. Randomized evaluation of the safety and efficacy of enoxaparin versus unfractionated heparin in high-risk patients with non-ST-segment elevation acute coronary syndromes receiving the glycoprotein IIb/IIIa inhibitor eptifibatide. Circulation. 2003;107:238–44.

26. Blazing MA, de Lemos JA, White HD, Fox KA, Verheugt FW, Ardissino D, et al. Safety and efficacy of enoxaparin vs unfractionated heparin in patients with non-ST-segment elevation

acute coronary syndromes who receive tirofiban and aspirin: a randomized controlled trial. JAMA. 2004;292:55–64.

27. Antman EM, McCabe CH, Gurfinkel EP, Turpie AG, Bernink PJ, Salein D, et al. Enoxaparin prevents death and cardiac ischemic events in unstable angina/non-Q-wave myocardial infarction. Results of the thrombolysis in myocardial infarction (TIMI) 11B trial. Circulation. 1999;100:1593–601.

28. Ferguson JJ, Califf RM, Antman EM, Cohen M, Grines CL, Goodman S, et al. Enoxaparin vs unfractionated heparin in high-risk patients with non-ST-segment elevation acute coronary syndromes managed with an intended early invasive strategy: primary results of the SYNERGY randomized trial. JAMA. 2004;292:45–54.

29. Stone GW, McLaurin BT, Cox DA, Bertrand ME, Lincoff AM, Moses JW, et al. Bivalirudin for patients with acute coronary syndromes. N Engl J Med. 2006;355:2203–16.

30. Fifth Organization to Assess Strategies in Acute Ischemic Syndromes Investigators, Yusuf S, Mehta SR, Chrolavicius S, Afzal R, Pogue J, et al. Comparison of fondaparinux and enoxaparin in acute coronary syndromes. N Engl J Med. 2006;354:1464–76.

31. Petersen JL, Mahaffey KW, Hasselblad V, Antman EM, Cohen M, Goodman SG, et al. Efficacy and bleeding complications among patients randomized to enoxaparin or unfractionated heparin for antithrombin therapy in non-ST-segment elevation acute coronary syndromes: a systematic overview. JAMA. 2004;292:89–96.

32. Peterson ED, Roe MT, Rumsfeld JS, Shaw RE, Brindis RG, Fonarow GC, et al. A call to ACTION (Acute Coronary Treatment and Intervention Outcomes Network): a national effort to promote timely clinical feedback and support continuous quality improvement for acute myocardial infarction. Circ Cardiovasc Qual Outcomes. 2009;2:491–9.

33. Eikelboom JW, Mehta SR, Anand SS, Xie C, Fox KA, Yusuf S. Adverse impact of bleeding on prognosis in patients with acute coronary syndromes. Circulation. 2006;114(8):774–82.

34. Yusuf S, Collins R, MacMahon S, Peto R. Effect of intravenous nitrates on mortality in acute myocardial infarction: an overview of the randomised trials. Lancet. 1988;1:1088–92.

35. ISIS-4 (Fourth International Study of Infarct Survival) Collaborative Group. ISIS-4: a randomised factorial trial assessing early oral captopril, oral mononitrate, and intravenous magnesium sulphate in 58,050 patients with suspected acute myocardial infarction. Lancet. 1995;345:669–85.

36. Gruppo Italiano per lo Studio della Sopravvivenza nell'infarto Miocardico. GISSI-3: effects of lisinopril and transdermal glyceryl trinitrate singly and together on 6-week mortality and ventricular function after acute myocardial infarction. Lancet. 1994;343:1115–22.

37. Henrikson CA, Howell EE, Bush DE, Miles JS, Meininger GR, Friedlander T, et al. Chest pain relief by nitroglycerin does not predict active coronary artery disease. Ann Intern Med. 2003;139:979–86.

38. Diercks DB, Boghos E, Guzman H, Amsterdam EA, Kirk JD. Changes in the numeric descriptive scale for pain after sublingual nitroglycerin do not predict cardiac etiology of chest pain. Ann Emerg Med. 2005;45:581–5.

39. Roberts R, Rogers WJ, Mueller HS, Lambrew CT, Diver DJ, Smith HC, et al. Immediate versus deferred beta-blockade following thrombolytic therapy in patients with acute myocardial infarction. Results of the Thrombolysis in Myocardial Infarction (TIMI) II-B Study. Circulation. 1991;83:422–37.

40. Van de Werf F, Janssens L, Brzostek T, Mortelmans L, Wackers FJ, Willems GM, et al. Short-term effects of early intravenous treatment with a beta-adrenergic blocking agent or a specific bradycardiac agent in patients with acute myocardial infarction receiving thrombolytic therapy. J Am Coll Cardiol. 1993;22:407–16.

41. Freemantle N, Cleland J, Young P, Mason J, Harrison J. beta Blockade after myocardial infarction: systematic review and meta regression analysis. BMJ. 1999;318:1730–7.

42. Chen ZM, Pan HC, Chen YP, Peto R, Collins R, Jiang LX, et al. Early intravenous then oral metoprolol in 45,852 patients with acute myocardial infarction: randomised placebo-controlled trial. Lancet. 2005;366:1622–32.

43. Yusuf S, Wittes J, Friedman L. Overview of results of randomized clinical trials in heart disease. II. Unstable angina, heart failure, primary prevention with aspirin, and risk factor modification. JAMA. 1988;260:2259–63.
44. Ellis K, Tcheng JE, Sapp S, Topol EJ, Lincoff AM. Mortality benefit of beta blockade in patients with acute coronary syndromes undergoing coronary intervention: pooled results from the Epic, Epilog, Epistent, Capture and Rapport Trials. J Interv Cardiol. 2003;16:299–305.
45. Newby LK, Kaplan AL, Granger BB, Sedor F, Califf RM, Ohman EM. Comparison of cardiac troponin T versus creatine kinase-MB for risk stratification in a chest pain evaluation unit. Am J Cardiol. 2000;85:801–5.
46. Farkouh ME, Smars PA, Reeder GS, Zinsmeister AR, Evans RW, Meloy TD, et al. A clinical trial of a chest-pain observation unit for patients with unstable angina. Chest Pain Evaluation in the Emergency Room (CHEER) Investigators. N Engl J Med. 1998;339:1882–8.

# Provocative Testing

**Ezra A. Amsterdam, Sandhya Venugopal, Muhammad Majid, and Edris Aman**

## 1  Introduction

Patients with low-risk chest pain (CP) presenting to the emergency department (ED) remain a common and perplexing group responsible for approximately eight million ED visits annually in the US [1]. It was usual practice until several decades ago for many of these low-risk patients to undergo costly hospitalization which frequently resulted in negative findings [1]. More recently, major efforts to improve clinical understanding of this large patient population have demonstrated the following findings: (1) low-risk patients comprise a majority of those presenting to the ED with CP; (2) the current description of low risk in these patients is based on the likelihood of no major adverse cardiac events (MACE) within 30 days of presentation; (3) low risk can be estimated by risk stratification using clinical data; and (4) a wide array of diagnostic procedures has furthered our understanding of this challenging group of patients. The results of these endeavors have promoted safe, accurate, efficient, and cost-effective management of low-risk patients presenting to the ED with CP. One of the most important advances in this setting has been evolution of their evaluation from a day or more to several hours in many centers [1–7]. An important factor in this achievement has been the result of noninvasive provocative cardiac testing, which is the subject of this chapter.

E. A. Amsterdam (✉) · S. Venugopal · M. Majid · E. Aman
Division of Cardiovascular Medicine, Cardiology and Internal Medicine, UC Davis Medical Center, Sacramento, CA, USA
e-mail: eaamsterdam@ucdavis.edu



M. Pena et al. (eds.), *Short Stay Management of Chest Pain*, Contemporary Cardiology, https://doi.org/10.1007/978-3-031-05520-1_14

## 2 Recognition of Low-Risk Patients

This aspect of patient evaluation is essential not only for diagnostic purposes but also for enhancing the safety of provocative testing. The rationale of early cardiac testing in these patients is that low risk in patients with CP is not "no risk" and warrants further evaluation, especially prior to provocative testing. Low clinical risk can be estimated by a focused evaluation to which the electrocardiogram (ECG) and cardiac injury markers (preferably high sensitivity cardiac troponin) provide pivotal information [1–7]; clinical risk scores are also useful in this setting and the numerous relatively benign causes of CP must also be considered. Of utmost importance is exclusion of three potentially lethal cardiovascular entities that present with CP: acute coronary syndromes (ACS), acute aortic conditions, and pulmonary embolism. In the absence of an acute process, provocative testing can usually be considered within several hours following patient presentation.

## 3 Provocative Cardiac Testing

Provocative cardiac testing provides inferential evidence of myocardial ischemia and coronary artery disease (CAD) in low-risk CP patients presenting with nondiagnostic findings, including a nonischemic electrocardiogram (ECG) and negative cardiac injury markers. This approach includes several types of tests based on induction of myocardial ischemia in a controlled setting by exercise testing or a pharmacologic agent. Ischemia can be detected by non-imaging methodology (exercise ECG [ETT]) or imaging studies (stress echocardiography [SE], myocardial perfusion imaging [MPI], or cardiac magnetic resonance [CMR]). These noninvasive methods have had major roles in identifying low-risk patients who are appropriate candidates for discharge from the ED or observation unit (ED/OU). Because the tests are based on provoking ischemia in patients with potential ACS, they require appropriate patient selection, judicious implementation, prudent discontinuation, and skilled interpretation. Precautions and considerations associated with provocative tests are indicated in Table 1.

### *3.1 Exercise Treadmill Testing*

#### 3.1.1 Methods

Criteria for ETT are a normal baseline ECG (isoelectric ST segments or ≤0.5 mm depression) and ability to exercise. ETT in the ED/OU is usually performed according to the Bruce protocol or its modified version with supervision by cardiologists or other trained clinicians, including non-MD health professionals. The standard

**Table 1** Considerations before performing provocative testing

| **General** |
| --- |
| Stable patient |
| Normal rhythm, Resting SBP 100–140 mmHg |
| Nonischemic ECG |
| Normal cardiac injury markers (high sensitivity cardiac troponin preferred) |
| **Exercise Treadmill Test** |
| Ability to exercise |
| **Stress Echocardiography** |
| Ability to exercise unless pharmacologic stress utilized |
| Adequate echo windows |
| **MPI (with adenosine, regadenosine)** |
| Adequate heart rate, no AV Block |
| Adequate pulmonary function |
| **CMR** |
| Same as for MPI if vasodilator agents used |
| Adequate renal function if gadolinium used |

*AV* atrioventricular, *CMR* cardiac magnetic resonance, *ECG* electrocardiogram, *MPI* myocardial perfusion imaging, cardiac magnetic resonance, *SBP* systolic blood pressure

Bruce protocol, which is the most frequently employed of multiple protocols [8], utilizes progressive 3-min stages of treadmill speed and grade, starting at 1.7 mph and 10% grade (unless the modified Bruce protocol is used, which begins at 1.7 mph and 0 grade). Although a diagnostic ETT in elective outpatients requires attainment of an exercise-induced heart rate $\geq$85% of age-predicted maximum, we have found that in assessing low-risk CP patients, a heart rate $\geq$80% of age-predicted maximum is associated with a negative post-discharge course [2].

Abnormal test criteria suggesting consideration of further evaluation include horizontal ischemic ST segment shift ($\geq$1.0 mm) (Fig. 1), fall in systolic blood pressure, significant arrhythmias, undue dyspnea, chest pain in the first stage of the protocol, or failure to achieve an exercise capacity of $\geq$5 METs [8, 9]. The latter indicates marked impairment of functional capacity, a powerful prognostic indicator [8]. It is prudent to terminate a stress test at the initial appearance of ischemic ST shift ($\geq$1.0 mm) even if there are no other abnormalities. A rare but ominous ECG response is exercise-induced ST elevation, which localizes a severe coronary artery obstruction or spasm (Fig. 2), and indicates the ischemic myocardial region [10]. This finding is usually an indication for invasive coronary angiography.

Although the sensitivity and specificity of ETT to detect CAD are approximately 60% and 70%, respectively, these rates are related exclusively to the ST segment response to exercise. In assessing an ETT, the entire spectrum of subjective and objective data (symptoms, ECG, hemodynamic, and rhythm responses) is considered in determining the appropriateness of the patient for early discharge or additional assessment; an abnormal response in any of these parameters can suggest CAD, occult ACS, and other cardiac or noncardiac conditions.

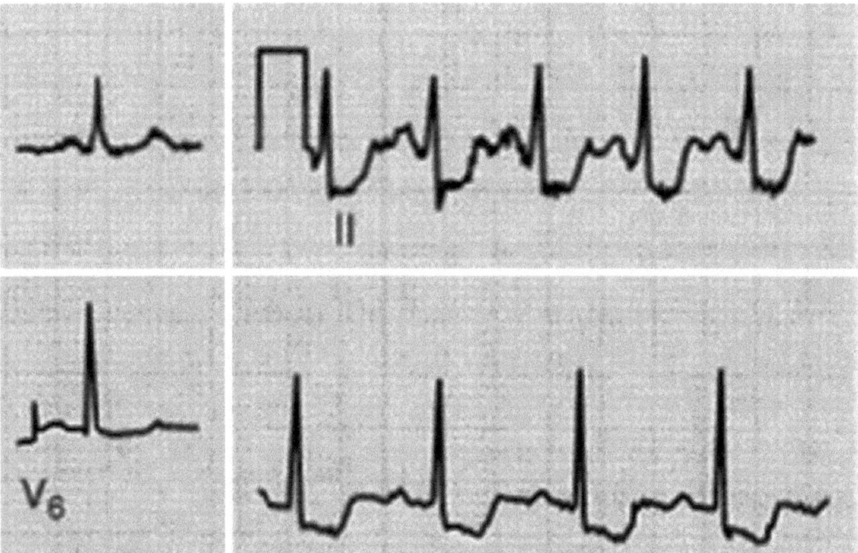


**Fig. 1** Examples of ST-segment responses during exercise testing. The top row demonstrates horizontal depression of 3.0 mm that is markedly positive for ischemia. The second row reveals downsloping ST segment depression. There is J point depression of >2.0 mm with further depression of the ST segment after the J point. (Chaitman BR: Exercise electrocardiographic stress testing. In Beller GA [ed]: Chronic Ischemic Heart Disease. In Braunwald E [series ed]: Atlas of Heart Diseases. Vol 5. Chronic Ischemic Heart Disease. Philadelphia, Current Medicine, 1995, pp 2.1–2.30. Adapted from reference [9] with permission from Elsevier [STM Guidelines])

Absence of abnormal ETT findings associated with failure to reach at least 80% of age-predicted maximum heart rate is designated a nondiagnostic test. Abnormal and nondiagnostic ETTs suggest the need for further evaluation while a negative ETT is an indication to consider early discharge. Of note, failure to achieve an adequate ETT (≥80% of predicted maximum heart rate) to induce CP markedly lowers the likelihood that CAD is the cause of the CP prompting the ED visit. The diagnostic utility of ETT can be enhanced by use of an integrated ETT score such as the Duke Treadmill Score. However, we have found that in the contemporary era this score has lost some of its predictive value for cardiac events which is likely related to therapeutic advances that have reduced cardiovascular risk in the decades since the score was developed [11].

### 3.1.2 Utility

ETT is one of the most frequently utilized tests in determining the safety of early discharge for low-risk patients. It is applicable in stable patients with a normal baseline ECG and ability to exercise. The utility of ETT in this setting was initially validated by multiple studies that included approximately 3000 patients who underwent ETT after ≤12 h of an initial negative clinical evaluation for ACS and were discharged directly from the ED/OU within hours in many cases [1]. No adverse effects

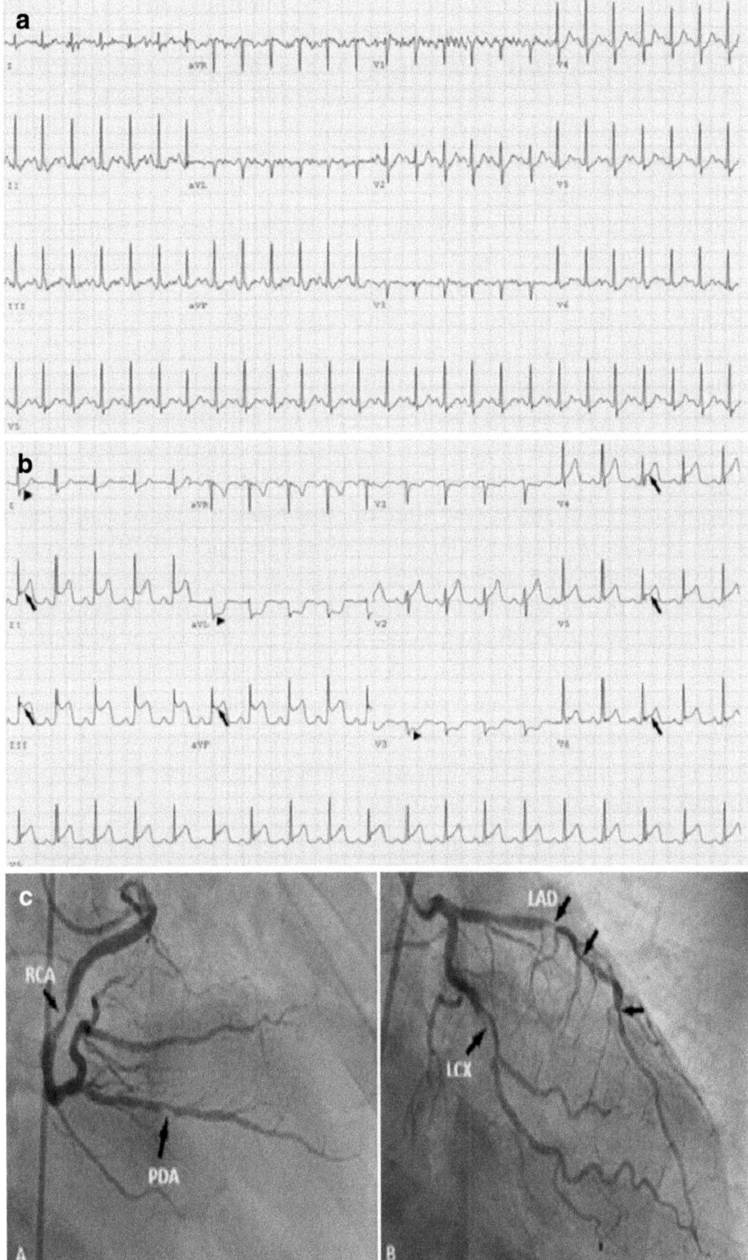

**Fig. 2** (**a**) 12-lead exercise electrocardiogram showing sinus tachycardia (maximum heart rate 153/min and no exercise-induced abnormalities). (**b**) Post-exercise electrocardiogram (1.5 min of recovery) showing 3–4 mm ST elevation in leads 2, 3, aVF (arrows) and 1–2 mm ST elevation in leads V4-V6 (arrows). There is also ST-depression in I, aVL and V3 (arrowheads). (**c**) Coronary angiogram of the patient showing multiple coronary artery stenoses (arrows) in the left anterior descending coronary artery (LAD), left circumflex artery (LCX) and right coronary artery (RCA). (From Takahashi N, et al. Reference [10], with permission from Elsevier)

of the method were reported. During follow-up comprising up to 17 months, there was only one reported cardiac death and the incidence of ACS and revascularization were 0% and 2%, respectively. In patients with normal ETT who were discharged early, the negative predictive value (NPV) was ≥99% for subsequent cardiac events during short- or intermediate-term assessment. A concurrent study of 400 patients who received early discharge after either a negative ETT or stress imaging test reported similar findings [12].

Cost-effectiveness of early ETT has been demonstrated in comparisons of this strategy with regular care involving hospital admission of low-risk CP patients. These benefits have included both reduced length of stay and lower cost [1, 12, 13]. The outcomes of these investigations have been similar in both women and men, young, and older patients, and in those with and without a history of CAD, ACS, revascularization, and cardiac co-morbidities [1–7, 12, 13].

The continuing evolution of care for low-risk CP patients has recently resulted in evidence that predischarge testing by ETT (or other methods currently in use) is not a prerequisite for early discharge in all low-risk patients. When testing was limited to physician discretion, there were similarly low rates of clinical events at 30 days in patients assessed with and without predischarge testing [3, 5–7]. Absence of testing is also associated with shorter ED/OU length of stay with favorable cost implications [3, 6, 7]. In this regard, absence of predischarge cardiac testing has recently become a more frequent approach in the assessment of low-risk patients for early discharge [3, 5–7]. Shared decision making in this process is now recognized as an integral part of the interaction between patient and physician regarding management. Thus, the management of low-risk patients has evolved further from shorter length of stay to support for less frequent predischarge testing, which has also been increasingly supported in recent literature [14–17].

## 4 Cardiac Stress Imaging Tests

Noninvasive cardiac imaging in low-risk CP ED/OU patients has been primarily performed by SE and MPI; CMR has had limited use in this setting except in centers with special capability. All three methods can utilize exercise or pharmacologic stress. Indications for these studies include whether a patient is able to exercise, baseline ECG abnormalities, as well as physician preference and institutional expertise. They have greater accuracy for detection of CAD/ischemia than ETT. The approximate sensitivity and specificity of these methods for revealing obstructive CAD are: ETT—60% and 75%, respectively; SE—80% and 85%, respectively; MPI 85% and 80%, respectively; and CMR 90% and 75%, respectively. These values vary with the prevalence of CAD in the populations tested [9]. The imaging techniques also convey valuable data on the site and extent of myocardial ischemia and the involved coronary artery, as well as depicting global ventricular function and regional contractile abnormalities. However, despite their superiority for revealing CAD/ischemia, it is noteworthy that the NPV of ETT for predicting post-discharge adverse cardiac events is *comparable* to those of SE and MPI [1]; data for CMR are insufficient for this comparison.

## 4.1 Stress Echocardiography

### 4.1.1 Methods

Myocardial ischemia induces a regional wall motion abnormality within 20 s and SE can usually detect this contractile impairment close to its onset. In SE provocative testing, the stressor can be dobutamine or exercise, but preference in ED/OU patients has favored the catecholamine because echocardiographic observation is continuous during drug infusion rather than performed "immediately" after exercise. Continuous echocardiography during drug administration has the advantage of "on-line" cardiac observation and also offers a slight advantage in sensitivity for CAD compared to the short delay ($\leq$30 s) in transit to supine position and initiation of recording after termination of exercise.

Dobutamine is a positive beta-adrenergic agent that increases myocardial contractility, systolic blood pressure, and heart rate, thereby augmenting myocardial oxygen demand which increases coronary blood flow in normal vessels. This effect is blunted in obstructed (>50% narrowed) coronary arteries, resulting in regional ischemia and segmental ventricular wall motion abnormalities disclosed on echocardiography from which the involved coronary artery can also be inferred. Contractile abnormalities detected by echocardiography are also reflected by decreased systolic segmental wall thickening and excursion. Dobutamine is administered by graded doses in 3-min stages at 5-, 10-, 20-, 40-mg/kg body weight/min until target heart rate (85% of 220-age) is reached or signs/symptoms occur. These endpoints are similar to those assessed during ETT. If target heart rate is not achieved with dobutamine, atropine is added (0.25–0.50 mg/min to total of 1–2 mg). The echocardiogram and ECG are continuously observed, and blood pressure is measured at each stage of the infusion. A disadvantage of dobutamine is that it can induce arrythmias and impart a subjective sense of uneasiness.

Echocardiography does not involve radiation, can be performed at the patient's bedside, and can also disclose evidence of nonischemic causes of patients' symptoms, including valvular heart disease, cardiomyopathy, pericardial disease, and pulmonary embolism. Limitations include inadequate imaging windows in obese patients and those with severe pulmonary disease.

### 4.1.2 Utility

Although SE has not been as widely utilized as ETT and MPI in low-risk patients presenting with CP, it has been similarly effective in identifying low-risk patients suitable for early discharge. In three of four early investigations with dobutamine

SE [1], the NPV for post-discharge adverse cardiac events was 96% in 351 patients at 6 months, 100% in 87 patients after 2 months, and 98% in 130 patients at 3 months. In the fourth and smallest study of 80 patients with negative SEs, NPV was 89% [1]. The positive predictive value was 29–53% in three of the four studies, reflecting the low prevalence of CAD and ACS in the populations tested, as has also been true of ETT and MPI. In an innovative study published over two decades ago, dobutamine SE was performed by specially trained nurses and sonographers in low-risk patients and the data were transmitted to cardiologists by telemetry [18]. The NPV in 139 patients followed for 3 months was 98.5%. Dobutamine SE was completed within 6 h of patient presentation to the ED. The test was discontinued because of ventricular ectopy, dyspnea or nonspecific symptoms in 6.3% of patients. The authors published a subsequent report of this technique that revealed its sustained value in over 700 patients in which it proved safe and accurate [19].

The results of SE have remained comparable to other ED/OU cardiac tests to identify low-risk patients who warrant early, safe discharge. This was demonstrated in a study of low-risk CP patients in a national insurance database of >48,000 patient records [20]. Utility of SE and MPI were compared on post-discharge clinical outcomes and downstream resource utilization after >6 months. Compared to MPI, SE was associated with significantly lower rates of repeat ED visits, cardiac catheterization, and revascularization procedures. There were no differences in repeat testing or myocardial infarction, but the cost of downstream care was higher with MPI ($2194 vs. $1631, $p < 0.0001$).

SE also compared favorably with coronary computed tomography angiography (cCTA) in 400 women reporting to the ED with intermediate risk CP [21]. Patients were randomized to SE or cCTA and events analyzed during index visit and at a median follow-up of 24 months. Index visit events: 19% cCTA patients were hospitalized vs. 11% of SE patients ($p < 0.03$); median length of ED stay: 5.4 h for cCTA vs. 4.7 h for SE ($p < 0.001$); MACE at 24 months: $n = 11$ and 7 for cCTA and SE, respectively (ns). Total radiation exposure with cCTA was greater than tenfold that for SE ($p < 0.001$). Thus, SE resulted in lower rates of hospitalization, shorter length of stay, less radiation, and maintenance of safety.

In a study of patients presenting to the ED with low-risk CP, the utility of SE ($n = 117$) was compared to usual care ($n = 109$) [22]. There were no differences in patients receiving revascularization, median time to discharge was significantly less with SE (573 min vs. 1466 min), cost was significantly lower with SE ($4381 vs. $6192), and no MACE reported at 1 or 6 months related to SE or early discharge.

A recent comparison assessed the utility of exercise SE and dobutamine SE in 705 patients [23]. During an average follow-up of >4.5 years, the NPV was 89.2% for dobutamine SE and 96.5% for exercise SE ($p = 0.001$). These findings suggest that the latter approach, if feasible, may be more accurate in identifying patients appropriate for early discharge because of its higher NPV. Because there is a single report of myocardial infarction during dobutamine SE in stable outpatients [24], we do not exceed a maximum dose of 40 µg/kg/min. SE does not disclose the age or etiology of a wall motion abnormality, which can be related to ischemia and acute or old MI. However, prior MI may be suggested by segmental myocardial thinning with decreased systolic thickening.

## 4.2 Myocardial Perfusion Imaging

### 4.2.1 Methods

The major MPI methods employed in low-risk patients presenting with CP are (1) single photon emission computed tomography (SPECT) with the technetium 99m ($Tc^{99m}$) radionuclides, sestamibi, and tetrafosmin, and (2) positron emission tomography (PET), which employs rubidium 82 ($RB^{82}$). These isotopes are transported in blood and their myocardial distribution reflects coronary perfusion, which is homogeneous in the presence of normal coronary arteries. Obstructed vessels prevent elevation of flow in response to cardiac stressors, resulting in a maldistribution of perfusion that is reflected by reduced regional radioactivity on the cardiac scan (Figs. 3 and 4). The region of diminished radioactivity typically localizes the obstructed coronary artery.

Stress can be imposed by coronary vasodilators (adenosine or regadenosine) or by inotropic stimulation with exercise or dobutamine. In addition to identifying a perfusion defect, MPI also indicates the extent of the perfusion abnormality, and with ECG gating, can reveal segmental wall motion function and left ventricular ejection fraction. SPECT MPI has maintained an important role in assessing low-risk ED/OU patients although MPI with PET $Rb^{82}$ has demonstrable advantages in image quality, greater sensitivity, and more reliable attenuation correction. However, these gains are associated with increased cost and SPECT MPI remains the more frequent approach in most centers.

Because early redistribution of the $Tc^{99m}$ radionuclides is negligible, they have provided a unique approach to detection of perfusion defects in CP patients on arrival to the ED. With these radionuclides, a perfusion defect present at the time of their injection persists for 3–4 h, allowing patient stabilization and subsequent imaging [25]. Thus, this method provides a "snapshot" of myocardial perfusion at the time of injection. It may also be applied in patients whose symptoms have abated before reporting to the ED because an ischemic perfusion defect may be maintained for a few hours following cessation of symptoms. In these strategies, the patients' symptoms provide the "stress phase" of the study.

### 4.2.2 Utility

Normal rest MPI is associated with a very low rate of MACE and thereby a high NPV following early discharge from the ED/OU. In multiple studies performed in the 1990s, the NPV of SPECT rest MPI in low-risk ED patients with CP was $\geq$99% and sensitivity for ischemia was >90% [1]. In an early multicenter randomized, prospective trial (ERASE) of 2475 low-risk ED patients, outcomes were compared in patients receiving usual care ($n = 1260$) and those managed according to results of SPECT rest MPI ($n = 1215$) with $Tc^{99m}$ sestamibi [26]. Early discharge after negative MPI was associated with significantly fewer unnecessary admissions (42% vs. 52%, $p = 0.002$) with no increase in ischemic events at 30 days. Additionally, the

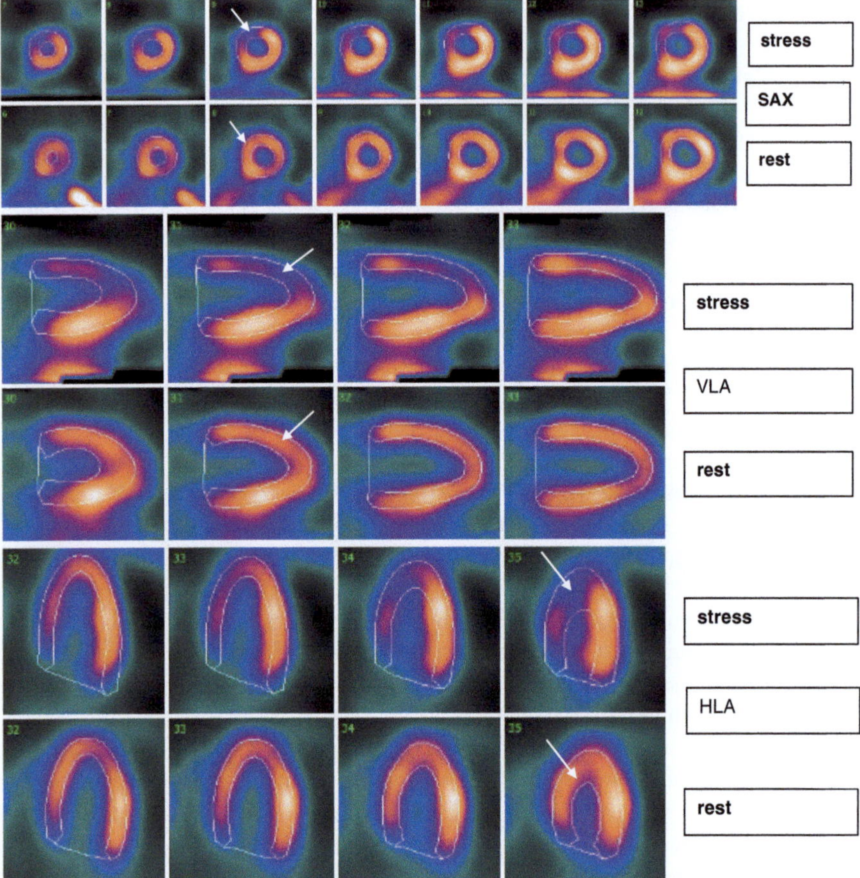

**Fig. 3** Large, moderate-severe, nearly fully reversible perfusion defect detected by SPECT (single photon emission computed tomography) Technetium 99m stress/rest study of the left ventricular anterior wall and septum reflecting obstruction of the left anterior descending coronary artery territory. *SAX* short axis, *VLA* vertical long axis, *HLA* horizontal long axis. Arrows indicate the defects during stress and reperfusion during rest

risk ratio for a cardiac ischemic event at 30 days was almost 4 times higher ($p < 0.001$) in patients with equivocal/abnormal scans than in those with a normal scan. Another prospective randomized investigation reported that SPECT MPI compared favorably with cCTA in 598 low-intermediate risk CP patients in terms of time to diagnosis, length of stay, and cost, with improved prognostic accuracy and less radiation exposure [27]. Based on the highly reliable findings with stress MPI in low-risk patients with acute CP, the American College of Radiology and American College of Cardiology rated this method "appropriate" for this clinical context in a joint document [28]. The findings of a comparative analysis of the value of ETT with and without MPI in 680 propensity-matched low-risk CP patients are of

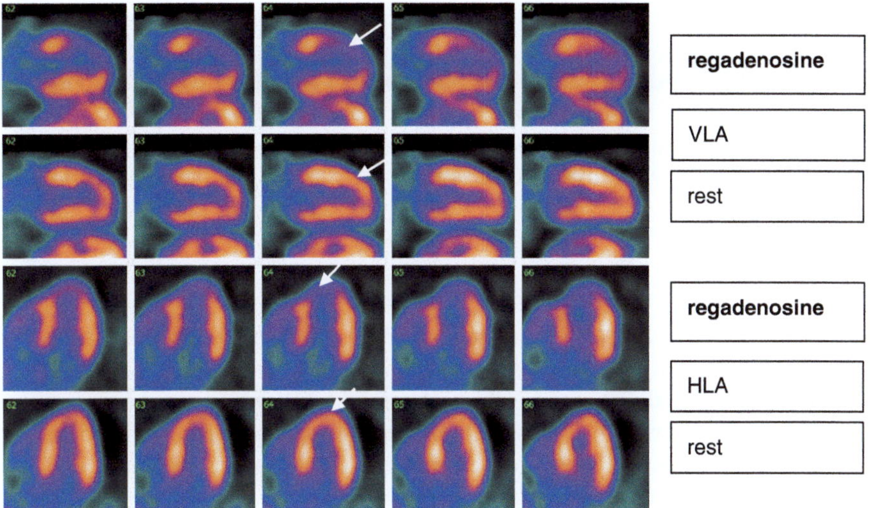



**Fig. 4** Large, severe perfusion defect in the mid-anterior left ventricular wall detected by Rubidium-82 positron emission tomography (PET) during regadenosine stress. There is almost complete reversibility of the defect with rest. *VLA* vertical long axis, *HLA* horizontal long axis. Arrows indicate area of defect during stress with reversibility at rest, indicating an area of ischemia related to a lesion in the left anterior descending coronary artery

interest [29]. There was no difference between groups in occurrence of MACE at 3 days and 1 year. Although cost was 30% higher for the MPI group, they were event-free longer than the ETT group.

MPI is an accurate method for confirming low clinical risk in patients presenting with acute undifferentiated CP. It is noninvasive and can demonstrate extent of ischemia and ventricular function. However, it does involve radiation, and vasodilator stress requires caution to ensure the patient has an adequate heart rate and atrioventricular conduction, and no significant bronchospastic disease as adenosine and regadenosine can produce bradycardia, heart block, and bronchospasm.

## *4.3 Cardiac Magnetic Resonance*

### 4.3.1 Method

CMR provides comprehensive anatomical and functional analysis of the heart, as well as information on blood flow within the coronary circulation and total flow to and from the heart. Acute and chronic myocardial tissue injury as in ischemia and infarction can be defined, and because this technique can image the spectrum of the ischemic cascade, subendocardial, and transmural infarct can be distinguished. Stress CMR can be performed with dobutamine, adenosine, or regadenosine; and gadolinium delayed enhancement can reveal ischemia and its pathophysiologic outcomes. Despite these remarkable attributes, CMR has a number of limitations which preclude its widespread application for rapid evaluation of low-risk CP patients: the method requires transfer of the patient from the ED/OU, the patient is inaccessible during the examination, imaging times are prolonged, and cost is high. Nonetheless, current studies provide a perspective on the potential utility of the method in patients with suspected ischemia.

### 4.3.2 Utility

The diagnostic value of CMR was demonstrated in an early study carried out in a community hospital [30]. Adenosine stress CMR was performed 72 h after admission on 135 low-risk patients in whom abnormal CMR was defined as a regional wall motion abnormality, adenosine-induced perfusion defect, or gadolinium delayed enhancement. Patients were followed for 1 year for incidence of CAD reflected by angiography, abnormal correlative stress test, myocardial infarction, or death. Perfusion abnormalities were 100% sensitive and 93% specific for predicting clinical outcome. These results were considered "striking" by the authors, especially considering the high specificity in this low-risk group in which clinical probability of CAD was <15%. Although excellent predictive accuracy of CMR was demonstrated in this small study, delay of the test until several days after admission did not address its utility for rapid evaluation of low-risk patients. Subsequent application of CMR was reported in a study in which 103 low-risk CP patients received adenosine stress CMR within 24 h of presentation [31]. CMR was negative in 89 patients (86.4%) and during follow-up of 277 days, none of this group reached a primary endpoint (cardiac death, nonfatal acute infarction, re-hospitalization for chest pain, obstructive CAD or revascularization), reflecting an NPV of 100%. These findings were extended in a subsequent investigation of 60 patients with intermediate risk CP in which the utility of stress CMR (adenosine) was compared with dobutamine SE [32], an established method. All patients underwent both tests in random order initiated within 12 h of presentation to the ED. Endpoints included evidence of CAD (>50% stenosis, infarction, or death) during a mean follow-up of 14 months. There were no significant differences in the NPV and PPV for adenosine CMR vs. dobutamine SE, but multivariable logistic regression analysis showed that adenosine CMR was the strongest independent predictor of the clinical endpoints ($p = 0.002$). This investigation demonstrated achievability of early CMR and favorable diagnostic efficacy compared with an established noninvasive method.

Although CMR is considered the most comprehensive imaging technique for anatomic and functional evaluation of the heart and does not involve radiation, its widespread application in patients with acute CP has important obstacles. In addition to its aforementioned limitations in this clinical setting, others include: cardiac and respiratory motion artifacts, patient factors such as claustrophobia, cardiac devices (e.g., pacemakers, implantable cardioverter defibrillators), certain intracranial aneurysm clips, arrhythmias, and advanced chronic kidney disease in which administration of gadolinium is contraindicated because of its association with nephrogenic systemic fibrosis [33]. Several of these drawbacks have been diminished by recent technological advances, but at present, the accuracy and versatility of other noninvasive methods have provided more readily available and less costly methods to achieve excellence in diagnosis and prognosis of low-risk patients presenting with CP. Thus, CMR in patients presenting with low-risk CP at present is largely the province of centers with special interest, capability, and expertise with this method.

# 5  Summary

During the last several decades, continuing advances have resulted in major improvement in the management of low-risk patients presenting to the ED with chest pain. It is now appreciated that a minority of these patients have ACS or other life-threatening conditions. Among the methods that have enhanced clinicians' expertise in affording low clinical risk and appropriate early patient discharge, noninvasive provocative cardiac testing has been widely utilized with excellent results. These approaches have helped reduce length of stay from days to hours while maintaining safety as indicated by a very low event rate at $\geq 30$ days, as well as lowering cost. The test methods are variable and versatile with selection depending on type of patient, availability of test, clinician preference, and institutional expertise. The major test methods include exercise treadmill test, stress echocardiography, and myocardial perfusion imaging. Cardiac magnetic resonance, although the most robust and complete cardiac diagnostic method, has significant obstacles that preclude current widespread application.

# References


1. Amsterdam EA, Kirk JD, Bluemke DA, Diercks D, Farkouh ME, Garvey JL, Kontos MC, McCord J, Miller TD, Morise A, Newby LK, Ruberg FL, Scordo KA, Thompson PD. Testing of low-risk patients presenting to the emergency department with chest pain: a scientific statement from the American Heart Association. Circulation. 2010,122:1756–76.
2. Amsterdam EA, Kirk JD, Diercks DB, Lewis WR, Turnipseed SD. Immediate exercise testing to evaluate low-risk patients presenting to the emergency department with chest pain. J Am Coll Cardiol. 2002;40:251–6.
3. Stauber SM, Teleten A, Li Z, Venugopal S, Amsterdam EA. Prognosis of low-risk young women presenting to the emergency department with chest pain. Am J Cardiol. 2015;117:36–9.
4. Prasad P, Sharma A, Vipparla N, Majid M, Daniela A, Howell S, Wilson M, Amsterdam EA. Identification and management of intermediate risk patients in the chest pain unit. Crit Pathw Cardiol. 2019;19:26–9.
5. Eddin M, Venugopal S, Chatterton B, Thinda A, Amsterdam EA. Long-term prognosis of low-risk women presenting to the emergency department with chest pain. Am J Med. 2017;130:313–7.

6. Howell SJ, Bui JB, Balasingam T, Amsterdam EA. Utility of Physician Selection of Cardiac Tests in a Chest Pain Unit to Exclude Acute Coronary Syndrome Among Patients Without a History of Coronary Artery Disease. Am J Cardiol. 2018;121:825–9.

7. Howell SJ, Prasad P, Vipparla NS, Venugopal S, Amsterdam EA. Usefulness of predischarge cardiac testing in low risk women and men for safe, rapid discharge from a chest pain unit. Am J Cardiol. 2019;123:1772–5.

8. Amsterdam EA, Takahashi N, Majid M, Taha S, Alismail Y, Venugopal S. Chapter "Exercise electrocardiographic stress testing". In: Wong N, Amsterdam EA, Toth PP, editors. ASPC manual of preventive cardiology. 2nd ed. New York, NY: Humana Press; 2020.

9. Chaitman BR. Exercise electrocardiographic stress testing. In: Beller GA, editor. Chronic ischemic heart disease. In Braunwald E (series ed), Atlas of heart diseases. Vol 5. Chronic Ischemic Heart Disease. Philadelphia, Current Medicine; 1995. p. 2.1–2.30.

10. Takahashi N, Gall E, Fan D, Majid M, Amsterdam EA. ST elevation during recovery phase of exercise test. Am J Med. 2020;133:1287–90.

11. Beri N, Dang P, Bhat A, Venugopal S, Amsterdam EA. Usefulness of excellent functional capacity in men and women with ischemic exercise electrocardiography to predict a negative stress imaging test and very low late mortality. Am J Cardiol. 2019;124:661–5.

12. Farkouh M, Smars PA, Reeder GS, Zinsmeister AR, Evans RW, Meloy TD, Kopecky SL, Allison TG, Gibbons RJ, Gabriel SE. A clinical trial of a chest-pain observation unit for patients with unstable angina. NEJM. 1998;339:1882–8.

13. Gomez MA, Anderson JL, Labros AK, Muhlestein JB, Mooders FB. An emergency department-based protocol for rapidly ruling out myocardial ischemia reduces hospital time and expense: results of a randomized study (ROMIO). J Am Coll Cardiol. 1996;28:25–33.

14. Amsterdam EA, Aman E. The patient with chest pain. Low risk, high stakes. JAMA Intern Med. 2014;174:553–4.

15. Winchester DE, Brandt J, Schmidt C, Allen B, Payton T, Amsterdam EA. Diagnostic yield of routine noninvasive cardiovascular testing in low-risk acute chest pain patients. Am J Cardiol. 2015;116:204–7.

16. Amsterdam EA, Venugopal S. Utility of simplicity for low-risk chest pain patients. Eur Heart J Acute Cardiovasc Care. 2018;7:285–6.

17. Booth J, Thomas JJ. Provocative testing for low-risk chest pain patients, must we continue? J Nucl Cardiol. 2019;26:1647–9.

18. Trippi JA, Lee KS, Kopp G, Nelson DR, King GY, Cordel WH. Dobutamine stress tele- echocardiography for evaluation of emergency department patients with chest pain. J Am Coll Cardiol. 1997;30:627–32.

19. Trippi JA, Lee KS. Dobutamine stress tele-echocardiography as a clinical service in the emergency department to evaluate patients with chest pain. Echocardiography. 1999;16:179–85.

20. Davies R, Liu G, Sciamanna C, Davidson WR Jr, Leslie DL, Foy AJ. Comparison of the effectiveness of stress echocardiography versus myocardial perfusion imaging in patients presenting to the emergency department with low-risk chest pain. Am J Cardiol. 2016;118:786–1791.

21. Levsky JM, Haramati LB, Spevack DM, Menegus MA, Chen T, Mizrachi S, Brown-Manhertz D, Selesny S, Lerer R, White DJ, Tobin JN, Taub CC, Garcia MJ. Coronary computed tomography angiography versus stress echocardiography in acute chest pain: a randomized controlled trial. JACC Cardiovasc Imaging. 2018;11:1288–97.

22. Jasani G, Papas M, Patel AJ, Jasani N, Levine B, Zhang Y, Marshall ES. Immediate stress echocardiography for low-risk chest pain patients in the emergency department: a prospective observational cohort study. J Emerg Med. 2018;54:156–64.

23. Samiei N, Parsaee M, Pourafkari L, Tajlil A, Pasbani Y, Rafati A, Nader ND. Value of negative stress echocardiography in predicting cardiovascular events among adults with no known coronary disease. J Cardiovasc Thorac Res. 2019;11:85–94.

24. Lewis WR, Arsna FJ, Galloway MT, Bommer WJ. Acute myocardial infarction associated with dobutamine stress echocardiography. J Am Soc Echocardiogr. 1997;10:576–8.

25. Henzlova MJ, Duvall WL, Einstein AJ, Travin MI, Verberne HJ. ASNC imaging guidelines for SPECT nuclear cardiology procedures: stress, protocols, and tracers. J Nucl Cardiol. 2016;23:606–39.
26. Udelson JE, Beshansky JR, Ballin DS, Feldman JA, Griffith JL, Handler J, Heller GV, Hendel RC, Pope JH, Ruthazer R, Spiegler EJ, Woolard RH, Selker HP. Myocardial perfusion imaging for evaluation and triage of patients with suspected acute cardiac ischemia: a randomized controlled trial. JAMA. 2002;288:2693–7000.
27. Nabi F, Kassi M, Muhyieddeen K, Chang SM, Xu J, Peterson L, Wray N, Shirkey B, Ashton C, Mahmarian J. Optimizing evaluation of patients with low-to-intermediate-risk acute chest pain: a randomized study comparing stress myocardial perfusion tomography incorporating stress-only imaging versus cardiac CT. J Nucl Med. 2016;2016(57):378–84.
28. Rybicki FJ, Udelson JE, Peacock WF, Goldhaber SZ, Isselbacher EM, Kazerooni E, Kontos MC, Litt H, Woodard PK, Emergency Department Patients With Chest Pain Rating Panel; Appropriate Utilization of Cardiovascular Imaging Oversight Committee. ACR/ACC/AHA/ AATS/ACEP/ASNC/NASCI/SAEM/SCCT/SCMR/SCPC/SNMMI/STR/STS. J Am Coll Cardiol. 2016;67:853–9.
29. Amirian J, Javdan O, Misher J, et al. Comparative efficiency of exercise stress testing with and without stress-only myocardial perfusion imaging in patients with low-risk chest pain. J Nucl Cardiol. 2018;25:1274–82.
30. Ingkanisorn PW, Kwong RW, Bohme NS, Geller NL, Rhoads KL, Dyke CK, Paterson DI, Mushabbar AS, Aletras AH, Arai AE. Prognosis of negative adenosine stress magnetic resonance in patients presenting to an emergency department with chest pain. J Am Coll Cardiol. 2006;47:1427–32.
31. Lerakis S, McLean DS, Anadiotis AV, Janik M, Oshinski JN, Alexopoulos N, Zaragoza-Macias E, Veledar E, Stillman AE. Prognostic value of adenosine stress cardiovascular magnetic resonance in patients with low-risk chest pain. J Cardiovasc Magn Reson. 2009;11:37.
32. Heitner JF, Klem I, Rasheed D, Chandra A, Kim HW, Van Assche LM, Parker M, Judd RM, Jollis JG, Kim RJ. Stress cardiac MR imaging compared with stress echocardiography in the early evaluation of patients who present to the emergency department with intermediate-risk chest pain. Radiology. 2014;271:56–64.
33. Balfour PC Jr, Gonzalez JA, Kramer CM. Non-invasive assessment of low- and intermediate-risk patients with chest pain. Trends Cardiovasc Med. 2017;27:182–9.

# Use of Multislice CT for the Evaluation of Patients with Chest Pain

Vijaya Arun Kumar and Brian O'Neil

## 1 Overview of CT Technology

The advent of helical/spiral CT imaging technology and the dramatic advances in the temporal and spatial resolution of CT [3] have made it possible to visualize the coronary arteries with systems that are able to synchronize the image reconstruction with the cardiac phase [4, 5]. Images with high temporal and spiral resolution in all directions can be obtained with multiple-row detector CT scanners and expressed as isotropic spatial resolution [6]. The advances in technology have considerably decreased the gantry rotation time to as low as 330–370 ms, and based on the acquisition mode, the temporal resolution can range from 80 to 250 ms [6]. Improved detector and collimator hardware now provide submillimeter image resolution (0.4–0.5 mm). The high resolution sixty-four slice scanners have become standard for CCTA [7]. Such scanners decrease breath-hold time and reduce cardiac motion artifacts which have increased the overall percentage of "interpretable" scans, and allowed imaging without the need for beta blockade in many patients. Challenges remain in imaging patients with heavily calcified coronary arteries, coronary artery stents, and markedly obese patients. Although 320-slice machines are now available, these are not widely diffused and the existing published evidence is specific to 64-slice scanners [8].

V. A. Kumar · B. O'Neil (✉)
Department of Emergency Medicine, Wayne State University, Detroit, MI, USA
e-mail: vkumar@med.wayne.edu; boneil@med.wayne.edu



M. Pena et al. (eds.), *Short Stay Management of Chest Pain*, Contemporary
Cardiology, https://doi.org/10.1007/978-3-031-05520-1_15

## 2 Accuracy of Coronary CT Angiography

The main requirement for CCTA to be an acceptable tool for evaluation of patients suspected for coronary artery disease (CAD) includes the complete visualization of all therapeutic relevant coronary arteries [9]. The need to exclude life threatening causes such as acute coronary syndrome (ACS) among patients presenting to the ED with chest pain (CP) is crucial, since an estimated 2% of these patients are inappropriately sent home and suffer higher morbidity than admitted patients [10, 11]. The ability of CCTA to quantitate coronary artery lesion severity correlates well with invasive coronary angiography (Pearson correlation, $r = 0.72$) [7, 12–14]. The considerable standard deviation in these early studies, however, limits its quantitative accuracy (see Fig. 1).

Figure recreated from a diagnostic accuracy study of 64-slice coronary computed tomography angiography (CCTA) in 70 consecutive patients who underwent elective invasive coronary angiography for suspected coronary artery disease [7]. Bland–Altman analysis of the differences of percent diameter stenosis measured by CCTA versus quantitative coronary angiography (QCA) during invasive catheterization, compared to the average percent diameter stenosis by the two methods. The mean difference was $1.3 \pm 14.0\%$ (central line). A total of 94% of the values lie within 1.96 standard deviations of the mean (outer lines). There was no significant correlation between stenosis difference and stenosis severity (Spearmen correlation = $-0.07$, $p = 0.59$).

There have been several studies that have evaluated the safety and diagnostic accuracy of 64-slice CCTA for triage of ED patients with acute chest pain. Overall, these studies suggest that CCTA can identify a subset of ED chest pain patients who can be safely discharged home on the basis of CT findings [15–17]. In the study by Goldstein et al., a randomized control trial of 197 low-risk acute chest

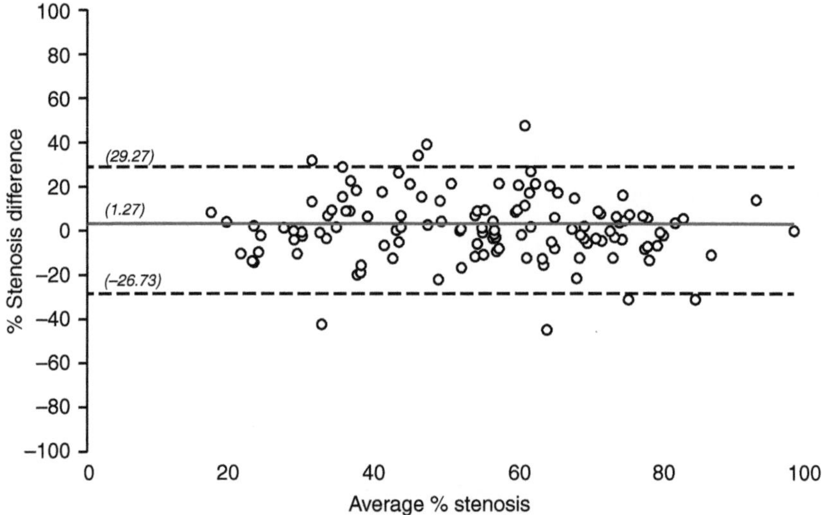


**Fig. 1** Diagnostic accuracy of noninvasive coronary angiography using 64-slice spiral computed tomography. Adapted from Raff et al. [14]

pain patients was evaluated by either early CCTA ($n = 99$) or a standard diagnostic protocol ($n = 98$) [18]. Patients randomized to early CCTA were eligible for discharge with normal or minimally abnormal results (<25% stenosis), patients with severe stenosis (>70%) were referred for immediate invasive angiography, whereas patients with intermediate-grade stenosis underwent additional stress testing. The two groups were compared for safety, diagnostic accuracy and efficiency. Among patients randomized to CCTA, 75% had decisive triage by CCTA alone (67% immediately discharged and 8% referred for immediate catheterization, which revealed significant disease in 7 of 8 referred cases). Importantly, CCTA alone was not considered adequate for diagnosis in 24 of 99 cases, owing either to lesions of unclear hemodynamic significance (stenosis = 26–70%) in 13 of these patients or to nondiagnostic quality scans in 11 patients (all 24 underwent noninvasive stress testing) (see Fig. 2). Among the patients discharged immediately, none had a major adverse cardiac event (MACE) or subsequent diagnosis of CAD over a 6-month follow-up period (see Table 1). The overall diagnostic accuracy of CCTA was 94%, and the negative predictive value (NPV) was 100%. Diagnostic efficiency, defined

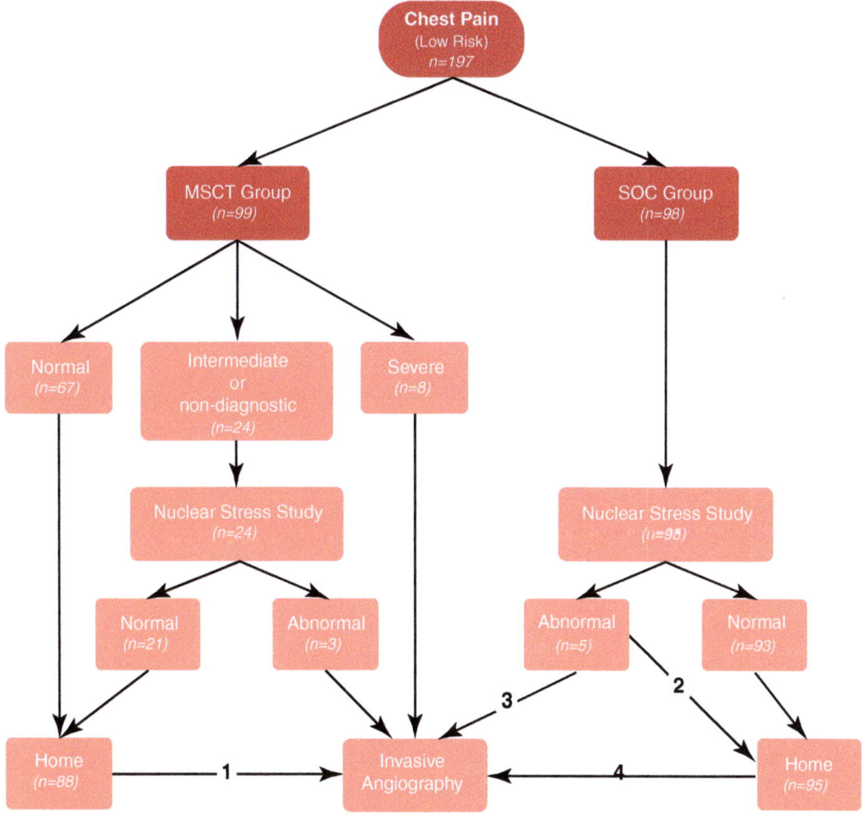


**Fig. 2** A randomized controlled trial of multislice coronary computed tomography for evaluation of acute chest pain. Adapted from Goldstein et al. [17]

**Table 1** Early and 6-month clinical outcomes in the study by Goldstein et al.

| | MSCT<br>$N = 99$ | SOC<br>$N = 98$ | $P$ value |
|---|---|---|---|
| Index visit outcomes | | | |
| Test complications | 0 (0%) | 0 (0%) | NA |
| Direct ED discharges | 88 (88.1%) | 95 (96.9%) | 0.03 |
| Acute Myocardial infarction | 0 (0%) | 0 (0%) | NA |
| Death | 0 (0%) | 0 (0%) | NA |
| In-hospital diagnostic cath | 11 (11.1%) | 3 (3.1%) | 0.03 |
| Positive cath | 9 (9.1%) | 1 (1%) | 0.02 |
| In-hospital PCI | 3 (3.0%) | 1 (1.0%) | 0.62 |
| In-hospital CABG | 2 (2.0%) | 0 (0%) | 0.50 |
| 6-month outcomes | | | |
| Test complications | 0 (0%) | 0 (0%) | NA |
| Unstable angina | 0 (0%) | 0 (0%) | NA |
| Myocardial infarction | 0 (0%) | 0 (0%) | NA |
| Death | 0 (0%) | 0 (0%) | NA |
| Late ED R/O ischemia | 6 (6.1%) | 6 (6.1%) | 1.00 |
| Late office R/O ischemia | 2 (2.0%) | 2 (2.0%) | 1.00 |
| Late diagnostic Cath | 1 (1.0%) | 4 (4.1%) | 0.21 |
| Late stress/MSCT test | 1 (1.0%) | 3 (2.0%) | 0.37 |
| Cath cumulative | 12(12%) | 7 (7.1) | 0.24 |
| True-positive cumulative | 8/12 (67.7%) | 1/7 (14.3%) | 0.06 |
| True-positive cumulative | 1/12 (8.3%) | 4/7 (57.1%) | 0.04 |
| False-positive cumulative | 3 (25%) | 2 (28.5%) | 1.00 |
| False-negative cumulative | 0 (0%) | 0 (0%) | NA |
| Cath-accuracy cumulative | 9 (75%) | 5 (71.4%) | 1.00 |
| Clinically correct diagnosis | 96/99 (97.0%) | 96/98 (98.0%) | 1.00 |
| Late tests cumulative | 2 (2.0%) | 7 (7.1%) | 0.10 |
| Diagnostic efficacy | 94/99 (94.9%) | 89/98 (90.8%) | 0.26 |
| PCI cumulative | 4 (4%) | 1 (1.0%) | 0.37 |
| CABG cumulative | 2 (2.0%) | 0 (0%) | 0.50 |

*CABG* coronary artery bypass grafting, *Cath* cardiac catheterization/invasive coronary angiography, *ED* emergency department, *MSCT* multislice computed tomography, *PCI* percutaneous coronary intervention, *R/O* rule out
Adapted from Goldstein et al. [17]

as time from randomization to definitive diagnosis, showed that the CCTA approach was more rapid (3.4 vs. 15.0 h) and reduced costs by 15%. The American College of Cardiology Foundation in their 2006 guidelines mentioned that the clinical application of CTCA for acute chest pain can only be considered "appropriate" when its application is limited to patients with intermediate pretest probability without EKG and serial biomarker changes [16].

In this Diagnostic algorithm, patients in the multislice computed tomography group with normal scans were eligible for immediate discharge. Patients with severe stenosis on MSCT (over 70%) were referred for invasive angiography, whereas those with intermediate lesions or radio diagnostic scans were referred for nuclear stress scans. Patients in the standard diagnostic group underwent nuclear stress scans and were eligible for discharge if normal or refused for invasive angiography if abnormal. SOC = standard of care diagnostic evaluation.

In the blinded observational trial: rule out myocardial infarction using computer assisted tomography (ROMICAT), 368 chest pain patients with normal troponin and nonischemic EKGs were enrolled. The results showed that 50% of patients who presented with acute chest pain to the ED and were at low to intermediate likelihood of ACS had no CAD by coronary CTA, a finding that had a 100% NPV but limited positive predictive value (PPV) for the subsequent diagnosis of ACS and MACE. In addition, the results indicate that while the NPV remains excellent (98%), the exclusion of significant coronary stenosis by coronary CTA (>50%) had a limited sensitivity (77%) for the detection of ACS [19]. Kim et al., in their prospective observational study of 296 "CCTA eligible" acute chest pain patients presenting to the ED with "low to intermediate clinical risk profile," showed the overall accuracy of CCTA for ACS was 88.5% (sensitivity), 85.1% (specificity), 60.7% (positive predictive value), and 96.6% (negative predictive value) [17].

## 3   Cost-Effectiveness of Coronary CT Angiography

There is some concern that injudicious use of CCTA may result in increased health-care cost. A study by Otero et al. evaluated the cost-effectiveness of CCTA, stress echocardiography, and myocardial single-photon emission computerized tomography (SPECT) for 10,000 simulated patients. Using reported imaging test characteristics, prevalence and risk of CAD, and Medicare reimbursement schedules, the study reported that the clinical application of CCTA may significantly reduce the overall observation period and total health-care cost [20].

## 4   Safety Concerns of Coronary CT Angiography

The primary safety concern associated with CCTA is the potential carcinogenicity from radiation exposure. The effective radiation dose of a scan is calculated as the dose-length product (measured and displayed by the scanner on each patient) multiplied by the European Commission thoracic conversion factor (0.017) to yield the effective dose in milliSieverts (mSv). Thus, the radiation dose is directly proportional to the scan length in centimeters. The dose estimates from CCTA have been found to range from 7 to 13 mSv, while dose estimates from coronary angiogram have been found to be 3–25 mSv. The cancer risk from 100 mSv was estimated to be six out of 1000 people by the International Commission on Radiation Protection. Using appropriate CCTA protocol and techniques has been found to substantially reduce patient radiation dose [8].

## 5 Calcium Scoring in Addition to the CCTA

The inclusion of the calcium score into the chest pain protocol is controversial. CT calcium scoring allows detection and quantification of coronary artery calcification. The prospective multicenter Assessment by Coronary Computed Tomographic Angiography of Individuals Undergoing Invasive Coronary Angiography (ACCURACY) trial by Budoff et al. conducted at 16 centers enrolling 230 patients compared the diagnostic accuracy of coronary arterial calcium (CAC) by 64-row CT to invasive coronary angiography, and concluded that CAC demonstrates a high sensitivity and low specificity for the presence of coronary artery stenosis [21]. Abnormal levels of calcium may place patients into a higher risk group, but does not always help with the clinical diagnosis, particularly in the presence of diffuse moderate coronary atheroma. A zero-calcium score (ZCS) is associated with an excellent prognosis in healthy patients [22]. As the calcium score rises above zero and patients have symptoms of ACS, so does the prevalence of CAD and risk of death.

A recent study by Hulten et al. reported up to a 2% prevalence rate among symptomatic patients with ZCS using CCTA [23]. Prior studies have demonstrated high sensitivity but poor specificity of positive CAC to detect obstructive CAD ($\geq$50% stenosis by invasive coronary angiography) among patients with stable chest pain. Conversely, a CAC of 0 provides high specificity but poor sensitivity to identify obstructive CAD among patients with acute chest pain. In this regard, CAC might be a gatekeeper to identify low risk patients; however, CAC cannot reliably exclude obstructive CAD in subjects with acute chest pain seen in the ED [24].

## 6 Coronary CTA and Identification of Unstable Plaques

Goldstein et al., in their study, also showed that CCTA has the ability to recognize vulnerable plaques and provide additional relevant information beyond angiography alone [18]. Complex plaque morphology is the angiographic hallmark of unstable coronary lesions. Invasive, complex lesions are characterized by haziness, border irregularity, frank ulceration, intraplaque contrast persistence, and luminal filling defect. CCTA features of plaques in patients with ACS are just being identified. However, the CCTA correlates of angiographically diagnosed, complex unstable coronary lesions have not been fully delineated. The CCTA-documented lesion morphology is strikingly similar to invasive angiographic features indicative of plaque disruption, including lesion haziness, irregularity, ulceration, and intraplaque contrast penetration (See Fig. 3). On CCTA images, complex lesions

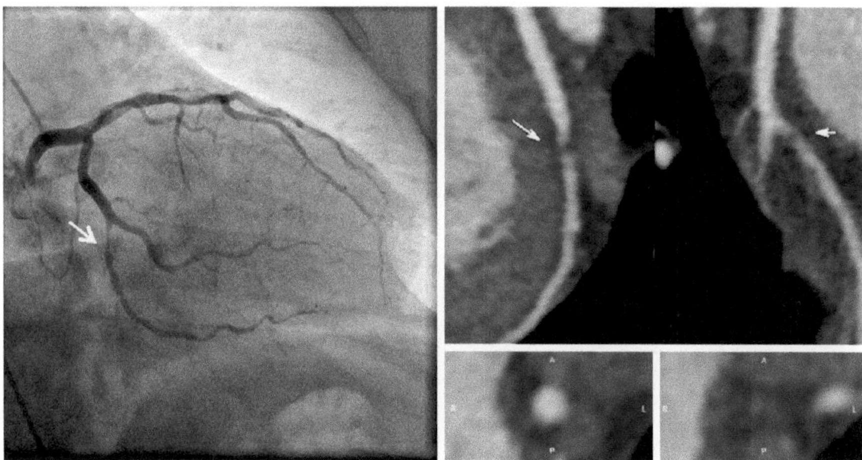

**Fig. 3** A very concerning unstable plaque. A 50-year-old male patient with unstable (resting) chest pain, and normal ECG × 2 and troponin panel. CCTA shows subtotal (99%) mostly soft plaque-formed Distal LCX stenosis *(white arrows)*. Personal history of poorly controlled diabetes × 10 years and family history of CAD. (Images obtained courtesy of Dr. Aiden Abidov)

typically appeared bulky, hypodense, eccentric, and positively remodeled with features similar to complex ruptured plaque seen by intravascular ultrasound (see Fig. 4). Given the increasing use of CCTA to evaluate acute chest pain, characterization of plaque instability has considerable clinical implications [25].

The CCTA can identify more than 1 complex plaque apart from the angiogram-identified culprit vessel. A fair amount of data shows that patients with ACS may have multiple complex plaques this may be detectable by CCTA (see Fig. 4), but significant plaque extension is underappreciated by invasive angiography.

# 7 CT for Diagnosis of Pulmonary Embolism

The 64-slice CT scan reduces examination time, collimation, and partial-volume averaging, and increases total volume scanned. There are several acquisition protocols for CT scanning in pulmonary embolism (PE) where breath holding is required between 4 and 40 s based on the clinical status and CT technology. Using MSCT, almost every patient is able to maintain a strict breath holding spell of a minimum 5 s which is sufficient to comply with the fastest protocol. Different protocols of contrast medium administration are available and can be either low concentration–high volume or high concentration–low volume, thus creating a balance between quality of vascular enhancement and total amount of iodine injected.

Direct demonstration can be made using vascular signs of acute PE on spiral CT pulmonary angiography (SCTPA) and these include (1) central partial intravascular defect surrounded by contrast medium, (2) eccentric partial filling defect or mural

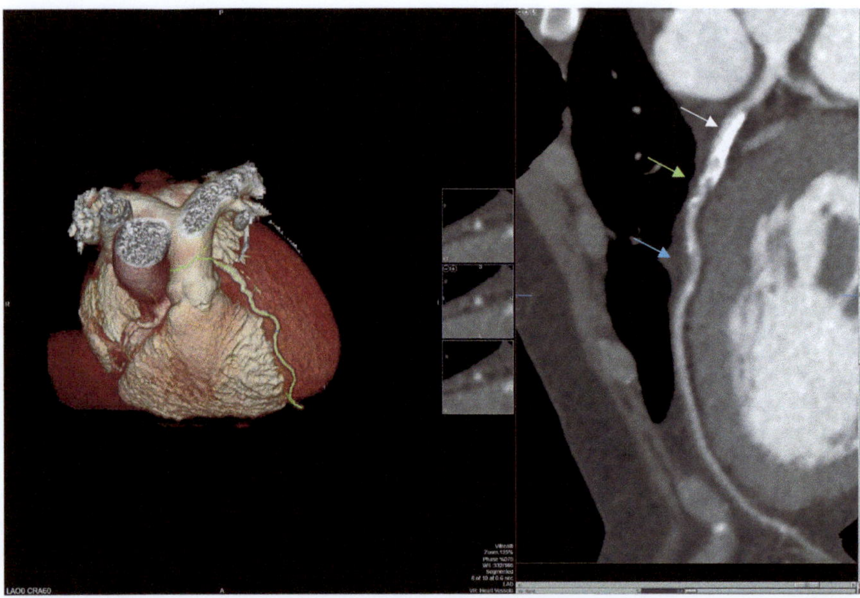

**Fig. 4** CCTA can identify more than 1 complex plaque. A 46-year-old male patient with progressive exertional angina, normal ECG and biomarkers and evidence of obstructive predominantly calcified (white arrow) proximal LAD plaque, obstructive mixed (calcified and noncalcified proximal-mid LAD plaque (green arrow) and high grade (95%) soft mid LAD plaque (blue arrow). The patient has strong family history of CAD, and personal history of heavy smoking (40 pack/ years) and untreated hyperlipidemia. (Images obtained courtesy of Dr. Aiden Abidov)

defect surrounded by contrast medium presenting an acute angle with the vessel wall, and (3) complete filling defect not surrounded by contrast medium and occupying the entire arterial vessel section (see Fig. 5). Ancillary findings related to PE included wedge-shaped pleural-based consolidation, "vascular sign" which is thickened vessel leading to the apex of the consolidation and usually indicating an infarction, oligemia, and dilatation of central arteries [26]. The acute dilatation of the right ventricle (RV) can be a useful sign to assess the severity of PE though RV strain or failure and is best detected by echocardiography; however, SCTPA can quantify some morphological abnormalities [27]. Positive results for PE on SCTPA are widely accepted as a valid demonstration of PE, but a negative result has been viewed with skepticism by many physicians. The clinical validity of a negative CT scan in a patient suspected of PE was evaluated in a systematic review of fifteen studies that showed an overall negative likelihood ratio of a venous thromboembolism after a negative SCTPA was 0.07 (95% confidence interval [CI], 0.05–0.11) and the NPV was 99.1% (95% CI, 98.7–99.5%) [28]. These results clinically validated that the use of SCTPA to rule out PE is similar to that reported for conventional pulmonary angiography, and patients with negative results need no further evaluation or treatment.

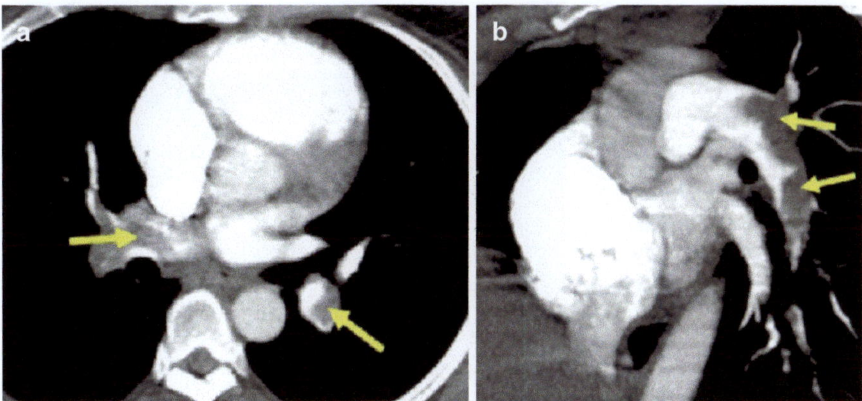

**Fig. 5** (**a, b**) Bilateral pulmonary embolism in a patient presenting with circulatory collapse and chest pain (**a**) Reconstructed axial CT angiograms (1.25 mm thick) obtained with Multislice CT demonstrate multiple clots. Acute clots (*yellow arrows*) in the left and right pulmonary arteries present as filling defects in the column of contrast material, that form an acute angle with the vessel wall. (**b**) Coronal oblique view with large pulmonary embolism in left pulmonary artery (yellow arrow) (images obtained courtesy of Dr. Samuel Johnson)

## 8   CT for Diagnosis of Aortic Dissection

Aortic dissection (AD) is the most frequent and fatal aortic emergency, and with the newer imaging modalities including the MSCT scan, we are able to identify entry tears and involvement of visceral branches, making it helpful to make management decisions in the ED. A better understanding of the complex mechanisms involved with dissection and the development of endovascular techniques has made the management of AD more likely to be successful [29].

When AD is suspected, the examination must explore the entire thoracic and abdominal aorta together with the iliac and common femoral arteries. The MSCT scanners permit this extended exploration with multiplanar reformatting to clarify certain details that are difficult to analyze in the conventional transverse and axial sections [30]. The cardinal sign of AD is the appearance of a detached intimal flap in the form of a fine, hypodense band in the opacified aortic lumen. This indicates the extent of dissection in the aortic wall and thus distinguishes the true channel (true aortic lumen) from the false channel (blood circulating in the wall of the aorta) [31, 32].

"Cobwebs" are residual ribbons of media between the damaged aortic wall and the intima; these structures thus identify the false channel. In CT angiography, they appear as fine, hypodense, linear strips attached to the damaged aortic wall and may or may not rejoin the intima (see Fig. 6). The abdominal branches of the descending aorta and iliac arteries may trigger malperfusion of the organs due to the dissection

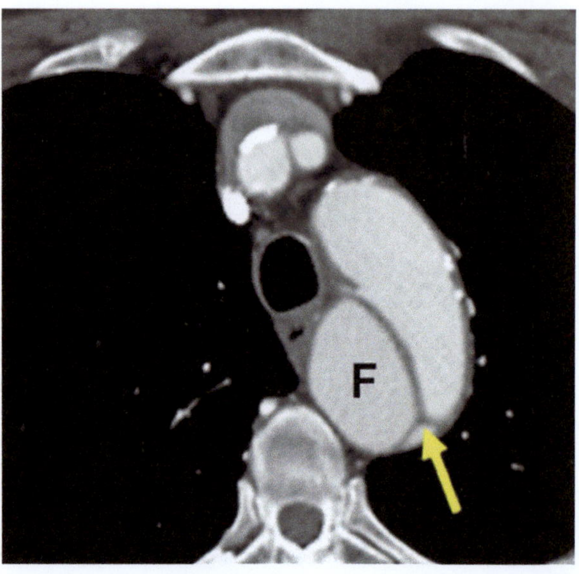

**Fig. 6** Chronic aortic dissection. CT-scan obtained in descending aorta showing web like intimal flap from chronic dissection. Outer wall calcification surrounding the true lumen (*F*). Visualization of an aortic cobweb between the intimal flap and the outer wall (yellow *arrow*). (Images obtained courtesy of Dr. Samuel Johnson)

during the acute phase or on follow-up (see Fig. 7) [33]. Although transesophageal echocardiography (TEE) is still useful in AD, the rapid availability of MSCT scan, nonreliability on an operator, and ability to detect malperfusion syndrome makes MSCT a much better option to be used in the ED.

## 9   The "Triple Rule Out" CT Protocol

CCTA has shown diagnostic accuracy in excluding ACS in ED patients and proven clinical accuracy for diagnosis of AD [33–36] and PE [26, 28, 37–39]; therefore, a "triple rule-out" (TRO) scan protocol to simultaneously exclude all three potentially fatal causes of acute chest pain with a single scan has come to be an attractive option. Once 64-slice CT scanners became widely available, the technical limitations of combined simultaneous evaluation of all three vascular areas have been largely overcome. A conventional CCTA "field of view" already includes the anatomy between the carina and the diaphragm. The technical challenge of a TRO scan protocol is to obtain high and consistent contrast intensity in all three vascular beds. A combined simultaneous evaluation for the pulmonary and coronary vessels and thoracic aorta requires a carefully tailored imaging and injection protocol (see Fig. 8). In evaluating one such protocol, Vrachliotis et al. prospectively imaged 50 ED chest pain patients who underwent single-acquisition 64-slice CT angiography to evaluate the enhancement of the coronary, pulmonary, and thoracic vasculature [40]. A "triphasic" injection protocol was used that delivered the standard 100 mL of iodinated contrast at 5 mL/sec typical for CCTA examinations, followed by an additional 30 mL at 3 mL/s to maintain pulmonary artery opacification, followed by

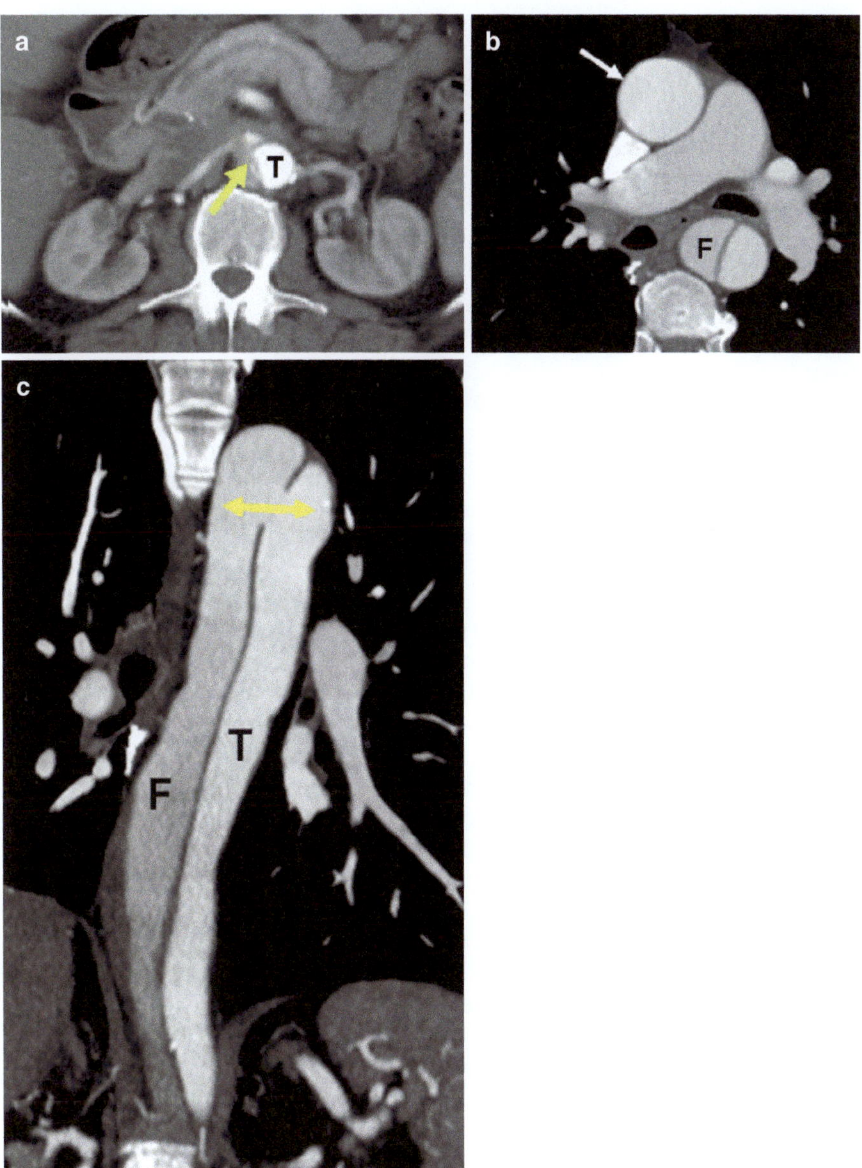

**Fig. 7** (**a–c**) Acute dissection with extension along the abdominal aorta. (**a**) Axial CT scan section at the level of the left renal artery shows dissection extend into abdominal aorta (Yellow arrow) with both renal arteries supplied by true lumen (*T*: true lumen) with normal perfusion. (**b**) Transverse image shows normal ascending aorta (white arrow) and dissection in descending with lower enhancement in the false lumen (*F* false lumen). (**c**) Coronal view shows communication (yellow double end arrow) between true (*T* true lumen) and false (*F* false lumen) lumen. (Images obtained courtesy of Dr. Samuel Johnson)

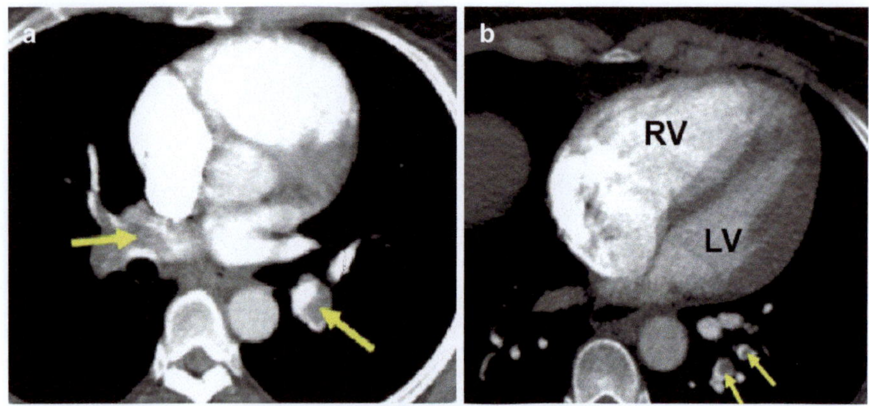

Fig. 8 (a, b) "Triple rule out" scan acquisition in a patient with acute chest pain (a) Bilateral large pulmonary emboli are seen, as well as (b) right heart strain, RV > LV (RV = right ventricle, LV = left ventricle); pulmonary embolism in left lower lobar branches (yellow arrows). The patient was also noted to have >50% mixed calcified and noncalcified plaque in the proximal left anterior descending coronary artery). (Images obtained courtesy of Dr. Samuel Johnson)

a standard saline flush injection. This protocol is easy to achieve with commercially available radiographic injectors. Importantly, a caudal–cranial scan acquisition was used (as opposed to the standard CCTA cranial–caudal technique) to scan the distal pulmonary arteries at the base of the lung earlier, as these are the most subject to problems with low contrast intensity. Mean coronary artery, pulmonary artery, and aortic enhancement values were consistently higher than 250 Hounsfield Units, and right atrial enhancement did not interfere with interpretation of the coronary arteries [40].

## 10 Dedicated Coronary Vs. "Triple Rule Out" Scan Protocol: Radiation Dose Considerations

In spite of these technical advances, important radiation safety concerns remain that should limit indiscriminate application of a TRO scan protocol. Compared to the usual radiation dose of a standard CCTA (generally ranging from 7 to 13 mSv, depending on body habitus, gender, and scan protocol), the effective radiation dose of a TRO CT scan is often increased by 50%, simply due to the greater anatomic coverage and thus increased field of view [41]. Further, among patients who undergo CCTA as a primary triage test in the ED, there is a subset who also require a noninvasive stress test (often a radionuclide test), followed in some cases by diagnostic and interventional invasive angiographic procedures. This combined radiation dose is a cause for concern; however, changing the 0.6 mm high-resolution used for CCTA to 2 mm for scanning the upper lung fields (since pulmonary angiography does not require submillimeter resolution) in theory can significantly reduce radiation dosage. Innovative imaging protocols involving tight heart rate control and "prospective gating" can drastically reduce radiation exposure (to under 5 mSV) but these are difficult to apply in ED patients and not currently being utilized in these patients.

In addition, the TRO CT also has a slightly higher intravenous contrast load to opacify both the right and left sided circulations [41, 42]. A recently conducted systematic review and meta-analysis of eleven studies showed that TRO CT had comparable image quality to CCTA and is highly accurate in detecting CAD, but the low prevalence of PE and AD (<1% in the studies) and the increased risk of radiation and contrast exposure make TRO CT not recommendable at the moment for this indication [42].

## 11 Assessment for Noncardiac, Extravascular Pathology

Well over 50% of acute chest pain is caused by noncardiac conditions [43]. In patients who undergo a dedicated CCTA, images of noncardiac thoracic structures are contained in the field of view and therefore available to the expert reader. Diseases that can be detected (in addition to aortic and pulmonary arterial pathology) include pericardial thickening and/or effusions, esophageal pathology, pneumonia, pulmonary nodules, pneumothoraces, mediastinal masses, pleural effusions and masses, as well as chest-wall abnormalities. Previous studies have demonstrated that up to 1 in 6 patients without coronary abnormalities detected on CT were diagnosed with noncardiac findings that could explain their presenting symptoms [44]. These findings suggest that for patients with acute chest pain, a comprehensive review of the thoracic, cardiac, and noncardiac structures should be undertaken.

There has been an ongoing debate about whether to use a more limited approach to imaging so that it raises fewer false alarms or a broader approach so that serious pathological conditions are not missed. In the study by Johnson et al. comparing the two approaches, it was shown that almost one-fourth of all patients who underwent CCTA had extra cardiac findings [45]. When CCTA were viewed in a limited, or focused way, the result was substantially reduced sensitivity for pathologic findings outside the mediastinum and heart. Serious pathologic conditions were missed, but many false-positive diagnoses were avoided. Use of the broader view approach led to downstream workup of 10.2% of the findings, and a later follow-up of 50.6% of the patients demonstrated little or no new clinical consequence to the patient. After small hiatal hernia, lung nodules were the most common extra cardiac finding (6.2% of the patients). In another study by Lee et al., most extra cardiac findings were indeterminate pulmonary nodules [46]. Until more studies clarify the benefits and risks of identifying early lung neoplasms, we cannot say for certain whether it is prudent to report incidental extra cardiac findings on CCTA. A conservative approach of careful comparison of incidental findings with prior studies, providing clear follow-up recommendations, and proper interphysician communication will be key to preventing unnecessary utilization of medical resources.

## 12 Coronary CTA Limitations and Protocol Considerations

Coronary CTA has several important limitations that affect its usefulness in the triage of ED patients with acute chest pain. There are two major limitations for reliable assessment of all coronary segments: motion artifacts and severe coronary calcifications [9]. It has been convincingly shown that the heart rate and regularity of the rhythm is closely related to motion artifact, image quality, and thus accuracy of coronary stenosis estimation [7]. It is common practice to premedicate patients who have resting heart rates >65 beats/min with beta blocking drugs, and to administer sublingual nitroglycerin to patients to enhance image quality. If available, dual-source CCTA obviates the need for beta blocker administration in most patients. At this time, most facilities do not perform CCTA in patients with irregular rhythms; however, recent hardware and software improvements allow for imaging of patients with irregular rhythms including atrial fibrillation [47, 48]. A second major limitation is that CCTA presently provides data regarding anatomical lesions only, not their physiologic impact on coronary blood flow.

It is also essential to screen patients in the ED for a history of iodine allergy and to avoid administration of contrast in patients with diminished creatinine clearance. Finally, the importance of a team approach to implementation of a CCTA ED triage protocol cannot be overstated. Emergency physicians, radiologists and cardiologists must be well educated regarding the application and inherent limitations of CCTA, and a complete review of cardiac and adjacent structures available from the CT data should be performed by physicians with appropriate backgrounds and level of experience.

There are now over 30 published studies comparing CCTA to quantitative invasive coronary angiography, encompassing over 2000 patients [7, 12, 49–52]. Among the 18 studies in which per-patient analyses are available (involving 1329 patients, using either 16 or 64-slice CT), the mean subject-weighted sensitivity and specificity for the detection of obstructive CAD was 97% and 84% respectively [7]. An analysis of just the 64-slice studies revealed a sensitivity and specificity of 98% and 93%, respectively. Importantly, the combined results from all 18 studies demonstrated a mean per-patient NPV of 97%. These data support the hypothesis that a low risk CCTA may obviate the need for invasive angiography in properly selected clinical circumstances. These studies validate that patients at the opposite ends of the disease spectrum (i.e. those with <25% vs. >70% maximal luminal stenosis) can be accurately triaged by CCTA alone, while patients with lesions of intermediate severity (25–70% stenosis) may require functional testing.

## 13 Conclusions

Computed tomography has evolved over the past three decades into a powerful imaging tool that has proven clinical accuracy for the diagnosis of AD and PE. CCTA has been recently validated as a highly sensitive and reliable technique to confirm or exclude significant coronary stenosis in patients with suspected CAD. Initial experience suggests that CCTA is an accurate and efficient test for the triage of appropriately selected acute chest pain patients to early discharge or further inpatient diagnosis and treatment. Patients presenting the ED with a low to intermediate pretest likelihood of CAD and nonsignificant cardiac biomarkers and EKGs are best suited for CCTA-based triage. Technical advances now permit acquisition of well-opacified images of the coronary arteries, thoracic aorta, and pulmonary arteries from a single CCTA scan protocol. While this TRO technique can potentially exclude fatal causes of chest pain in all three vascular beds, the resultant higher radiation dose of this method precludes its routine use, except when there is sufficient support for the diagnosis of either AD or PE. Having good interphysician communication about the incidental findings on the CCTA scan is vital in making sure that important findings are not missed and there is appropriate utilization of medical resources.

**Acknowledgements**  Images obtained courtesy Samuel Johnson MD (Interim Chair, Department of Radiology, Wayne State University, Detroit, Michigan, USA) and Aiden Abidov MD PhD (Section Chief, Cardiology, VA Hospital Detroit, Michigan, USA. Department of Medicine/ Division of Cardiology, Wayne State University, Detroit, Michigan, USA).

# References


1. McCaig LF. National Hospital Ambulatory Medical Care Survey 2003: emergency department summary: advance data from vital and health statistics, No. 358. National Center for Health Statistics; 2005.
2. Bhuiya FA, Pitts SR, McCaig LF. Emergency department visits for chest pain and abdominal pain: United States, 1999-2008. NCHS Data Brief. 2010;43:1–8.
3. Kalender WA, Seissler W, Klotz E, Vock P. Spiral volumetric CT with single-breath-hold technique, continuous transport, and continuous scanner rotation. Radiology. 1990;176(1):181–3.
4. Ohnesorge B, Flohr T, Becker C, Kopp AF, Schoepf UJ, Baum U, et al. Cardiac imaging by means of electrocardiographically gated multisection spiral CT: initial experience. Radiology. 2000;217(2):564–71.
5. Achenbach S, Ulzheimer S, Baum U, Kachelriess M, Ropers D, Giesler T, et al. Noninvasive coronary angiography by retrospectively ECG-gated multislice spiral CT. Circulation. 2000;102(23):2823–8.
6. Mahesh M. Search for isotropic resolution in CT from conventional through multiple-row detector. Radiographics. 2002;22(4):949–62.
7. Raff GL, Goldstein JA. Coronary angiography by computed tomography: coronary imaging evolves. J Am Coll Cardiol. 2007;49(18):1830–3.
8. Medical AS. 64-slice computed tomographic angiography for the diagnosis of intermediate risk coronary artery disease: an evidence-based analysis. Ont Health Technol Assess Ser. 2010;10(11):1–44.
9. Mollet NR, Cademartiri F, Nieman K, Saia F, Lemos PA, McFadden EP, et al. Multislice spiral computed tomography coronary angiography in patients with stable angina pectoris. J Am Coll Cardiol. 2004;43(12):2265–70.
10. Lee TH, Goldman L. Evaluation of the patient with acute chest pain. N Engl J Med. 2000;342(16):1187–95.

11. Pope JH, Aufderheide TP, Ruthazer R, Woolard RH, Feldman JA, Beshansky JR, et al. Missed diagnoses of acute cardiac ischemia in the emergency department. N Engl J Med. 2000;342(16):1163–70.
12. Mollet NR, Cademartiri F, van Mieghem CA, Runza G, McFadden EP, Baks T, et al. High-resolution spiral computed tomography coronary angiography in patients referred for diagnostic conventional coronary angiography. Circulation. 2005;112(15):2318–23.
13. Leber AW, Knez A, von Ziegler F, Becker A, Nikolaou K, Paul S, et al. Quantification of obstructive and nonobstructive coronary lesions by 64-slice computed tomography: a comparative study with quantitative coronary angiography and intravascular ultrasound. J Am Coll Cardiol. 2005;46(1):147–54.
14. Raff GL, Gallagher MJ, O'Neill WW, Goldstein JA. Diagnostic accuracy of noninvasive coronary angiography using 64-slice spiral computed tomography. J Am Coll Cardiol. 2005;46(3):552–7.
15. Gallagher MJ, Raff GL. Use of multislice CT for the evaluation of emergency room patients with chest pain: the so-called "triple rule-out". Catheter Cardiovasc Interv. 2008;71(1):92–9.
16. Hollander JE, Litt HI, Chase M, Brown AM, Kim W, Baxt WG. Computed tomography coronary angiography for rapid disposition of low-risk emergency department patients with chest pain syndromes. Acad Emerg Med. 2007;14(2):112–6.
17. Kim J, Lee H, Song S, Park J, Jae H, Lee W, et al. Efficacy and safety of the computed tomography coronary angiography based approach for patients with acute chest pain at an emergency department: one month clinical follow-up study. J Korean Med Sci. 2010;25(3):466–71.
18. Goldstein JA, Gallagher MJ, O'Neill WW, Ross MA, O'Neil BJ, Raff GL. A randomized controlled trial of multi-slice coronary computed tomography for evaluation of acute chest pain. J Am Coll Cardiol. 2007;49(8):863–71.
19. Hoffmann U, Bamberg F, Chae CU, Nichols JH, Rogers IS, Seneviratne SK, et al. Coronary computed tomography angiography for early triage of patients with acute chest pain: the ROMICAT (rule out myocardial infarction using computer assisted tomography) trial. J Am Coll Cardiol. 2009;53(18):1642–50.
20. Otero HJ, Rybicki FJ. Reimbursement for chest-pain CT: estimates based on current imaging strategies. Emerg Radiol. 2007;13(5):237–42.
21. Budoff MJ, Jollis JG, Dowe D, Min J. Diagnostic accuracy of coronary artery calcium for obstructive disease: results from the accuracy trial. Int J Cardiol. 2013;166(2):505–8.
22. Shaw LJ, Giambrone AE, Blaha MJ, Knapper JT, Berman DS, Bellam N, et al. Long-term prognosis after coronary artery calcification testing in asymptomatic patients: a cohort study. Ann Intern Med. 2015;163(1):14–21.
23. Hulten E, Bittencourt MS, Ghoshhajra B, O'Leary D, Christman MP, Blaha MJ, et al. Incremental prognostic value of coronary artery calcium score versus CT angiography among symptomatic patients without known coronary artery disease. Atherosclerosis. 2014;233(1):190–5.
24. Rubinshtein R, Gaspar T, Halon DA, Goldstein J, Peled N, Lewis BS. Prevalence and extent of obstructive coronary artery disease in patients with zero or low calcium score undergoing 64-slice cardiac multidetector computed tomography for evaluation of a chest pain syndrome. Am J Cardiol. 2007;99(4):472–5.
25. Goldstein JA, Dixon S, Safian RD, Hanzel G, Grines CL, Raff GL. Computed tomographic angiographic morphology of invasively proven complex coronary plaques. JACC Cardiovasc Imaging. 2008;1(2):249–51.
26. Ghaye B, Remy J, Remy-Jardin M. Non-traumatic thoracic emergencies: CT diagnosis of acute pulmonary embolism: the first 10 years. Eur Radiol. 2002;12(8):1886–905.
27. Reid JH, Murchison JT. Acute right ventricular dilatation: a new helical CT sign of massive pulmonary embolism. Clin Radiol. 1998;53(9):694–8.
28. Quiroz R, Kucher N, Zou KH, Kipfmueller F, Costello P, Goldhaber SZ, et al. Clinical validity of a negative computed tomography scan in patients with suspected pulmonary embolism: a systematic review. JAMA. 2005;293(16):2012–7.

29. Khayat M, Cooper KJ, Khaja MS, Gandhi R, Bryce YC, Williams DM. Endovascular management of acute aortic dissection. Cardiovasc Diagn Ther. 2018;8(1):97–107.
30. Novelline RA, Rhea JT, Rao PM, Stuk JL. Helical CT in emergency radiology. Radiology. 1999;213(2):321–39.
31. Williams DM, Joshi A, Dake MD, Deeb GM, Miller DC, Abrams GD. Aortic cobwebs: an anatomic marker identifying the false lumen in aortic dissection–imaging and pathologic correlation. Radiology. 1994;190(1):167–74.
32. LePage MA, Quint LE, Sonnad SS, Deeb GM, Williams DM. Aortic dissection: CT features that distinguish true lumen from false lumen. AJR Am J Roentgenol. 2001;177(1):207–11.
33. Willoteaux S, Lions C, Gaxotte V, Negaiwi Z, Beregi JP. Imaging of aortic dissection by helical computed tomography (CT). Eur Radiol. 2004;14(11):1999–2008.
34. Yoshida S, Akiba H, Tamakawa M, Yama N, Hareyama M, Morishita K, et al. Thoracic involvement of type A aortic dissection and intramural hematoma: diagnostic accuracy–comparison of emergency helical CT and surgical findings. Radiology. 2003;228(2):430–5.
35. Hamada S, Takamiya M, Kimura K, Imakita S, Nakajima N, Naito H. Type A aortic dissection: evaluation with ultrafast CT. Radiology. 1992;183(1):155–8.
36. Shiga T, Wajima Z, Apfel CC, Inoue T, Ohe Y. Diagnostic accuracy of transesophageal echocardiography, helical computed tomography, and magnetic resonance imaging for suspected thoracic aortic dissection: systematic review and meta-analysis. Arch Intern Med. 2006;166(13):1350–6.
37. Anderson DR, Kovacs MJ, Dennie C, Kovacs G, Stiell I, Dreyer J, et al. Use of spiral computed tomography contrast angiography and ultrasonography to exclude the diagnosis of pulmonary embolism in the emergency department. J Emerg Med. 2005;29(4):399–404.
38. Prologo JD, Gilkeson RC, Diaz M, Asaad J. CT pulmonary angiography: a comparative analysis of the utilization patterns in emergency department and hospitalized patients between 1998 and 2003. AJR Am J Roentgenol. 2004;183(4):1093–6.
39. Ghanima W, Almaas V, Aballi S, Dorje C, Nielssen BE, Holmen LO, et al. Management of suspected pulmonary embolism (PE) by D-dimer and multi-slice computed tomography in outpatients: an outcome study. J Thromb Haemost. 2005;3(9):1926–32.
40. Vrachliotis TG, Bis KG, Haidary A, Kosuri R, Balasubramaniam M, Gallagher M, et al. Atypical chest pain: coronary, aortic, and pulmonary vasculature enhancement at biphasic single-injection 64-section CT angiography. Radiology. 2007;243(2):368–76.
41. Burris AC, Boura JA, Raff GL, Chinnaiyan KM. Triple rule out versus coronary CT angiography in patients with acute chest pain: results from the ACIC Consortium. JACC Cardiovasc Imaging. 2015;8(7):817–25.
42. Ayaram D, Bellolio MF, Murad MH, Laack TA, Sadosty AT, Erwin PJ, et al. Triple rule-out computed tomographic angiography for chest pain: a diagnostic systematic review and meta-analysis. Acad Emerg Med. 2013;20(9):861–71.
43. Gallagher MJ, Ross MA, Raff GL, Goldstein JA, O'Neill WW, O'Neil B. The diagnostic accuracy of 64-slice computed tomography coronary angiography compared with stress nuclear imaging in emergency department low-risk chest pain patients. Ann Emerg Med. 2007;49(2):125–36.
44. Onuma Y, Tanabe K, Nakazawa G, Aoki J, Nakajima H, Ibukuro K, et al. Noncardiac findings in cardiac imaging with multidetector computed tomography. J Am Coll Cardiol. 2006;48(2):402–6.
45. Johnson KM, Dennis JM, Dowe DA. Extracardiac findings on coronary CT angiograms: limited versus complete image review. AJR Am J Roentgenol. 2010;195(1):143–8.
46. Lee CI, Tsai EB, Sigal BM, Plevritis SK, Garber AM, Rubin GD. Incidental extracardiac findings at coronary CT: clinical and economic impact. AJR Am J Roentgenol. 2010;194(6):1531–8.
47. Andreini D, Pontone G, Mushtaq S, Conte E, Perchinunno M, Guglielmo M, et al. Atrial fibrillation: diagnostic accuracy of coronary CT angiography performed with a whole-heart 230-microm spatial resolution CT scanner. Radiology. 2017;284(3):676–84.

48. Mushtaq S, Conte E, Melotti E, Andreini D. Coronary CT angiography in challenging patients: high heart rate and atrial fibrillation. A review. Acad Radiol. 2019;26(11):1544–9.
49. Leschka S, Alkadhi H, Plass A, Desbiolles L, Grunenfelder J, Marincek B, et al. Accuracy of MSCT coronary angiography with 64-slice technology: first experience. Eur Heart J. 2005;26(15):1482–7.
50. Pugliese F, Mollet NR, Runza G, van Mieghem C, Meijboom WB, Malagutti P, et al. Diagnostic accuracy of non-invasive 64-slice CT coronary angiography in patients with stable angina pectoris. Eur Radiol. 2006;16(3):575–82.
51. Ropers D, Rixe J, Anders K, Kuttner A, Baum U, Bautz W, et al. Usefulness of multidetector row spiral computed tomography with 64- × 0.6-mm collimation and 330-ms rotation for the noninvasive detection of significant coronary artery stenoses. Am J Cardiol. 2006;97(3):343–8.
52. Hamon M, Morello R, Riddell JW, Hamon M. Coronary arteries: diagnostic performance of 16- versus 64-section spiral CT compared with invasive coronary angiography–meta-analysis. Radiology. 2007;245(3):720–31.

# Use of Magnetic Resonance Imaging for Evaluation of Patients with Chest Pain


Vijaya Arun Kumar and Brian O'Neil


## 1 Overview of CMR Technology

The MRI process involves the use of a very strong static magnetic field, time-varying (gradient) fields and radiofrequency energy which leads to exquisite soft tissue delineation. CMR allows for the study of cardiac shape, size, and function along with myocardial perfusion. It also helps with the detection of scar tissue, thrombus formation, and at-risk myocardium. All these features cannot be cumulatively detected by other imaging modalities and can certainly aid in risk stratification [1]. Cine steady-state free precession (SSFP), T2-weighted and late gadolinium enhancement (LGE) sequences comprise the cornerstone of CMR protocols in patients with CP. For detection of myocardial edema, the hallmark of acute injury, T2-weighted CMR is mandatory, T2 weighted CMR increases the accuracy of detecting acute myocardial infarction (AMI) in the ED from 84 to 93% [2]. Regional ventricular function can be analyzed on the basis of wall motion abnormalities and wall thickness at end diastole, which aids in differentiating acute from chronic MI. The wall motion index is calculated by dividing the sum of the semiquantitative AHA classification score of each segment by the number of segments being evaluated. One of the main limitations for the implementation of CMR in the ED is the duration of testing, particularly in critical patients. Recent strategies for reducing the acquisition time have been implemented making CMR more accessible to patients.


V. A. Kumar · B. O'Neil (✉)
Department of Emergency Medicine, Wayne State University, Detroit, MI, USA
e-mail: vkumar@med.wayne.edu; boneil@med.wayne.edu



© The Author(s), under exclusive license to Springer Nature Switzerland AG 2022

M. Pena et al. (eds.), *Short Stay Management of Chest Pain*, Contemporary Cardiology, https://doi.org/10.1007/978-3-031-05520-1_16

## 2 Safety Concerns

Though CMR is one of the safer imaging techniques, it is not without safety issues, including effects of contrast agents, and effects of magnetic fields and radiofrequencies on the body [3]. The safety in pregnancy has been debated and seems to be related to its effect at a cellular level due to thermogenesis during first trimester and the high level of acoustic noise generated in second and third trimester. Overall consensus seems to be that the benefit of MRI outweighed the risk for clinically imperative indications throughout pregnancy [4]. Other potential risks that have been documented include claustrophobia and its potential for tinnitus [3]. A review by Ponrartana et al. showed well-documented risks associated with gadolinium-based contrast agents (GBCAs) including acute adverse reactions which are both idiosyncratic and anaphylactoid, nephrogenic systemic fibrosis, and gadolinium deposition [5] The incidence of severe reaction is estimated at 1 in 350,000–450,000 for GBCAs which is considerably lower than that of iodinated contrast agents, both ionic and nonionic [6]. The small overall risk must always be weighed against the additional diagnostic information that is obtained with CMR.

## 3 CMR in Acute Coronary Syndrome

CMR imaging in ACS patients can be classified into three stages: initial workup for diagnosis of CP, early after repolarization and late after repolarization. In patients with symptoms suggestive of ACS, non-ST elevation on electrocardiogram (EKG) and negative serum biomarkers (troponin) cardiac imaging can be performed in the ED or shortly after discharge. In this low-risk group CMR has the advantage of assessing myocardial function, perfusion, and viability all in one session [2]. The AHA guidelines on ACS recommend a noninvasive approach for patients with severe comorbidities and a low likelihood of ACS [7]. CMR may be an alternative when echocardiography is inconclusive or of suboptimal quality. Stress testing, including adenosine stress CMR, can be used to evaluate myocardial ischemia and viability even with multivessel disease [8]. The utilization of CMR in the ED triaging of CP patients may also help to reduce hospital admissions and costs [2, 9]

A review of the evidence to date shows that CMR has promise both as an anatomical and a functional assay of the CP patients with non-ST elevation MI (non-STEMI). Kwong et al. studied 161 consecutive non-STEMI ACS patients presenting with at least 30 min of CP and an abnormal serial troponin-I (>1.96 µg/dl) with a temporal pattern consistent with AMI and any clinical evidence of coronary artery disease (CAD). Qualitative MRI included rest MRI with perfusion, left ventricular (LV) function, and gadolinium enhancement for MI. Confirmation of unstable angina required a 70% epicardial coronary stenosis or true positive abnormal stress test performed during the index hospitalization or subsequent 6–8-week follow-up period. Qualitative MRI readings showed a sensitivity of 84% and specificity of

85% in detecting ACS which was superior to the use of strict EKG criteria for ischemia. The test took on average 38 min ± 12 min to complete [2].

The use of adenosine stress CMR was studied by Ingkanisorn et al., in 135 ED patients with 30 min of chest discomfort, negative troponin >6 h after last episode of discomfort, and a nondiagnostic EKG. The outcome was the 1 year incidence of death, AMI, stenosis >50%, or abnormal correlative stress test. Twenty patients (14.8%) experienced an outcome: 15 had >50% stenosis, 2 abnormal stress, 1 AMI, and 1 death. None of the patients with a normal Adenosine CMR had an adverse outcome at 1 year. Cardiac risk factors and CMR were both significant predictors of the defined outcome by Kaplan–Meier analysis [10]. Heitner et al., in their prospective study of patients with CP presenting to the ED, showed that adenosine stress CMR performed within 12 h of presentation is safe and potentially has improved performance characteristics compared to stress echocardiography [11].

Multiple studies have compared multidetector computed tomography angiography (CTA) and MRI utilizing 3D navigator for stenotic accuracy. Kefer et al. in 52 patients scheduled for catheterization (cath.) received both MRI and 16 slice CTA. CTA had better sensitivity and equivalent specificity and diagnostic accuracy as MRI with correlation of 0.6 for MRI and 0.75 CTA for the prediction of degree of coronary artery stenosis [12]. Gerber et al. evaluated 27 patients undergoing cath.; CTA and MRI had high negative predictive value for segmental stenosis: 93% (168 of 180 segments) for CT and 90% (198 of 220 segments) for MRI. However, the overall diagnostic accuracy favored MRI 80% (234/294 segments) versus CTA 73% (214/294 segments, $P < 0.05$) [13].

The use of magnetic resonance angiography (MRA) for the detection of CAD has been studied by a few small observational trials. Muller et al. showed in 35 patients with significant stenosis >50%, MRA had a positive predictive value of 87% and a negative predictive value of 93% [14]. Kim et al. found that in 109 patients undergoing cath., with 636 out of 759 proximal and middle distal segments interpretable, there was a low specificity of 42% and a diagnostic accuracy of 72%. Testing took an average 70 min to complete [15]. Further, Kessler et al. found that in 73 patients the sensitivity was 65% and specificity 88% [16]. Nikolaou et al., utilizing the same criteria in 20 patients, showed multidetector computed tomography (MDCT) compared to MRA had better sensitivity (85% vs. 79%) and specificity (77% vs. 70%) [17]. Liu et al. compared 64-slice MDCT and MRA in 18 patients with elevated calcium scores >100. Coronary MRA had higher image quality for coronary segments with nodal calcification than for coronary segments with diffuse calcification.

## 4 CMR in Myocarditis

Tornvall et al. performed a meta-analysis showing that acute myocarditis is present in 33% of patients presenting with AMI and unobstructed coronary arteries [18]. With the association of myocarditis with COVID 19 mRNA vaccines [19] and COVID 19 infection, it is important to be able to make a rapid diagnosis of these cases. Myocardial edema affects myocardial function and may be the expression of diffuse myocardial inflammation due to a systemic immune response, direct myocardial damage from severe acute respiratory syndrome virus 2 (SARS-CoV-2), or vascular leakage due to endothelial damage [20]. Although endomyocardial biopsy is the gold standard, CMR allows for diagnosis of up to 79% of cases of pathology-proven myocarditis [8]. CMR is important for assessment of severity and risk stratification [21]. LGE cardiac MRI is the best indicator for all-cause mortality and cardiac mortality and is superior to conventional prognostic biomarkers [21].

## 5  CMR in Myocardial Infarction with Nonobstructed Coronary Arteries (MINOCA)

The underlying mechanism of MINOCA is the pathophysiology that is responsible for type 1 (involvement of epicardial coronary arteries) and type 2 (microvascular involvement) AMI as per the third universal definition of MI. MINOCA comprises 5–20% of type 1 acute MIs with plaque rupture as the predominant mechanism [8]. CMR identifies subendocardial or transmural scar that follows the distribution of an involved coronary artery during LGE MRI [21]. In addition, T2-weighted MRI allows differentiation of acute, subacute and chronic disease, because the presence of extensive areas of myocardial edema, with or without small areas of necrosis suggest a transient compromise of the coronary flow in a large vessel that is related to plaque rupture with secondary thrombosis or coronary spasm [8].

## 6  CMR in Takotsubo Cardiomyopathy

Cardiomyopathy (CM) is the third most common cause of suspected ACS with unobstructed coronary arteries. Takotsubo cardiomyopathy is the most frequent CM and has been seen in increasing frequency among postmenopausal women who usually present with an elevated troponin. It is defined by its characteristic wall motion abnormalities that are reversible and transient without any underlying coronary artery disease [22]. CMR is usually performed as a second line test, when 2D echocardiography is suboptimal. The pathophysiology involves initial myocardial edema which resolves in 2–3 months and is difficult to detect after the first 2 weeks. Edema is associated with the dyskinetic portions of the LV showing dyskinetic myocardial segments that create a ballooning pattern on cine images and is not related to a single coronary artery territory. LGE disappears after myocardial edema and is associated with heart failure and severe wall motion abnormality [21].

## 7 MRA in Aortic Dissection

In patients with contraindications to CTA, MRA provides a rapid and reliable alternative and can be performed both with and without contrast enhancement. The MRA findings are similar to CTA and is characterized by a curvilinear intraluminal filling defect that extends along a variable length of the aorta. MRA provides important information like location and extent of dissection, location of intimal tears, size of the aorta and the relative filling of true and false lumen, all of which are important for the management. In a meta-analysis by Shiga et al., MRA had a sensitivity of 91–100% and specificity of 94–100% [23].

## 8 MRA in Pulmonary Embolism

In the Prospective Investigation of Pulmonary Embolism Diagnosis (PIOPED) II study, up to 24% of the enrolled patients had a contraindication for CTA [24]. In patients with suspected pulmonary embolism (PE) and contraindication for CTA both ventilation–perfusion scintigraphy and MRA are alternative imaging options. Another benefit of MRA compared to CTA is the ability to repeat MRA with a GBCA if there was a suboptimal imaging initially because radiation exposure and contrast-induced nephropathy are not a concern. GBCA has been used as the contrast agent with different injection rates and typically PE presents as a central hypointense filling defect and peripheral wedge-shaped pulmonary perfusion defects as a secondary sign of PE. In PIOPED III the sensitivity and specificity of contrast enhanced MRA for the detection of PE were 78% and 99%, respectively [25]. The sensitivity was low mainly due to artifacts or insufficient vascular enhancement as shown in the study by Revel et al., where 28–30% of the studies were inconclusive [26].

## 9 Conclusions

In summary, the pros of CMR are they provide excellent details of cardiac ischemia and viability, provide excellent evaluation of myocardial function, and can also visualize aorta and lungs with a sensitivity and specificity comparable to nuclear imaging, without radiation exposure. The cons of CMR are it does not visualize the coronary anatomy, there is limited experience and availability, no clinically proven advantage over nuclear stress/echocardiography, it is more expensive, and gadolinium exposure can lead to adverse reaction and nephrogenic systemic fibrosis. The use of CMR for the detection of CAD displayed only fair sensitivity and specificity when compared to cardiac catheterization. In the small studies comparing MDCT to MRA, MDCT appeared superior; however, MRA may be useful in patients with nodal calcification and potentially coronary stents. Adenosine stress testing CMR has been studied in ED chest pain patients and shown to be effective. Although the overall utility of MRI and MRA in the ED is unclear due to few studies, the wide array of imaging sequences and applications CMR permits a better understanding of the different pathophysiological features that occur not only in patients with ACS but in patients with chest pain from alternate etiologies presenting to the ED. When performed early, CMR may help with risk stratification and identification of patients with atypical clinical features with or without significant CAD like myocarditis, MINOCA, aortic dissection, Takotsubo cardiomyopathy, or pulmonary embolism.

# References


1. Broncano J, Bhalla S, Caro P, Hidalgo A, Vargas D, Williamson E, et al. Cardiac MRI in patients with acute chest pain. Radiographics. 2021;41(1):8–31.
2. Kwong RY, Arai AE. Detecting patients with acute coronary syndrome in the chest pain center of the emergency department with cardiac magnetic resonance imaging. Crit Pathw Cardiol. 2004;3(1):25–31.
3. Chung SM. Safety issues in magnetic resonance imaging. J Neuroophthalmol. 2002;22(1):35–9.
4. Patenaude Y, Pugash D, Lim K, Morin L, Diagnostic Imaging C, Lim K, et al. The use of magnetic resonance imaging in the obstetric patient. J Obstet Gynaecol Can. 2014;36(4):349–63.
5. Ponrartana S, Moore MM, Chan SS, Victoria T, Dillman JR, Chavhan GB. Safety issues related to intravenous contrast agent use in magnetic resonance imaging. Pediatr Radiol. 2021;51(5):736–47.
6. Carr JJ. Magnetic resonance contrast agents for neuroimaging. Safety issues. Neuroimaging Clin N Am. 1994;4(1):43–54.
7. Gibler WB, Cannon CP, Blomkalns AL, Char DM, Drew BJ, Hollander JE, et al. Practical implementation of the guidelines for unstable angina/non-ST-segment elevation myocardial infarction in the emergency department: a scientific statement from the American Heart Association Council on Clinical Cardiology (Subcommittee on Acute Cardiac Care), Council on Cardiovascular Nursing, and Quality of Care and Outcomes Research Interdisciplinary Working Group, in Collaboration With the Society of Chest Pain Centers. Circulation. 2005;111(20):2699–710.
8. Agewall S, Beltrame JF, Reynolds HR, Niessner A, Rosano G, Caforio AL, et al. ESC Working Group position paper on myocardial infarction with non-obstructive coronary arteries. Eur Heart J. 2017;38(3):143–53.
9. Shapiro MD, Guarraia DL, Moloo J, Cury RC. Evaluation of acute coronary syndromes by cardiac magnetic resonance imaging. Top Magn Reson Imaging. 2008;19(1):25–32.
10. Ingkanisorn WP, Kwong RY, Bohme NS, Geller NL, Rhoads KL, Dyke CK, et al. Prognosis of negative adenosine stress magnetic resonance in patients presenting to an emergency department with chest pain. J Am Coll Cardiol. 2006;47(7):1427–32.
11. Heitner JF, Klem I, Rasheed D, Chandra A, Kim HW, Van Assche LM, et al. Stress cardiac MR imaging compared with stress echocardiography in the early evaluation of patients who present to the emergency department with intermediate-risk chest pain. Radiology. 2014;271(1):56–64.
12. Kefer J, Coche E, Legros G, Pasquet A, Grandin C, Van Beers BE, et al. Head-to-head comparison of three-dimensional navigator-gated magnetic resonance imaging and 16-slice computed tomography to detect coronary artery stenosis in patients. J Am Coll Cardiol. 2005;46(1):92–100.

13. Gerber BL, Coche E, Pasquet A, Ketelslegers E, Vancraeynest D, Grandin C, et al. Coronary artery stenosis: direct comparison of four-section multi-detector row CT and 3D navigator MR imaging for detection--initial results. Radiology. 2005;234(1):98–108.
14. Muller MF, Fleisch M, Kroeker R, Chatterjee T, Meier B, Vock P. Proximal coronary artery stenosis: three-dimensional MRI with fat saturation and navigator echo. J Magn Reson Imaging. 1997;7(4):644–51.
15. Kim WY, Danias PG, Stuber M, Flamm SD, Plein S, Nagel E, et al. Coronary magnetic resonance angiography for the detection of coronary stenoses. N Engl J Med. 2001;345(26):1863–9.
16. Kessler W, Achenbach S, Moshage W, Zink D, Kroeker R, Nitz W, et al. Usefulness of respiratory gated magnetic resonance coronary angiography in assessing narrowings > or = 50% in diameter in native coronary arteries and in aortocoronary bypass conduits. Am J Cardiol. 1997;80(8):989–93.
17. Nikolaou K, Huber A, Knez A, Becker C, Bruening R, Reiser M. Intraindividual comparison of contrast-enhanced electron-beam computed tomography and navigator-echo-based magnetic resonance imaging for noninvasive coronary artery angiography. Eur Radiol. 2002;12(7):1663–71.
18. Tornvall P, Gerbaud E, Behaghel A, Chopard R, Collste O, Laraudogoitia E, et al. Myocarditis or "true" infarction by cardiac magnetic resonance in patients with a clinical diagnosis of myocardial infarction without obstructive coronary disease: a meta-analysis of individual patient data. Atherosclerosis. 2015;241(1):87–91.
19. Abu Mouch S, Roguin A, Hellou E, Ishai A, Shoshan U, Mahamid L, et al. Myocarditis following COVID-19 mRNA vaccination. Vaccine. 2021;39(29):3790–3.
20. Rafiee MJ, Babaki Fard F, Friedrich MG. COVID-19, myocardial edema and dexamethasone. Med Hypotheses. 2020;145:110307.
21. Dastidar AG, Rodrigues JC, Ahmed N, Baritussio A, Bucciarelli-Ducci C. The role of cardiac MRI in patients with troponin-positive chest pain and unobstructed coronary arteries. Curr Cardiovasc Imaging Rep. 2015;8(8):28.
22. Madhavan M, Prasad A. Proposed Mayo Clinic criteria for the diagnosis of Tako-Tsubo cardiomyopathy and long-term prognosis. Herz. 2010;35(4):240–3.
23. Shiga T, Wajima Z, Apfel CC, Inoue T, Ohe Y. Diagnostic accuracy of transesophageal echocardiography, helical computed tomography, and magnetic resonance imaging for suspected thoracic aortic dissection: systematic review and meta-analysis. Arch Intern Med. 2006;166(13):1350–6.
24. Stein PD, Fowler SE, Goodman LR, Gottschalk A, Hales CA, Hull RD, et al. Multidetector computed tomography for acute pulmonary embolism. N Engl J Med. 2006;354(22):2317–27.
25. Stein PD, Chenevert TL, Fowler SE, Goodman LR, Gottschalk A, Hales CA, et al. Gadolinium-enhanced magnetic resonance angiography for pulmonary embolism: a multicenter prospective study (PIOPED III). Ann Intern Med. 2010;152(7):434–43, W142–3.
26. Revel MP, Sanchez O, Couchon S, Planquette B, Hernigou A, Niarra R, et al. Diagnostic accuracy of magnetic resonance imaging for an acute pulmonary embolism: results of the 'IRM-EP' study. J Thromb Haemost. 2012;10(5):743–50.

## Suggested Reading

Saremi F, Cardiac MR. Imaging in acute coronary syndrome: application and image interpretation. Radiology. 2017;282(1):17–32.
Baritussio A, Scatteia A, Bucciarelli-Ducci C. Role of cardiovascular magnetic resonance in acute and chronic ischemic heart disease. Int J Cardiovasc Imaging. 2018;34(1):67–80.

# New Technologies for the Evaluation of Acute Coronary Syndromes: Magnetocardiography—The Next Generation of Super Electrocardiogram?

Donatella Brisinda, Riccardo Fenici, and Peter Smars

## 1 Measuring Cardiac Activity

### *1.1 The Electrocardiogram*

The evolution of the ECG in clinical use has undergone a slow and steady evolution over the last approximately 100 plus years [1]. Electrical activity that correlated with cardiac activity was first discovered in frogs by August Waller in 1877. He used a capillary electrometer and electrodes that confirmed electrical activity relating to ventricular contraction. However, it was William Einthoven who first demonstrated a clinical use of ECG by demonstrating the PQRST wave complex using a refined electrometer in approximately 1895 and published his first papers on this discovery in 1901 and 1903. He used a bipolar method where electrodes were applied to the upper and left lower extremities to create a three-lead ECG. These leads are used today as leads I, II, and III.

The clinical use of the ECG made its first US debut in 1909 primarily used for diagnosing arrhythmias, such as atrial fibrillation. It took until 1930 before it was recognized that by evaluating the ST segment, one could diagnose an acute myocardial infarction (AMI). However, it was soon discovered that many AMIs were

D. Brisinda
Fondazione Policlinico Universitario A. Gemelli IRCCS, Università Cattolica del Sacro Cuore, Rome, Italy

Biomagnetism and Clinical Physiology International Center (BACPIC), Rome, Italy

R. Fenici
Biomagnetism and Clinical Physiology International Center (BACPIC), Rome, Italy

P. Smars (✉)
Emergency Medicine Department, Mayo Clinic, Rochester, USA
e-mail: Smars.Peter@mayo.edu



M. Pena et al. (eds.), *Short Stay Management of Chest Pain*, Contemporary Cardiology, https://doi.org/10.1007/978-3-031-05520-1_17

missed with this three-limb ECG because areas of the myocardium were considered "silent" or electrically undetectable. In an effort to improve on this, Frank N. Wilson developed a concept in 1934 where he used a central referenced terminal by combining limb electrodes to create a unipolar, or "grounded" lead system placed in a horizontal plane on the chest creating the V1–6 precordial leads. Emmanuel Goldberger added the frontal unipolar lead system in 1942 using the "Wilson central terminal," creating the three-limb aVL, aVF, and aVR leads, thus creating a limb-based unipolar system, further improving on the sensitivity of the ECG as a diagnostic tool [1].

These developments are the basis for the currently used ECG. Further development of ECG technology has continued up until today with smaller and more effective systems, but essentially, ECG sensitivity and specificity remain static. Examples of ECG improvements include increased ease of mobility, interoperability, as well as interface with today's electronic software computer-based systems. A significant improvement to general use has been the development of algorithms using gender-based and age-related criteria, generating a computer interpretation.

It is well recognized that electrically undetectable areas of the left ventricle are a significant limitation to ECG sensitivity and specificity. Body surface mapping to visualize the electrical activity of these previously known undetectable areas was explored but largely found to be difficult to interpret by providers due to the significant variability of body size, and application of the electrodes was also noted to be difficult [2]. This idea has since largely disappeared from clinical use perspective. Therefore, it is safe to say that the 12-lead ECG has reached peak or close optimum performance as a diagnostic tool.

Although the ECG remains the single most important initial diagnostic test and can be performed almost immediately upon a patient's arrival to the ED, many ACS presentations will not be apparent, diagnostic or even suggestive on the ECG. The ECG has been shown to be diagnostic in 50% or less of AMI cases [3]. There is a small subset, approximately 5%, of suspected ACS presentations that may show ST depression or dynamic ST-T wave changes with ischemia or infarction [4, 5].


## 1.2  *Magnetocardiography*


With the knowledge of inherent limitations of the ECG evolved the idea of developing a system that could overcome the limitations of electrical resistance, or impedance, and the resulting electrically undetectable areas, and improve on the sensitivity and specificity of recognizing an ACS. Similar to the development of the ECG over many decades, magnetocardiography (MCG) has also undergone a dramatic evolution, both from a technical and a diagnostic standpoint [6–12].

As early as 1820, Hans Oerstedt discovered and described the fact of physics that an electric current generates a magnetic field. Even though the electrical activity of the cardiac cycle is not a true electric current flow but rather a cellular level depolarization followed by the repolarization of the myocardial cells, at ventricular level it appears as a relatively slow current progressing along the bundle of His and extending into the myocardium itself, followed by the repolarization phase also as a slow electrical current directed from the epicardium to the endocardium and from the apex to the base of the heart. This depolarization–repolarization process also generates a magnetic field as it progresses through the cardiac cycle.

One advantage of the magnetic field measurement is that cardiac magnetic fields are not impaired by the different electric measurement limitations mentioned above and therefore by the distance from the source of magnetic fields. This distance from the source remains a significant limiting factor of MCG measurements because of the fact that the magnetic field weakens the further away it is from the electric current source, that is, the myocardium itself. In addition, the strength of the magnetic field that the cardiac cycle generates is very weak compared to other well-known environmental sources of magnetic fields. For example, the earth's magnetic field is in the magnitude of 30–60 Micro-Tesla (or $30$–$60 \times 10^{-6}$ Tesla). In contrast, magnetic resonance imaging (MRI) generates a magnetic field in the order of 0.5–3.0 Tesla. The cardiac magnetic field, on the other hand, is in the range of Pico- to Femto-Tesla (or $10^{-12}$ to $10^{-15}$ Tesla). Moreover, the world we live in is filled with multiple magnetic fields generated from a multitude of sources, including the electrical currents that provide light and power to numerous applications in our environment, and moving metallic object such as cars, elevators or moving wheelchairs.

The first magnetic field measurements shown to reflect the electrical field changes of the heart were first recognized and recorded by Baule and McFee at Syracuse University, New York, in 1963 and later reproduced by Safonov et al. in Moskov in 1967. There were significant limitations at that time preventing MCG use in clinical situations. For example, the magnetic sensor coils were large and cumbersome and could only measure a small area at a time. MCG research continued by Cohen et al. at MIT, who had developed a significantly smaller sensor device based on induction coils as well as a better shielding room that reduced the magnetic interference by a factor of about 1000 [13]. He further explored the possibility of interpreting normal versus abnormal magnetic cardiac field patterns. [14].

The milestone allowing for easier and more reliable MCG recording was the invention of an innovative sensor, the Superconducting Quantum Interference Device (SQUID) based on superconductivity, that was first explored in the 1950s [15], and further developed in the 1970s [16]. The SQUID provided a significant improvement in biological magnetic field sensitivity, or its ability to sense and measure the desired magnetic field, and the size of the sensors could be reduced. With this development, Cohen et al. carried out the first study of direct current magneto-cardiography (DC-MCG) recordings of magnetic field changes caused by experimental ischemia in dogs [17, 18]. Thereafter, numerous other laboratories developed custom single-channel SQUID devices.[1] However, sequential mapping of the MCG signal with a just one SQUID sensor was very time-consuming and even

---

[1] Single-channel SQUID device could, in principle, be compared to a single V-lead ECG system.

methodologically inappropriate unless electrophysiological events were sufficiently stable along the time required to complete the mapping procedure [8, 19].

The MCG remained "de facto" a research tool until the 1990s, when two other major technological milestones favored a new interest for MCG as a potential clinical tool: (1) the development of several high-quality large-scale instrumentations for multichannel MCG mapping working in magnetically shielded rooms (MSR),[2] and (2) the construction and commercial availability of more compact and budget-priced systems[3] (featuring 4–9 channels) for sequential MCG mapping, capable of operating in unshielded hospital rooms. The former systems provided the ideal environment to obtain very low-noise MCG maps in real time, capable to detect even weak transient electrophysiological changes and therefore adequate also for stress MCG testing [20, 21]. However, although the MCG showed a significant improvement in sensitivity and specificity compared to the ECG in detecting electrophysiological abnormalities, the need of specially designed expensive, claustrophobic and space consuming MSRs was not very practical for clinical use. Thus, the environmental magnetic field interference continued to be a significant limiting factor in applying MCG to the clinical environment.

To avoid the need of MSRs, a technological alternative, developed since the 1970s, was the coupling of the SQUID sensors to superconducting pick-up coils designed as second- or higher-order gradiometers that would primarily measure the magnetic field gradient closest to the source and ignoring magnetic fields from further away (e.g., the environmental noise). Now, unshielded MCG could be recorded in very low-noise rural laboratories, and even in a regular hospital room [22], reaching a signal resolution high enough to measure the magnetic field generated by atrial repolarization and His-bundle depolarization [19]. The validation of such pioneering unshielded MCG recordings was demonstrated by repeating the same measurements in the Berlin Magnetic Shielded Room in the early 1980s [23]. Since then, a number of different cryogenic instrumentation for MCG have been developed in academic laboratories around the world, with multichannel configuration for simultaneous mapping and visualization of the cardiac magnetic field dynamics. Most multichannel systems still need heavy electromagnetic shielding; however, significant developments for unshielded magnetocardiography have been and are being developed [19, 24–28]. A more detailed description of the history of MCG and instrumentation development can be found in previous reviews and book chapters [22, 29, 30].

---

[2] The Siemens KRENIKON 37-channel; the Philips 62-channel featuring a Twin-Dewar configuration, the Berlin's 49 MCG channels, the Helsinki's 4D Neuroimaging Vector View 99 Channel, the Bochum's 61-channels MAGNES 1300 C, the Ulm's and Chieti's 55-channel ATB ARGOS, the Iena's Argos 200 vector-gradiometer, Hitachi 6400 64-channel system, 64-channel KRISS (Daejeon, Korea); CS-MAG II (BMP GmbH, Hamburg, Germany). The 304 SQUIDs Vector Magnetometer System for Biomagnetic Measurements in the Berlin MSR.

[3] CMI-A3609 (CardioMag Imaging, Schenectady, NY), MCG4 (SQUID AG, Essen, Germany); 7-channel MCG-scanners "Cardiomagscan" V *3.1 (Company KMG, Ukraine);* Cardiomox-MCG9 *(Oxford Cardiomox Ltd).*

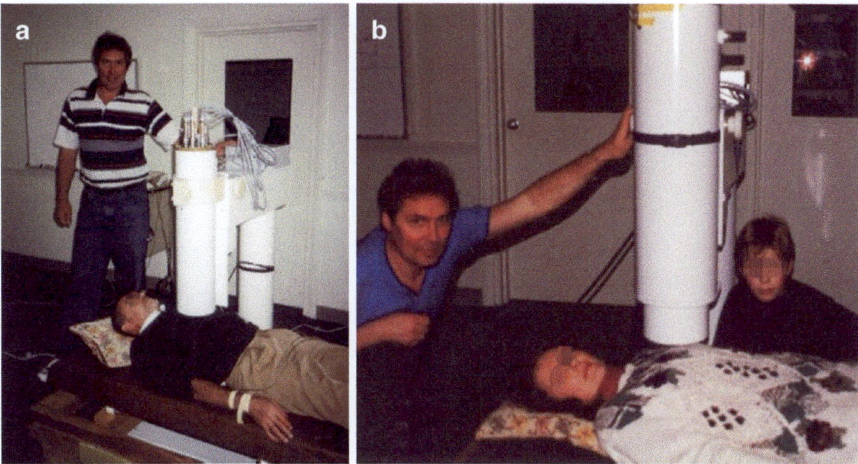

**Fig. 1** (**a**) The MCG of one of the authors (RF) is tested by Alexander Bakharev (also in the picture) with the 7-channel MCG prototype developed at CES (*Cryogenic Electronic Systems Corporation, Springfield*). (**b**) The Bakharev family with the prototype of the 9-channel system. (Courtesy of A. Bakharev)

## 2  Magnetocardiography Recording Devices

The 7-channel prototype for unshielded MCG developed by Alexander Bakharev and colleagues in 1996 was among the first multichannel MCG recording devices (Fig. 1a). This prototype featured an electronic noise suppression system (ENSS) residing in a gradiometer nearby a three-dimensional XYZ magnetometer that could measure the magnetic field "leakage" in all three dimensions and was placed in a large Helmholtz coil to create a very uniform magnetic field. The "leaks" could then be compensated for by sending out an electronic signal, again, three dimensional. This 7-channel prototype was soon followed by a 9-channel prototype (Fig. 1b).

The first generation of this technology was transferred to industry for commercial development of a 9-channel system (*CardioMag Inc.*), that was found to be clinically reliable [31] if it could be placed in a relatively magnetically quiet area (e.g., away from elevators or computers). This unit had nine sensors, each sensing an approximately 20 cm × 20 cm area. In order to cover the chest area of the average adult, the bed had to be moved four times to measure the entire chest area. The data from each area was then added together by software to visualize the entire heart. Each section of the chest took approximately 90 s to record; thus, the total time to scan each patient was approximately 10 min (Fig. 2a). In 2002, using the same technology, a custom 36-channel prototype for real-time unshielded MCG mapping[4] was constructed and installed at the Università Cattolica del Sacro Cuore (Rome),

---

[4] CMI-2436 (*CardioMag Imaging, Schenectady, NY*).

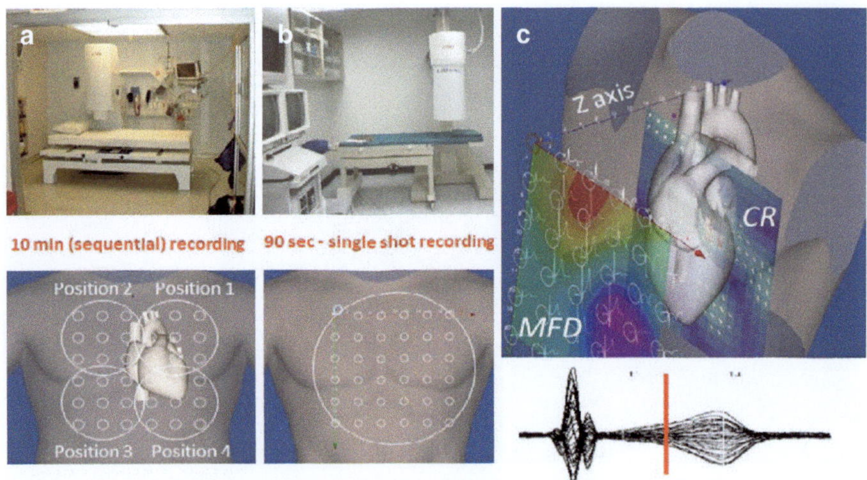



**Fig. 2** (**a**) CMI A3609 Unshielded 9-channel MCG system installed in the Mayo Clinic ED. (**b**) CMI 2436 Unshielded 36-channel MCG system installed in the amagnetic Cath-Lab of the *Biomagnetism and Clinical Physiology International Center* at the Università Cattolica del Sacro Cuore (Rome). (**c**) Three-dimensional oblique view (left cranial) showing the relationship between the magnetic field distribution (MFD) and the current reconstruction (CR) on the zeta plane, at a single instant of the ST segment (red bar on the "*butterfly*" MCG waveforms)

in the unshielded *Biomagnetism and Clinical Physiology International Center* (BACPIC), an amagnetic cath-lab fully equipped for intensive cardiac care where real-time MCG cardiac mapping in only 90 s was performed even during invasive electrophysiological interventions (Fig. 2b) [8, 11, 32–34]. This device, however, was never finalized for commercialization. Although the sensitivity and specificity of these systems were significantly better compared to the ECG, they were not yet considered sensitive enough to allow for safe discharge of patients presenting to the ED with chest pain [33, 35].

Most MCG equipment up to this point depended upon interpretation of the magnetic fields as measured in only a single plane, the Z-plane (Fig. 2c) Theoretically, this could possibly explain the fact that no system up to this point had demonstrated a sensitivity and specificity much more than 70–80%. Because only a single plane is evaluated, perhaps smaller areas further away from the central plane that are being measured and analyzed were magnetically leaked and lost, similar to the undetectable areas of an ECG. To correct for this limitation, single and multichannel instrumentations, most of them working in MSRs only [36, 37], were developed using vector magnetocardiography or vMCG [38–40], to measure the three components of a cardiac magnetic field simultaneously.

A novel cryogenic system for unshielded vMCG, the Avalon H90 system *(Mesuron LLC, US,)* features more than 70 smaller SQUIDs arranged in such a way that the three components of the cardiac magnetic field (*X*, *Y* and *Z*) can be simultaneously measured and is considered a true unshielded three-dimensional MCG imaging device of cardiac electrophysiological events (see Fig. 3a).

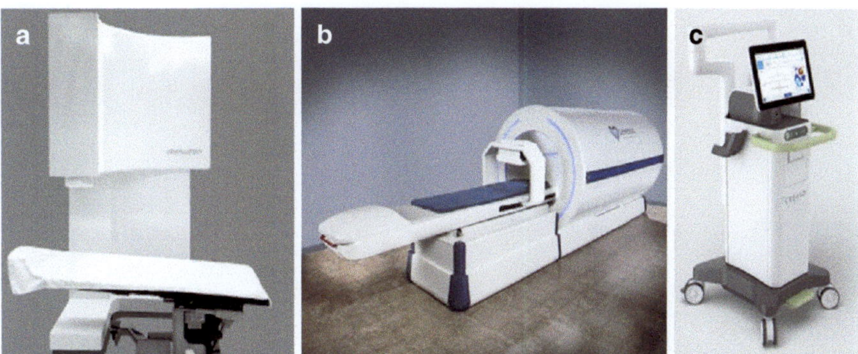

**Fig. 3** Most recent MCG technology developments: (**a**) Mesuron's Avalon-H90 (unshielded). (**b**) Genetesis' "CardioFlux" (shielded); (**c**) Creavo's "Corsens" (unshielded)

Noncryogenic alternatives to SQUID-based MCG systems intended for clinical use have been explored since the early 2000s [41, 42] and progressively developed to became clinically available, although still requiring heavy electromagnetic shielding. One of them, the CardioFlux (Genetesis, Inc., USA) features 36 magneto-optic sensors, which are shielded with the patient in a simplified tube-like magnetic shielding space to perform the MCG recording (see Fig. 3b). Also that system was originally designed within the Research Agreement between Genetesis and the Università Cattolica del Sacro Cuore, and features a similar sensors' grid geometry and analytic approach to facilitate comparison with the well validated SQUID-based 36-channel MCG mapping of that institution (Fig. 4). Accordingly, the novel CardioFlux cloud-based software system converts MCG data into dynamic images after a data acquisition time of 90 s, and provides a diagnostic report in approximately 5 min. The CardioFlux system is under validation with observational clinical trials as an alternative testing modality to identify chest pain patients that can be safely discharged from ED [43]. (*See the list of trials in the Appendix*).

Another noncryogenic alternative is the innovative MCG mapping device VitalScan/Corsens© (Creavo, UK) (Fig. 3c), which uses as magnetic field sensors inexpensive mini induction coils, was developed by Ben Varcoe at the University of Leeds, and could be ideal for clinical use, especially in EDs, because of its small size, portability at the patient's bedside, and capability to work in a regular unshielded hospital room [25]. This system is also under validation with observational clinical trials (See the list of trials in the Appendix).

## 3  Magnetocardiography for Evaluation of Chest Pain

Each year, approximately seven million US patients present to the ED with chest pain at an estimated cost of $5 billion [44, 45], although cardiovascular disease may be present in only about 20% of these patients, and less than 10% are ultimately

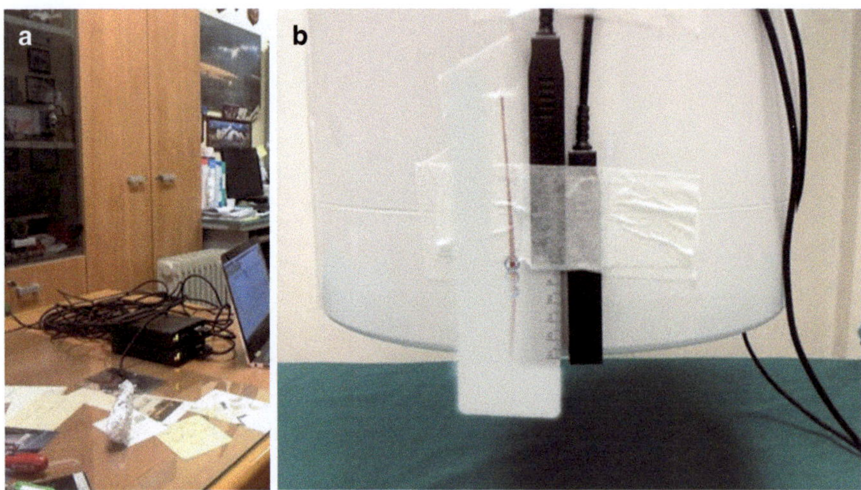


**Fig. 4** (**a**) Testing of QuSpin optically pumped magnetometers (OPM) in the unshielded biomagnetic catheterization laboratory of the BACPIC's, together with two Genetesis' researchers visiting, in 2017, within the Research Agreement with the Università Cattolica del Sacro Cuore. (**b**) Two QuSpin OPMs attached to the dewar of the CMI-2436 36-channel, to attempt a gradiometer configuration and evaluate their potential to work in unshielded environment

diagnosed with an ACS, with a total cost for testing between $10 and $13 billion annually [46, 47]. Current diagnostic testing for ACS includes testing that are non-invasive (stress testing, computed tomography coronary angiography, single-photon emission computed tomography [SPECT]) and/or invasive coronary angiography (CA) [48, 49], with sometimes unacceptable delays in time-to-cath in the case of true ACS, or unnecessary and expensive hospital length of stay and testing for those without a cardiac event. Thus, the need for novel, safe, noninvasive, and rapid alternative methods such as MCG to detect electrophysiological abnormalities induced by the early stage of myocardial ischemia and to effectively triage patients presenting with acute chest pain is unquestionable.

Magnetocardiography has been investigated and is emerging as a possible novel method to detect cardiac ischemia, because foundational theory and experimental research suggests ischemia in its early stage induces changes in the electrophysiological properties of the myocardium that can be detected by MCG but not ECG. This is because MCG is more sensitive to tangential currents, curl currents, transmural current flow, and closed-looped currents that are invisible to ECG [50–54]. Moreover, as mentioned above, cardiac magnetic fields are not attenuated or distorted by differences in the conductivity of body tissues or fluids and does not require skin-electrode contact.

Based on this knowledge, hundreds of patients with stable and/or acute IHD have been investigated around the world during the last three decades, but under very different experimental conditions that have impaired the integration of the available data and their univocal interpretation. Nevertheless, an attempt to pool results from these studies has been recently addressed in systematic review and meta-analysis papers [55, 56], providing reasonable evidence that rest-MCG has higher sensitivity than ECG, echocardiography, and conventional cardiac troponin assays to detect IHD in patients with stable coronary artery disease (CAD) or ACS. Therefore, the utilization of rest-MCG as a first-next level investigation following an undiagnostic ECG is currently under evaluation for rapid triage of patients presenting in the ED with acute chest pain and/or to provide noninvasive rule-out of IHD in ambulatory patients with cardiac abnormalities of uncertain diagnosis.

Although an average sensitivity, specificity and predictive accuracy around 80% has been reported in several studies [57–62], a cautious interpretation of previous results has been advocated, because the majority of these studies were investigating relatively small cohorts of selected and inhomogeneous patients' populations, including patients with or without documented stable CAD compared with healthy subjects, or even patients having chest pain of not cardiac origin. Thus, a more objective and unbiased validation on undifferentiated patients' cohorts is still lacking and deserve further investigation ideally in prospective randomised controlled clinical trials.

## 3.1 Clinical Evidence of Magnetocardiography to Detect Cardiac Ischemia

The first demonstration of the unique potential of MCG for the study of acute myocardial ischemia was provided by Cohen et al. in the 1970s who used experimental MCG measurements to reveal ischemic injury currents not detected by ECG and to verify the feasibility of such measurements in humans [17, 63, 64]. This provided the first demonstration that direct-current (DC) MCG was feasible and that it has the potential to provide a mechanistic differentiation between "apparent ST shift" (which in reality is a TQ shift) due to the injury current flowing due to the presence of ischemic myocardium, and "true ST shift" (an abnormal systolic event related to differences in action potential duration and timing). However, these pioneering studies were not followed up, likely because of technical difficulties foreseen by Savard et al. [63] to transfer such a complex investigational protocol from a MSR into environments more appropriate for clinical application. This is unfortunate because, if clinically available, DC-MCG could be also useful for better understanding not only of the arrhythmogenic mechanisms related to ischemia but also to those underlying the different kinds of "J-wave Syndromes" (e.g., Brugada and early repolarization syndromes) [65] and for their risk assessment.

Other research in the 1970s demonstrated the feasibility of clinical MCG measurements and attempted its interpretation by morphological comparison of the MCG waveforms with 12-lead ECG [66, 67]. In spite of prevalent skepticism, further studies attempting MCG measurements in a variety of clinical situations were conducted foreseeing contactless MCG as a novel tool with the potential to provide new information in patients with unclear or nondiagnostic ECG patterns [6, 7, 19, 68–70] and to simplify multisite mapping of cardiac electrophysiology compared with body surface electric mapping [2, 71].

Among such MCG devices, the CMI-A3609 9-channel system for unshielded sequential MCG was the first to receive the FDA clearance for human measurements[5] and was installed in academic hospitals of the United States (see the one installed in the Mayo Clinic ED (Rochester, Minnesota—(Fig. 2a and Europe [35, 72–75] to perform the first multicentre clinical trial *(See the list of clinical trials in the Appendix),* aiming to assess its reliability and to evaluate the predictive accuracy of MCG in detecting IHD in unshielded hospital environments.

## 3.2 Magnetocardiography Parameters and Methods for Ischemia Detection

MCG evaluation of IHD was initially based on the analysis of MCG ventricular repolarization waveforms and intervals duration [22–24]. However, since the early 1980s, isofield reconstruction of magnetic field distribution became available [76], followed by the development of more sophisticated mathematical algorithms, based on the inverse solution with the equivalent current dipole (ECD), the equivalent magnetic dipole (EMD), or other more sophisticated models [77], to investigate the spatial-temporal dynamics of equivalent cardiac sources.

To detect IHD, quantitative analysis of changes in the magnetic field during ventricular repolarization [78, 79] was mainly used, although other studies reported also ischemia-related abnormality of MCG QT interval dispersion [80] and of depolarization parameters [81].

In attempting a quantitative estimate and description of such abnormalities, different methods have been proposed; MCG parameters most frequently used to quantitatively assess ischemia-related ventricular repolarization abnormalities are summarized in Table 1 and will be discussed further below.

A common reproducible finding in patients with IHD, independent of the type of MCG system used and recording environment, is the loss of the stable dipolar configuration of the MFD during the ST segment interval and the T-wave [75, 82, 114] (Fig. 5a) typically observed in normal subjects (Fig. 5b), and/or the presence of an abnormal angle, between the direction of the largest gradient and the patient's right-left horizontal line, termed the *"α angle"* [78, 79, 116] (Fig. 6).

Hänninen et al., working in the BioMag Laboratory's MSR of the Helsinki University Central Hospital (HUCH), calculated the *α angle* of the maximum spatial gradient of the magnetic field pattern at the second quarter of the ST-segment and at the T-wave apex, and reported that its rotation induced by exercise was useful

---

[5]FDA approval CMI-A3609 (CardioMag Imaging, Schenectady, NY) July 2004 https://www.healthimaging.com/topics/diagnostic-imaging/cardiomag-sell-mcg-us-following-fda-approval

**Table 1**  Most used analytic methods to detect myocardial ischemia with MCG

| |
|---|
| Quantitative MCG parameters measured at rest/exercise from the ST integral and the T-wave peak [78, 79] |
|    Magnetic field orientation ($\alpha$ *angle*) measured at the 2° ST segment integral (ST$\alpha$) and at T-wave peak (T$\alpha$) |
| Quantitative MCG parameters measured at rest during the T wave from the $T_{max}/3$-$T_{peak}$ interval [74, 82, 83] |
|    Direction of the main vector from the plus to minus pole between −20° and +110° |
|    Change in the angle of the main vector ≥45° in a time interval of 30 ms between $T_{max}/3$-$T_{peak}$ |
|    Change in the distance separating the plus and minus poles ≥20 mm in a time interval of 30 ms between $T_{max}/3$-$T_{peak}$ |
|    Change in the ratio of the pole strengths ≥0.3 in a time interval of 30 ms between $T_{max}/3$-$T_{peak}$ |
| ST-Twave subtraction maps [84] |
| Isointegrap maps of tangential (Bxy) and normal (Bz) componet of QRST cardiac magnetic field [85, 86] |
| Kullback-Leibler (KL) entropy of QRST cardiac magnetic field [87] |
| Multilayer perceptron (MLP) neural network based on linear discriminant analysis of sample entropy of MCG QRS and ST intervals [59] |
| QT dispersion and smoothness indexes (SI) of the QT interval maps [58, 80, 88] |
| Machine learning of ST-Twave cardiac magnetic field [59, 61, 89, 90] |
| Probability density function [91] |
| ST-segment fluctuation score and T-wave non-dipole phenomenon [92, 93] |
| Bi-dimensional pseudo current reconstruction ("arrow-maps") [84, 94–100] |
| Three-dimensional current density imaging (CDI) [101–113] |

*MCG* magnetocardiography; *CAD* coronary artery disease; $T_{max}/3$ one-third of peak intensity; $T_{peak}$ peak intensity of the T-wave. $\alpha$ *angle* the angle between the direction of the largest gradient and the patient's right-left line

to differentiate patients with different coronary artery lesions [78, 79]. Brisinda et al. had similar results with unshielded MCG, comparing 27 patients with documented stable CAD and 33 healthy subjects [116, 117] at rest (Fig. 6) and, in another study, after exercise stress test [118].

Since ST parameters could be affected by the excessive noise of unshielded recordings, Park et al. used only parameters measured during the T-wave, during which the signal-to-noise (S/N) ratio is usually higher (Table 1) [74, 82, 83]. Comparing the performance of the two analytic methods on the same patient cohort, Brisinda et al. found that Hänninen's parameters [78] were less sensitive (76.1% vs. 80.9%, respectively) but more specific (92.3% vs. 84.6%, respectively) than those proposed by Park et al. [82]. Interestingly, in a subsequent study [89] aiming to validate automatic analysis of MCG with a machine learning method applied to the T-wave parameters, it was found that the predictive accuracy of MCG to detect IHD was in the order of 80% in untreated patients and dropped to 72% if patients investigated after PTCA were also included, a finding providing further evidence that MCG is sensitive to the presence of myocardial ischemia.

Other analytic methods have also been reported to identify IHD patients with MCG, such as: the subtraction maps [84], the isointegral maps [85, 86], the

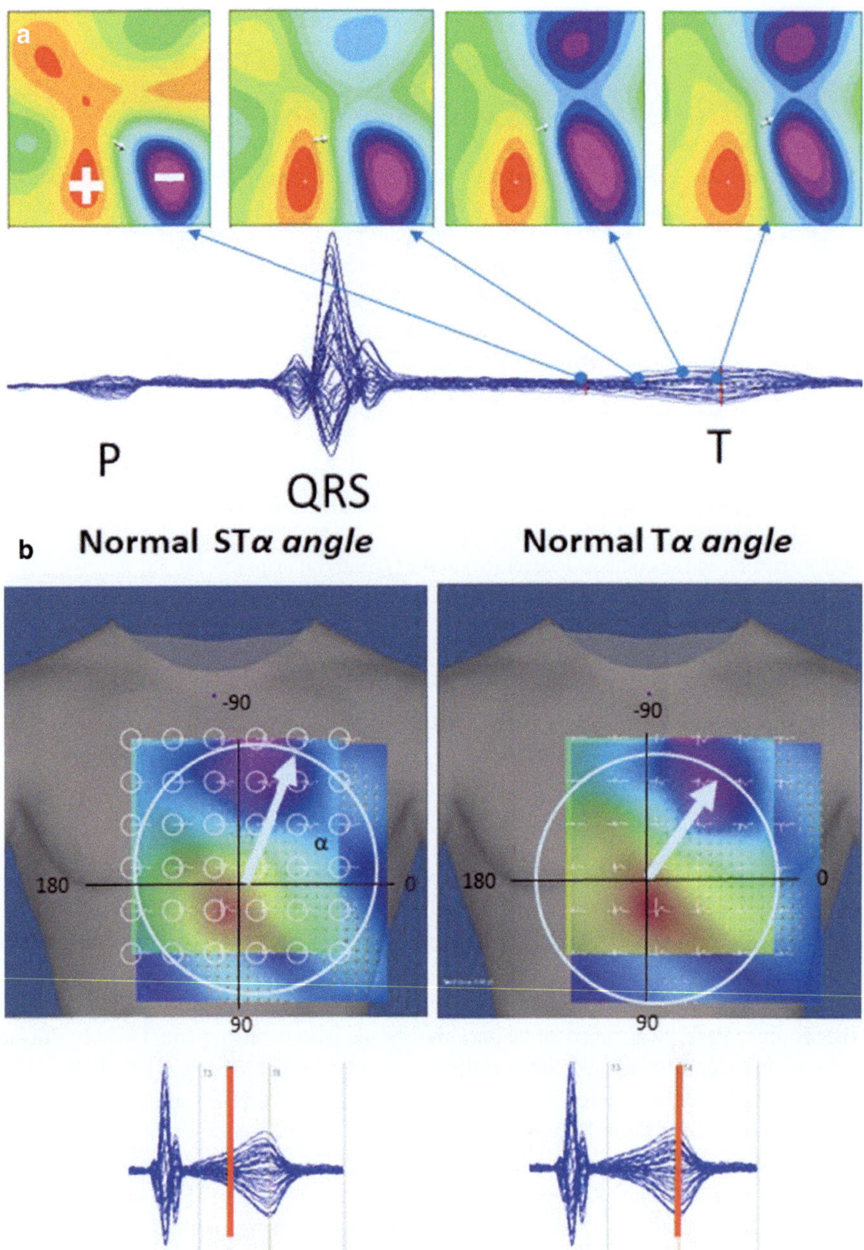


**Fig. 5** (**a**) Example of abnormal magnetic field distribution during the ST and the T wave peak in a patient with three vessel coronary artery disease. (Modified from reference [115]). (**b**) For comparison, normal ST and T-peak MFD and orientation of the α *angles*, calculated according to reference [78]

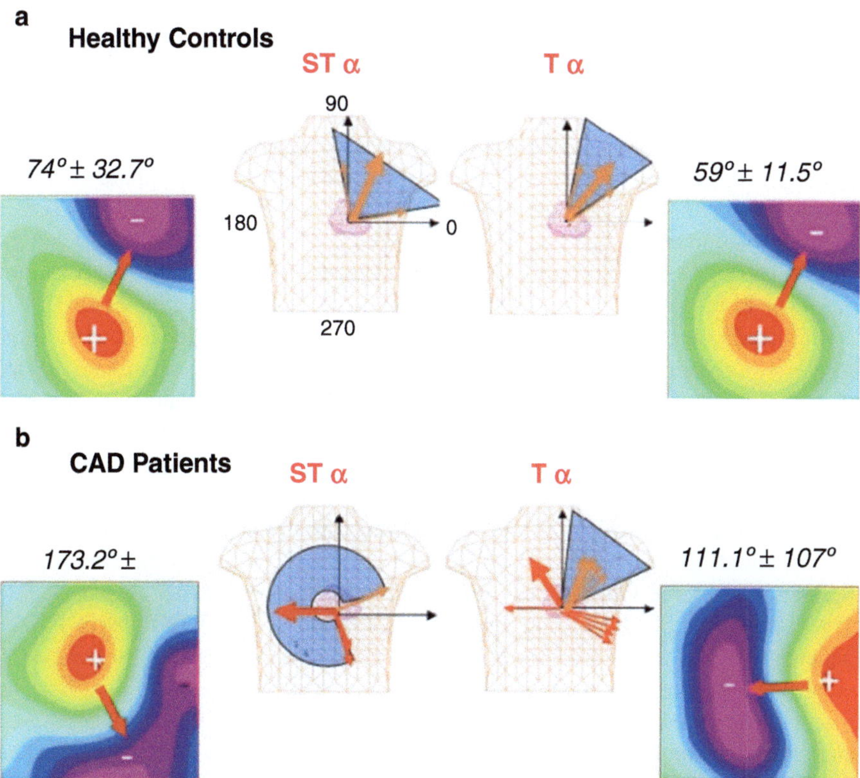



**Fig. 6** Example of normal magnetic field distribution (MFD) and magnetic field orientation ($\alpha$ *angle*), during the ST (ST$\alpha$) and at the T-wave peak (T$\alpha$) (**a**). In (**b**), example of abnormal multipolar MFD and $\alpha$ *angles* of patients with coronary artery disease (CAD). The central drawings show graphically the range of variability of ST and T $\alpha$ *angles* in normal and CAD patients. Average values ± SD of $\alpha$ *angles* are also shown. (Modified from reference [117])

Kullback–Leibler entropy [87], sample entropy [59], QTc heterogeneity and dispersion [58, 80, 88], the machine learning [61, 89, 90], the probability density function [91], the ST-segment fluctuation and T-wave nondipole phenomenon [92, 93], the Hosaka-Cohen transformation for current arrow maps [66, 94, 95] and the current density imaging [101, 102] (Table 1).

With the method of **subtraction maps**, a good correlation was found in IHD patients between the number of coronary artery lesion sites and the abnormal current distribution during the ST-T interval obtained by subtracting average normal magnetic ST-T fields from that of the investigated patient. Moreover, the different results observed in patients with myocardial infarction (MI) has demonstrated that using subtracted MCG ST-T waveforms makes it possible to estimate infarction size and coronary-artery lesions [84]. After experimental demonstration that **iso-integral maps** of de-repolarization phases are similar in healthy but not in ischemic hearts [85], clinical testing of this method showed that compared to healthy subjects, the integral value of repolarization is lower than that of depolarization in patients with myocardial ischemia due to Kawasaki disease [86]. Comparing cardiac magnetic field mapping of young healthy subjects with that of 59 CAD patients without previous MI, the best identification of CAD was achieved by Gapelyuk et al. using the **Kullback–Leibler (KL) entropy** of the repolarization phase (sensitivity/specificity of 85/80%), followed by the residual feature of the depolarization phase (85/75%) and the magnetic field orientation feature (80/73%) sets. The classification based on the combination of the first two parameters increased the sensitivity (88%) and the specificity (88%) for the differentiation of CAD patients from healthy controls (area under the ROC 94%) [87]. An automated method for the classification of CAD with a multilayer perceptron (MLP) neural network based on Linear Discriminant Analysis of sample entropy (SampEn) of MCG recordings was preliminarily tested in ten patients with coronary artery narrowing $\geq$ or $\leq 50\%$. The calculation of SampEn from rest MCG data provided 99% sensitivity, 97% specificity, 98% accuracy, 96% and 99% positive and negative predictive values for single heartbeats, with correct classification of all investigated patients [59]. In 2003, a new method was developed to quantify differences in **spatial distribution of QT interval** in CAD patients compared with healthy subjects on the basis of the **smoothness indexes (SI) of the QT interval maps** calculated from multichannel MCG [80]. The results suggested that abnormal values of QT SI at MCG identified CAD patients with still preserved left ventricular function and were useful for the assessment of post-MI arrhythmogenic risk [80]. Such evidence was also confirmed in recent studies investigating the usefulness of MCG to detect cardiac allograph vasculopathy [58] and obstructive CAD (defined as angiographic left main $\geq 50\%$ or maximum lesions of $\geq 70\%$ luminal stenosis in at least one of the primary coronary arteries and their major branches) in comparison with stress myocardial perfusion imaging calculation of the summed rest score (SRS), the summed stress score (SSS), and the summed difference score (SDS, which is the difference between SSS and SRS) [88]. In the latter study, using the combination of **QTc dispersion** $\geq$ 79 ms or SI-QTc $\geq$ 9.1 ms, the diagnostic performance of MCG was not significantly different in comparison with the cutoff values of SSS $\geq$ 4, SDS $\geq$ 4, or SSS > 8 semi-quantitative parameters calculated with myocardial perfusion imaging. However, myocardial perfusion imaging parameters were positively correlated with the number of stenosed coronary arteries, while MCG parameters were not.

Several efforts have also been carried out to find a reliable method for automated diagnosis of IHD from MCG ventricular repolarization parameters. The **machine learning method**, evaluated in a preliminary clinical study, provided 75% sensitivity, 85% specificity, 83% positive predictive value, 78% negative predictive value, and 80% predictive accuracy [89]. Similar results were obtained by Tantimongcolwat et al. in 2008 [90] with two types of machine learning techniques (sensitivity of 86.2%, specificity 72.7%, and accuracy of 80.4%). Higher diagnostic accuracy (above 90%) was reported by Steinisch et al. [59], and in a more recent study by Tao et al. [61], who extracted 164 features from MCG averaged T-wave segmentation and used four different machine learning classifiers [k-nearest neighbor, decision tree, support vector machine (SVM), and XGBoost].

Diagnostic accuracy for IHD above 80% was also obtained by Kwon et al. [91] by applying a different method to classify the diagnostic values of MCG based on the **probability density function** in 139 patients admitted to the hospital with chest pain. Rest MCG was found to have a sensitivity of 84% and specificity of 85%, compared to 44.7% and 73.5% respectively for rest ECG. The **ST-segment fluctuation score** is a quantitative parameter which was developed by Park et al. with the same signal-processing solution known as QRS fragmentation score [119, 120], that accurately (78.1%) predicted hemodynamically significant CAD when compared to fractional flow reserve [92]. In the same study, it was also found that the T-wave nondipole phenomenon was more accurate (88.5%) in detecting CAD than the change of ST-segment fluctuation score, and that their combination enhanced diagnostic performance for CAD detection (ROC area under the curve 0.93). Similar results were previously reported by Gapelyuk et al. [121].

Bi-dimensional **pseudo current reconstruction** (so called "arrow-maps") from MCG signals was initially developed by Cohen & Hosaka in the 1970s as a simple method to visualize the dipole sources underlying the component of the heart's magnetic field which is normal to the chest (Bz), especially those dipole combinations which produce very low body surface potentials but detectable Bz magnetic field component [94]. This method, since then refined to image the dynamics of cardiac electrophysiological events [96–98], has been widely used to investigate patients with IHD [95, 99], after successful percutaneous coronary interventions [100], and with malignant early repolarization pattern [122]. However, clinical experience has shown that the maximum values of pseudo-currents do not always coincide with the actual sites (especially in depth) where the electrophysiological currents are flowing. Therefore, **three-dimensional current density imaging (CDI)** has been a method used since the early 1990s [101, 102], and a first example of clinical application in a CAD patient after MI was published in 1998 [103]. Thereafter, a number of studies were carried out to validate the localization accuracy of the CDI method [104, 105] and its reliability to identify IHD patients with examination at rest [106–110], and after physical or pharmacological stress tests [111–113]. Interestingly, Chaikovsky et al. developed a software for polar map imaging of 3D current density distribution reconstructed from MCG and demonstrated that areas of the left ventricle with abnormal wall motion documented during dobutamine stress echocardiography are identified and localized by MCG as lower current density sites [107].

### 3.3  *Magnetocardiography Under Stress*

In 1974, Saarinen et al. were the first to report a depression of the ST segment in a CAD patient investigated with a single-channel MCG after exercise testing [67]. Almost 10 years later Cohen et al. studied one CAD patient with DC-MCG in a shielded room during a two-step exercise test. It was reproducibly demonstrated that the effort-induced depression of the ST segment was concomitant with a TQ segment (baseline segment) elevation at about 70% of the ST amplitude. After termination of exercise, the baseline TQ segment elevation disappeared somewhat more rapidly than the ST segment depression [64]. This one was the first and unique demonstrations that a stress-induced injury current could be measured noninvasively with DC-MCG in patients. However, despite demonstrated feasibility, the method was considered not practical for clinical purposes and abandoned. However, after almost 10 years, Brockmeier et al. demonstrated that both physical and pharmacological stress induced in normal subjects more distinct repolarization changes in multichannel MCG than in simultaneously recorded ECG [20, 54]. The authors suggested that the observed difference between electric and magnetic measurements could be due to exercise-induced vortex currents, which are not detectable with ECG [20, 54].

To understand the usefulness of MCG in tracking acute cardiac ischemic events from their onset, one must take into account that within less than a minute after the reduction of cardiac blood flow, the unmet metabolic demand induces electrophysiological alterations of the transmembrane action potential with consequent hypoxia-induced flow of abnormal (injury) currents [123, 124]. These currents have been experimentally detected with DC-MCG [17, 18] but may not be visible by ECG because of differences in the physical properties of magnetic and electrical fields [52, 99]. Based on experimental findings, it can be assumed that there are regional differences of myocardial current strength under stress due to flow-limiting stenosis in the corresponding vascular branch. Moreover, the ischemia-induced progressive decrement in the amplitude and the abnormal anisotropy of transmembrane action potentials is associated with asynchronous local depolarization sequence of functionally different cells, leading to conduction disturbances and fragmentation of the ventricular depolarization wavefronts [125] and fluctuation of the repolarization currents that is measurable with MCG [93].

Numerous articles have been published since the 1990s demonstrating the ability of multichannel MCG to detect stress-induced dynamic changes of cardiac magnetic fields during physical exercise or pharmacological interventions, and that the accuracy of MCG in detecting IHD is enhanced with stress testing [21, 78, 111, 112, 126–130]. Clinical experience has confirmed the experimental evidence that transient myocardial ischemia causes well-recognizable changes in a variety of MCG parameters [74, 92, 93, 112, 126, 128, 131, 132]. A detailed review of stress-MCG literature can be found in a recent article [56] that includes studies demonstrating that MCG may have wider clinical application in CAD diagnosis. For example, its use to detect functional ischemia and viability provides useful prognostic information for risk stratification, location and severity of postinfarction contractile abnormality, arrhythmogenesis, and prediction of MACE [83, 133, 134].

Most of the clinical research investigating stress MCG was carried out with multichannel instrumentation operating only in heavy MSRs, requiring the construction of dedicated amagnetic ergometers if exercise stress testing was performed [20, 21, 54, 113, 129, 135]. One of the earliest studies conducted in a shielded environment included seven CAD patients with ≥75% stenosis in at least one vessel, and showed that a 36-channel MCG could detect changes in the spatial distribution of QT dispersion at rest that were not evident on 12-lead ECG at rest or under stress [21]. Almost simultaneously, a series of Finnish studies demonstrated that exercise MCG carried out with an amagnetic bicycle-ergometer in the HUCH's MSR, was able to distinguish the CAD patients from the healthy subjects by the different orientation of the magnetic field gradient during the ST segment and at the T-wave apex [78]. Furthermore, the recording locations in multichannel MCG mapping were found sensitive enough to identify regional exercise-induced myocardial ischemia [79]. Using the simpler two-step Master exercise stress test, Kanzaki et al. reported higher diagnostic accuracy (83%) of multichannel MCG mapping in identifying CAD [130]. In that study, the maximal QRS integral change during the 40 ms centred on the R-wave peak, was significantly higher in the CAD patients and the best discriminator to differentiate them from control subjects. The significant difference of this parameter between the CAD patients and control subjects gradually decreased in the recovery phase after effort and improved also after successful PTCA [136].

Pharmacological stress was preliminarily reported by Brockmeier et al., who used orciprenalin and atropine in healthy subjects [54]. However, a more systematic prospective study using standardized dobutamine stress testing showed a higher diagnostic accuracy of multichannel MCG mapping (sensitivity 97.6% and specificity 82.8%) compared to stress-ECG (sensitivity 26.2% and specificity 82.8%) to identify coronary artery stenoses $\geq 70\%$. That study was initially conducted with the AtB Argos 55 MCG system [112] and continued with the CS MAG2 system [113]. It remains to be clarified the reasons underlying the contrasting results reported by Steinisch et al. [59], who obtained the best CAD diagnostic accuracy reported so far (above 98%) with their automatic MCG classifier based on SampEn when using data recorded at rest, but found a significant deterioration of the classification effectiveness when using MCG recorded during dobutamine-induced stress conditions. It could be speculated that the larger variability of SampEn (and consequent drop of the classifier performance) could be due to hidden nonlinear events enhanced by pharmacological effects, or to the interference of a higher level of noise, especially during the ST interval, to which entropy measurements are particularly sensitive.

MCG's reliability to assess myocardial viability after an acute MI was also evaluated by comparison with positron emission tomography (PET) and SPECT myocardial perfusion imaging (MPI) carried out in the same patients [111, 137]. In the study by Nenonen et al., current density reconstruction from MCG provided accurate imaging of viable myocardium compared with PET results, and provided evidence of good correspondence for segments of high and low amplitude in MCG current-density estimations and the viable and scar areas identified with PET after exercise-induced ischemia in patients with multivessel coronary artery disease [111]. In the subsequent study of Morguet et al., the amplitude of the R wave ($R_{max}$) and T wave ($T_{max}$ and $T_{min}$) were identified as parameters with the best selectivity at linear discriminant analysis to identify myocardial viability and to correctly classify the extension of myocardial scar within the viable tissues [137]. More recently, two other comparative studies [88, 138] confirmed previous findings [72], suggesting that even rest MCG is not inferior to stress SPECT MPI in identifying patients with CAD. Thus, it was suggested that an MCG scan could substitute for a nuclear scan in patients with low pretest probability of CAD. In fact, whereas stress nuclear MPI is recommended in patients with intermediate or high pretest likelihood of CAD [139, 140] the same indication cannot be applied to an unselected population of subjects with low pretest probability of CAD [140].

Overall, evidence has been provided that both physical and pharmacological stress tests may enhance the diagnostic accuracy of MCG to detect transient cardiac ischemia and may reach a diagnostic level comparable of that provided by nuclear scans, thus suggesting the use of MCG as a simpler, low-cost, radiation-free, and rapid first-level interventional diagnostic alternative when clinically required. Unfortunately, the complexity of installation and management of cryogenic multi-channel instrumentation requiring heavy magnetically shielding have made them available only in minority of academic hospitals, mostly as research tools, in spite of the potential clinical benefit of using MCG scan as a screening method. However, early evidence that stress (exercise) multichannel MCG is feasible and reliable within an unshielded hospital laboratory using a standard bicycle ergometer was demonstrated in 2004. In this pilot study, the stress-induced abnormal orientation of the ST magnetic field gradient correctly identified all investigated patients with CAD, five of whom did not show any evidence of stress-induced ischemia on the ECG (Fig. 7) [118]. Thus, with the present development of novel and less expensive technologies for unshielded MCG, the gap between research and routine clinical use of stress MCG may be soon filled.

Moreover, given the high three-dimensional localization accuracy of electro-physiological currents [104, 141, 142], MCG is foreseen to provide a single-stop-shop for noninvasive multimodal functional imaging and localization of ischemic areas and of arrhythmogenic mechanisms in IHD patients with malignant arrhythmias, enhancing the accuracy of risk assessment based on spatial-temporal quantification of de-repolarization heterogeneity [58, 95, 143], intra-QRS-fragmentation [119, 120, 144], and/or of late QRS activity [122] through the integration of the MCG findings within cardiac magnetic resonance imaging [145].

## *3.4 Magnetocardiography for the Triage of Emergency Department Patients with Acute Chest Pain*

While substantial advances have been made in MCG device technology and methods for automated unbiased analysis of ACS, only a relatively small number of studies have investigated the use of MCG to rule in/rule out suspected acute ACS. Results from systematic review and meta-analysis studies [55, 56] demonstrate that compared with other diagnostic tests (ECG, cardiac troponin I, and echocardiography), MCG has a higher sensitivity, comparable specificity, comparable PPV, and higher NPV in differentiating patients with acute chest pain due to hemodynamically significant CAD or ACS from those presenting with chest pain of noncardiac origin, independent of the different recording setups, and/or the qualitative or quantitative analytic methods used. Agarwal et al. [55] evidenced a pooled

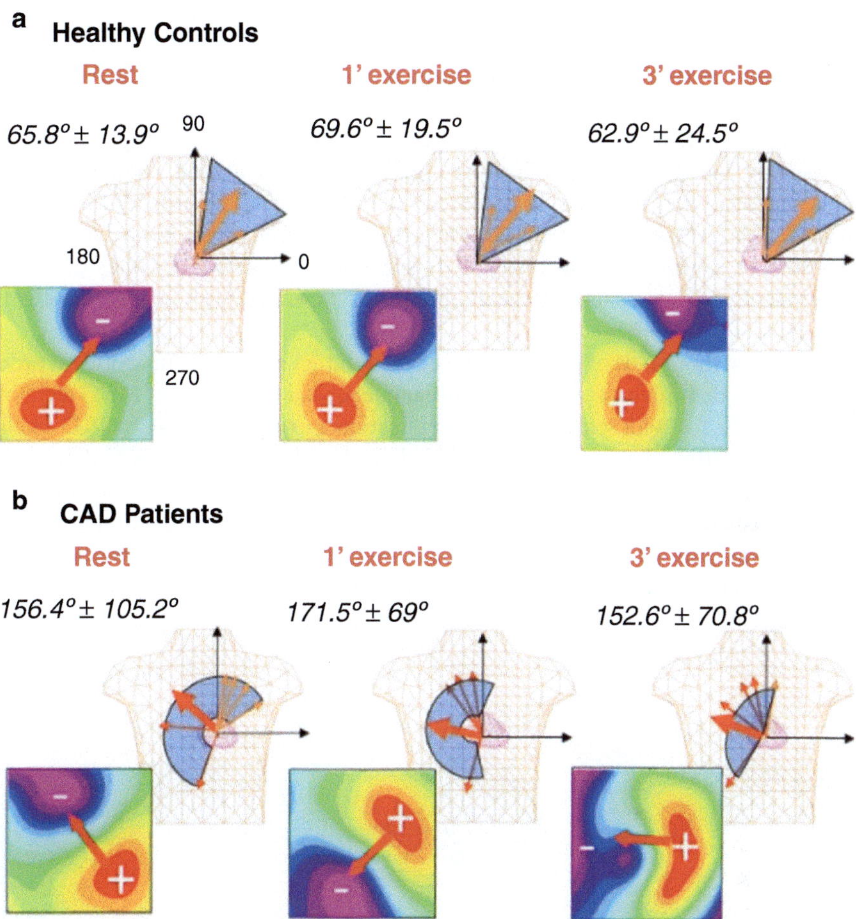



**Fig. 7** Example of normal (**a**) and abnormal (**b**) magnetic field distribution and rotation of ST$\alpha$ angle, at rest and 1 and 3 min after effort in healthy subjects and CAD patients. (Modified from reference [118])

sensitivity of 83% and a specificity of 77%, positive likelihood ratio 3.92 (95% CI 2.30–6.66) and negative likelihood ratio 0.20 (95% CI 0.12–0.35), but only two of the seven studies selected for the meta-analysis were related to MCG study of chest pain patients [55]. In the more recent review article by Camm et al. [56], 23 publications were identified related to the use of MCG for detection/rule-out of ACS in emergency settings; available data on the diagnostic performance of MCG as a rule-in/rule-out test for ACS has been summarized in the supporting Table 3 of reference [56]. In both of these articles, the wide heterogeneity was underlined among investigational conditions, including different recording setups and environments, unstandardized parameters and interpretation criteria, different clinical presentation of patients enrolled with acute chest pain (stable CAD, unstable angina, STEMI, or NSTEMI), and variable use of functional noninvasive testing or coronary angiography as gold standards for validation of MCG diagnostic accuracy. Therefore, validated MCG diagnostic criteria should be assessed in studies of unselected real-world cohorts, including patients with ACS, non-ACS, CAD, inducible ischemia, and non-ischemic chest pain, in order to establish the utility of MCG to differentiate among such clinical problems. On the other hand, despite such heterogeneity and lack of standardization regarding instrumentation, recording protocols, and analytical methods, both reviews [55, 56] seem to confirm that rest MCG provides an average diagnostic accuracy to detect IHD which is in the order of 75–80% or even better, especially if its sensitivity is enhanced with physical or pharmacological stress tests. Recently published papers are well in agreement with these findings [146–148].

Although thousands of patients have been investigated around the world, in order to provide a definitive answer to the multiannual question of whether MCG technology is ready for widespread clinical application in rule-out of ACS/CAD in the emergency setting, large-scale controlled clinical trials to validate MCG diagnostic accuracy in undifferentiated patient cohorts with standardized protocols and analytical methods are still needed. Moreover, there should be some caution in assuming abnormalities of the MCG parameters described are univocally diagnostic of CAD. In fact, similar abnormalities of ventricular repolarization have been observed in patients with essential hypertension (Fig. 8a) [149], mitral valve prolapse [150]

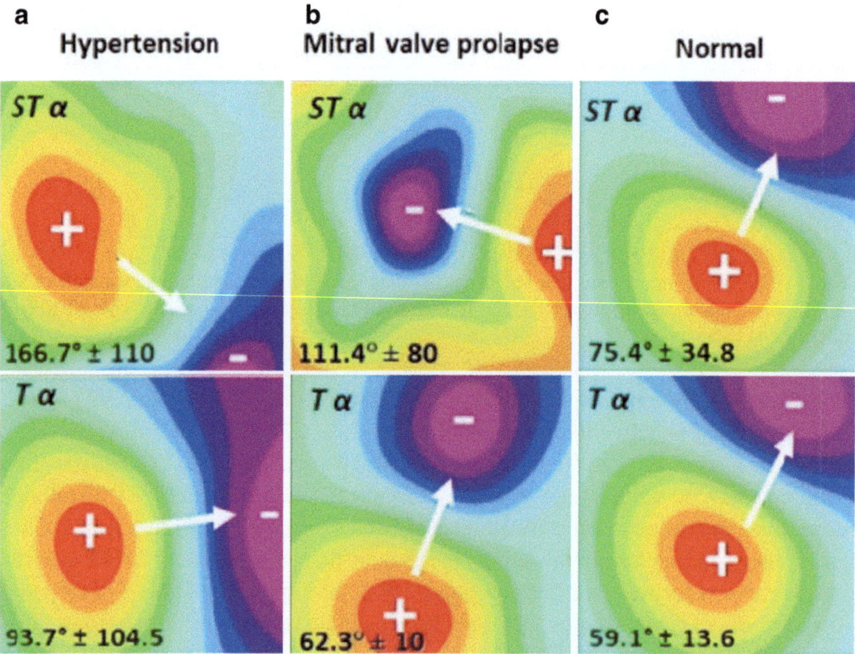


**Fig. 8** Examples of ischemia-like alterations of ST and T-peak MFD and *α angles* of patients with hypertension (**a**) and mitral valve prolapse (**b**). In (**c**) normal pattern, for comparison. Average values (in degrees) ± SD of *α angles* are also shown. (Modified from references [149, 150])

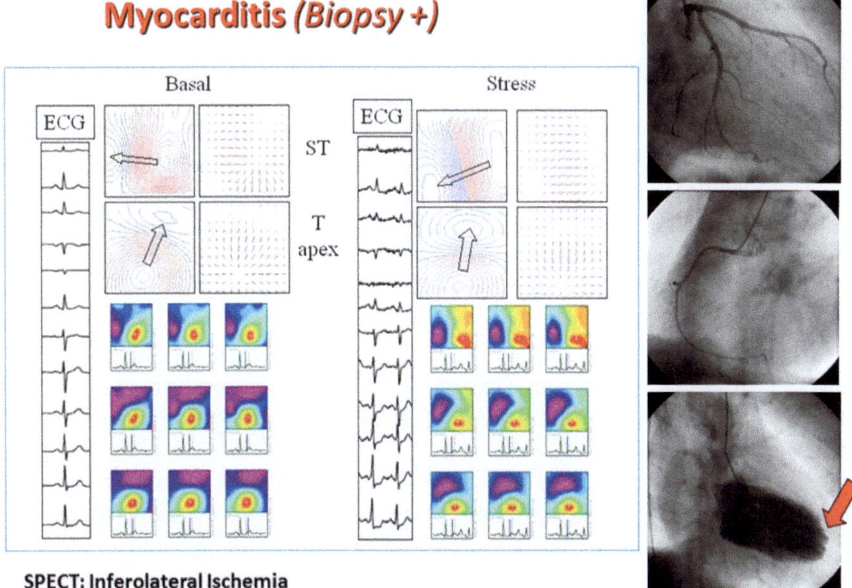



**Fig. 9** Example of MCG abnormality evidenced by exercise test, suggesting CAD in a 73-year-old patient with chest pain and ECG normal at rest and positive lateral ischemia under effort. Coronary angiography was normal. Left ventriculography and endomyocardial biopsy were diagnostic for subacute myocarditis. (Modified from reference [116])

(Fig. 8b), or other kinds of more severe myocardial injuries such as myocarditis (Fig. 9) and dilated cardiomyopathy [134, 151, 152].

On the other hand, one could speculate that such findings are further proof that MCG is very sensitive in detecting any sort of "myocardial ischemia," even when it is not determined by hemodynamically relevant stenoses of epicardial coronary arteries [150]. Indeed, an abnormal random current flowing during ventricular repolarization determined by inadequate oxygen supply [85] can also occur due to impairment of microcirculation, as seen in acute myocardial inflammation, papillary muscle strain, cardiomyopathy, or arterial hypertension, with consequent electrophysiological alteration initially detected by MCG only. One study has reported MCG parameters capable of differentiating between IHD and myocarditis [152]. Therefore, at the moment it might be more appropriate to assume that MCG is capable of ruling out any sort of "ischemic alteration" of the myocardium rather than to affirm that its abnormality is an index of CAD.

Present knowledge, however, does confirm that the accuracy of rest MCG in detecting an ischemic cardiac event is higher than that of rest ECG, and that a normal MCG provides a very high (although not absolute) negative predictive value useful to rule out the presence of a serious cardiomyopathy. Therefore, in order to reach clinical acceptance for MCG to be safely integrated in the workup of patients presenting in the ED with acute chest pain, more systematic MCG testing on undifferentiated patients is needed through appropriately designed multicenter controlled clinical trials, using, for example, the concept of the current European Society of Cardiology hs-cTnT/I 0/1-h algorithms [49] for validation. Recent results of the APACE trial, assessing the clinical performance of a point-of-care (POC)-hs-cTnI assay, have demonstrated that POC-hs-cTnI-TriageTrue assay provides high diagnostic accuracy (95% at presentation) in patients with suspected MI, excluding those with STEMI and kidney failure [153]. Thus, one might wonder if there is no longer a need, nor an acceptable cost-effectiveness in adding another diagnostic tool such as MCG, for the early rule-out of an ACS. However, one should consider that MCG has also proven useful for other diagnostic purposes such as fetal monitoring [154, 155], three-dimensional preinterventional imaging of arrhythmogenic substrates susceptible of ablation treatment [12, 156] and even for the noninvasive detection of partial mesenteric ischemia [157]. Thus, MCG may be considered a multipurpose diagnostic tool and return on investment shared among different clinical applications.

There are a few recent observational clinical trials that are currently investigating the diagnostic performance of the new generation of MCG devices designed to be deployed in emergency departments, or even portable for routine clinical use at the patient's bedside. A list of these can be found in the Appendix as well as at https://clinicaltrials.gov and https://ichgcp.net/registries. Three studies have been completed and their results recently published [43, 158, 159].

Two of these studies have been carried out to clinically test the reliability of a novel portable noncryogenic MCG mapping device, VitalScan (Creavo, UK) (Fig. 3c), in ruling-out ACS in patients with acute chest pain but had contradictory results. In the first study comparing MCG data of 70 IHD patients with those of 69 patients without IHD and those of 37 young healthy volunteers, a high sensitivity and a negative predictive value (> 95%) were found and the authors concluded that the portable unshielded magnetometer was adequate to assist in the triage of chest pain patients to rule out IHD [158]. However, the results of the second study, the MAGNET-ACS trial, a larger prospective multicenter observational study of 756 patients presenting to the ED with chest pain, showed very low diagnostic accuracy in adults with suspected ACS and the authors concluded that the MCG instrumentation used is currently unable to accurately rule out ACS and therefore not yet ready for use in clinical practice [159]. It remains to be understood why its performance was so different between the two studies. Examples of MCG imaging provided by the VitalScan device can be seen in figure 1 of reference [56].

The results of the third study, a single-center trial, testing the noncryogenic 36-channel MCG mapping system CardioFlux (Genetesis,—USA) (Fig. 3b) in 101 patients presenting to the ED with chest pain were also recently published [43]. The device, based on magneto-optic sensors (MOS), needs heavy electromagnetic shielding which was tentatively reduced to the minimum size of a tube the patient is slid into during the MCG recording. Examples of MCG imaging provided by the CardioFlux system can be seen in figure 3 of reference [43]. Unfortunately, the magnetic field sensitivity of the magneto-optic sensors MOS in such a reduced-scale MSR was not specified in the paper, nor are the waveforms shown for visual evaluation. The MCG device signal quality was evaluated by an automated function of the software and by the researchers before data analysis. Reported specificity (77.8%) and negative predictive value (89.7%) for coronary artery stenosis were well within the average [55, 56]. The authors concluded that a resting noninvasive, 90-s MCG scan using the novel imaging and analysis system shows promise in evaluating no high-risk chest pain patients which have a normal or nondiagnostic ECG and negative troponin results.

A very recent publication also suggests that MOS technology can provide very compact elliptically polarized laser-pumped Mx atomic magnetometers sensitive enough for clinical vector magnetocardiography (see figures 5–7 of reference [160]). However, the vMCG measurements were also carried out in a cylindrical five-layer 2 m-long magnetic shielding tube, that the patient slides into, which has some limitation for clinical use. In fact, Pena et al. reported that some patients with larger torsos had incomplete sensor capture likely due to sensor plate contact with the torso during scanning with CardioFlux and that about 3% of patients were not scanned due to claustrophobia [43]. Moreover, a mechanical barrier may not be desirable in high-risk chest pain patients with potential risk of sudden MACE. Unshielded MCG would be the most desirable option in these cases. Decades of clinical measurements have shown that SQUID-based systems featuring second- or higher-order gradiometers are reliable with adequate signal quality in unshielded hospital environments, as shown in a multicenter clinical trial reported by Tolstrup et al. [35], and also by other independent single-center studies [31, 57, 73, 146, 152, 161–163].

On the other hand, one major drawback of all cryogenic instrumentations has been the need for frequent (one to two times a week) refills of liquid helium to keep the system cool, implying related costs of helium and dedicated technical personnel. Such an expensive drawback has been overcome with the innovative technology of the Avalon-H90 3D MCG scanner system (*Mesuron LLC, US*) (Fig. 3a), which operates using a proprietary chamber with an integrated cooling system. Al the moment Mesuron's proprietary software focuses to visualize in the three dimensions the magnetic field vector movement throughout the T-wave ventricular repolarization phase (Fig. 10), aiming to use it for accurate detection of abnormalities generated by myocardial ischemia. In addition, a machine learning processing is used for automatic interpretation where minor nuances between normal variations versus abnormal or pathologic deviation changes can be differentiated. This system is currently being evaluated in a blinded clinical prospective observational study to assess the accuracy of magnetocardiography (MCG) as a tool for diagnosing acute coronary syndrome (ACS) in emergency department patients presenting with acute chest pain.

Based on previous experience [12, 164, 165], the configuration of the Avalon-H90 3D MCG is at the moment the only one MCG mapping system which has the potential to be used also during interventional procedures.

Finally, the development of new sensor technologies is foreseen to provide in the future more reliable portable and even wearable devices for noncontact MCG ambulatory monitoring of transient ischemic events [166]. Interestingly, the

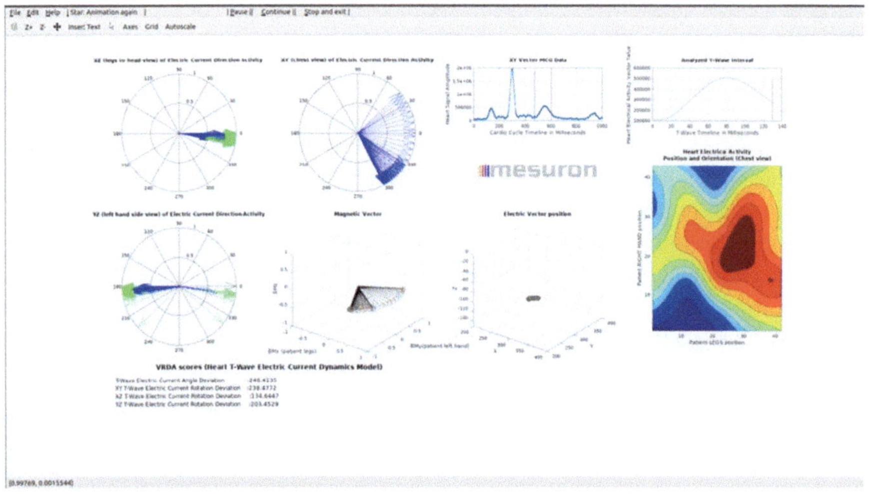

**Fig. 10** Example of Avalon-H90 3D imaging of T-wave current direction activity (each circle represent axial, frontal and sagittal heart views). Green arrows show the angle and blue ones show the relative strength of electrical current in a particular direction. In 3D charts you see direction deviation (on the left) and effective electrical current source displacement (on the right). Map shows an *XY* Vector value distribution. (Courtesy of A Bakharev, unpublished data)

reliability of a wearable MCG magneto-optic mapping prototype has been very recently reported, this innovative approach, however, is still needing electromagnetic heavy shielding [167].

## 3.5  *Potential Impact of MCG on the Management of Chest Pain in the Emergency Department*

The current typical management and workup of chest pain in the ED can be summarized as follows.

1. A brief history of chief complaint obtained at Triage.
2. Vitals taken and an ECG obtained.
3. Patients are taken to a room and seen by a provider for further history and a physical exam. A risk score assessment is commonly done and can further help define the likelihood of ACS as well as the risk level.
4. IV access is typically started during this initial phase.
5. If the ECG shows changes consistent with STEMI, or new/presumed new LBBB, the patient is either sent directly to the cath lab or to an institution that is equipped with a cath lab, or given thrombolytic therapy if "door to needle" time is estimated to be >90 min.

6. In the majority of patients with chest pain and ECG with normal or nonspecific ST T wave changes or unchanged LBBB from previous ECGs, a relative prolonged ED evaluation now begins. In summary this includes:

   (a) Baseline labs drawn including serial troponin at 0, 2, and 6 h. Results are typically returned in 20–45 min following the lab draw. Hence, the patient commonly will remain in the ED for a minimum of 3, but commonly up to 7 h following the initial lab draw.

   (b) The patient will be placed on a monitor and may be given stabilizing medications including nitroglycerin if ongoing pain while awaiting results of troponins and other lab tests.

   (c) If the patient remains stable and the troponin is either normal, or has a stable delta troponin, but clinical suspicion for unstable angina remains either by clinical judgment or by a reliable risk score assessment system such as the "Heart Pathway score," then the patient may be placed either in an ED observation unit or admitted under observation status to a monitored bed in the hospital. The workup during this phase will commonly include a stress test such as a standard ECG treadmill exercise test, or nuclear or echo stress test either by treadmill or pharmacologic induced stress.

   (d) A final disposition and plan is typically done at this point which may be either admission for cardiac catheterization or discharge with follow-up as an outpatient.

This relatively complex workup for these patients with suspected ACS is both time and resource consuming leading to a high cost, both for the individual and society. Further, a delay in treatment of an unrecognized ACS, may lead to further morbidity and mortality downstream.

So, what could the use of MCG potentially do in order to both improve the quality of care but also reduce resource consumption and cost? Potential changes in the management and workup of chest pain could instead be as follows:

1. If the accuracy of MCG could be shown to have a sensitivity approaching 98–100%, and if it is found to be normal while the patient is in the ED, then the patient could be assessed instead for other causes of their chest pain, for which the work-up in the majority of patients would be simpler, and the patient possibly discharged within 1–2 h after ED arrival. In addition, in patients with atypical symptoms or having an LBBB, early unpublished reports have suggested that MCG may accurately diagnose the presence or absence of ACS. This, however, remains to be proven.

2. For patients with a definitely positive MCG and a history and physical consistent with an ACS, the processes described under 6 above could be avoided and the patient sent directly for intervention to the cath lab or admitted to a monitored bed. This could avoid or minimize myocardial cell damage significantly. It also would reduce resource consumption significantly.

3. In addition, in the ED observation unit or outpatient setting, an MCG could potentially be used instead of nuclear or echo stress tests. These complex tests require many resources and highly trained personnel which may or may not be available in smaller hospitals. Instead, a highly accurate stress MCG could markedly improve on the accuracy of a standard stress test and potentially replace the standard ECG based stress test. As previously discussed, the single plane (Z plane) based MCG systems have not shown to have this needed degree of accuracy. Planned, and ongoing studies at this time may either prove or disprove this assumption with the technology currently available. However, further progress in software development for three- (and four-) dimensional volume rendering of current density reconstruction based on magnetic field mapping could theoretically provide higher degree of accuracy and bring the diagnostic power of MCG closer to that of nuclear scan.

# 4 Summary

Literature demonstrates that both shielded and unshielded MCG mapping can detect noninvasively electrophysiological abnormalities generated by hypoxia and ischemia of the myocardial fibers from the early stages of the ischemic event, thus adding a first-level additional quick diagnostic tool to evaluate cases with uncertain diagnosis. MCG has been proven reliable in differentiating cohorts of patients with ACS including NSTEMI, or patients with chronic stable IHD, from cohorts of healthy subjects or of patients with chest pain of noncardiac origin. However, the high sensitivity of MCG in detecting ischemia-related electrophysiological abnormalities might detect similar alterations due to other kind of cardiomyopathies, especially acute myocarditis, in the absence of CAD. At the moment no definite MCG criteria are available to differentiate among such clinical problems. On the other hand, a normal MCG scan has a very high negative predictive value in ruling-out the presence of a cardiomyopathy.

Large-scale prospective, multicenter observational studies of unselected undifferentiated patient cohorts are necessary to define the utility of MCG to rule out ACS in the emergency setting, and possibly to differentiate MCG abnormalities due to different pathogenic mechanisms. Standardization of MCG protocols, parameters, analytic methods, and further development of conversion software tools to a single output format, independent from the instrumentation and the recording environment used, will favor data pooling from multicenter studies [168].

**Acknowledgments** The authors would like to thank especially Alexander Bakharev for his help, comments, and pictures in the development of this chapter. He certainly also has been a major contributor and developer of MCG technology in the last 30 years.

# Appendix

### List of MCG clinical trials

1. https://clinicaltrials.gov/ct2/show/NCT02359773 **Quantum Imaging Limited;** Observational Pilot Study, MCG to Classify Non-Ischemic Chest Pain Patients and Myocardial Infarction Patients. Rule-out—ACS 70 pts—Principal Investigator: Mark Kearney, MBChB FRCP Leeds Teaching Hospitals NHS Trust. Results published in [158].

2. https://clinicaltrials.gov/ct2/show/NCT02921438 **Creavo UK;** Prospective Multi-centre Observational Study 756 chest pain patients. Rule-out ACS— "VitalScan MCG Rule-out Multi-centre Pivotal Study—UK (MAGNET-ACS)" Principal Investigator: Steve Goodacre, MB ChB MRCP DiplMC FCEM— University of Sheffield; Sheffield, UK. Results Completed—published in [159].

3. https://clinicaltrials.gov/ct2/show/NCT03255772?term=genetesis&rank=1 **Genetesis** Observational "Magnetocardiography Using a Novel Analysis System (Cardioflux) in the Evaluation of Emergency Department Observation Unit Chest Pain Patients." 101 chest pain patients—Rule-out ACS in ED—St. John Hospital Medical Center Detroit, Michigan, United States, 48,236. Completed—Results published in [43].

4. https://clinicaltrials.gov/ct2/show/NCT03546933 **Creavo US:** Prospective Multi-centre Observational Cohort Study: 651 chest pain patients. Rule-out ACS—"VitalScan MCG Rule-out Multi-centre Pivotal Study—US (MAGNET ACS)." Principal Investigator: Gregory J Fermann, MD—University of Cincinnati. Terminated (A correction needs to be made to the device's algorithm.)

5. https://clinicaltrials.gov/ct2/show/NCT04044391?term=genetesis&rank=2 **Genetesis Obervation cohort:** "Noninvasive Magnetocardiography Using the CardioFlux (TM) System in the Evaluation of Acute Coronary Syndrome Patients Going for Cardiac Catheterization." Intention to treat (Cath PCI)— Principal Investigator: Claire Pearson, M.D. Ascension St, John Medical Center. Terminated (Study was defunded.)

6. https://clinicaltrials.gov/ct2/show/NCT03968809?term=genetesis&rank=3 **Genetesis recruiting estimated completion day June 20, 2020** single-centre, prospective, Prospective Observational cohort 400 patients—"Role of Cardioflux in Predicting Coronary Artery Disease (CAD) Outcomes." Principal Investigator: Partho P Sengupta, MD—WVU Heart and Vascular Institute, J.W. Ruby Memorial Hospital. Recruiting.

7. https://clinicaltrials.gov/ct2/show/NCT00989924 *Research on the Correlation among Magnetocardiography Patterns and Known Cardiovascular Risk Factors in Diabetic Patients.* **—National Taiwan University Hospital— Observation 1100 Pts—Principal Investigator: Lee-Ming Chuang, MD. Ph.D.**

8. https://ichgcp.net/clinical-trials-registry/NCT04352816 **University Hospitals Coventry and Warwickshire NHS Trust** /Creavo UK. **Primary Completion Date: April 2021; Est study Completion Date: December 31, 2025**—Multi-centre Observational Cohort Trial Interventional—*MCG Parameters in the Prediction of Future ICD Therapy* 510 pts—Principal Investigator: **Faizel Osman, MD** FRCP FESC—University Hospital Coventry and Warwickshire. Recruiting.

9. https://www.clinicaltrials.gov/ct2/show/NCT00572442 **CardioMag Imaging/ Cedars-Sinai Medical Center**—MCG in Asymptomatic Individuals—Pilot Trial 40 HS—Withdrawn (sponsor funding) November 17, 2009—Principal Investigator: Kirsten Tolstrup, MDCedars-Sinai Medical Center.

10. https://clinicaltrials.gov/ct2/show/NCT00572949 **CardioMag Imaging/ Cedars-Sinai Medical Center**—MCG in the Diagnosis of Chest Pain Syndrome 398 pts—Withdrawn (sponsor funding) November 17, 2009—Principal Investigator: Kirsten Tolstrup, MD—Cedars-Sinai Medical Center.

11. https://www.clinicaltrials.gov/ct2/show/NCT00574561 **CardioMag Imaging/ Cedars-Sinai Medical Center**—MCG in Subjects Undergoing CT Angiography 300 pts—Withdrawn (sponsor funding) November 17, 2009—Principal Investigator: Kirsten Tolstrup, MD—Cedars-Sinai Medical Center.

12. https://clinicaltrials.gov/ct2/show/NCT00169975 **CardioMag Imaging Completed July 18, 2011** Observational—137 pts. MCG to diagnose ACS in ED—Principal Investigator:     Peter A. Smars, MD, EM—Mayo Clinic.

# References


1. Lüderitz B, de Luna AB. The history of electrocardiography. J Electrocardiol. 2017;50:539.
2. McClelland AJJ, Owens CG, Menown IBA, Lown M, Adgey AAJ. Comparison of the 80-lead body surface map to physician and to 12-lead electrocardiogram in detection of acute myocardial infarction. Am J Cardiol. 2003;92(3):252–7.
3. Dechamps M, Castanares-Zapatero D, Berghe PV, Meert P, Manara A. Comparison of clinical-based and ECG-based triage of acute chest pain in the Emergency Department. Intern Emerg Med. 2017;12(8):1245–51.
4. Fanaroff AC, Rymer JA, Goldstein SA, Simel DL, Newby LK. Does this patient with chest pain have acute coronary syndrome?: The rational clinical examination systematic review. JAMA. 2015;314(18):1955–65.
5. Kashyap R, Smars PA, Gartzen C, Bellolio MFRG. Incremental value of magnetocardiograph over electrocardiograph in diagnosing acute coronary syndrome inpatients presenting to the Emergency Department with high risk unstable angina. Ann Emerg Med. 2008;51:521.
6. Nakaya Y. [Magnetocardiography: a comparison with electrocardiography]. J Cardiogr Suppl. 1984;(3):31–40.
7. Mäkijärvi M, Korhonen P, Jurkko R, Väänänen H, Siltanen P, Hänninen H. Magnetocardiography. In: Macfarlane PW, van Oosterom A, Pahlm O, Kligfield P, Janse M, Camm J, editors. Comprehensive electrocardiology. London: Springer; 2010. p. 2007–28. https://doi.org/10.1007/978-1-84882-046-3_44.
8. Fenici R, Brisinda D, Meloni AM. Clinical application of magnetocardiography. Expert Rev Mol Diagn. 2005;5(3):291–313. http://www.tandfonline.com/doi/full/10.1586/14737159.5.3.291.

9. Yamada S, Yamaguchi I. Magnetocardiograms in clinical medicine: unique information on cardiac ischemia, arrhythmias, and fetal diagnosis. Intern Med. 2005;44(1):1–19.
10. Fenici R, Brisinda D, Venuti A, Sorbo AR. Thirty years of clinical magnetocardiography at the Catholic University of Rome: diagnostic value and new perspectives for the treatment of cardiac arrhythmias. Int J Cardiol. 2013;168(5):5113.
11. Sorbo AR, Lombardi G, La Brocca L, Guida G, Fenici R, Brisinda D. Unshielded magnetocardiography: repeatability and reproducibility of automatically estimated ventricular repolarization parameters in 204 healthy subjects. Ann Noninvasive Electrocardiol. 2018;23(3):1–12.
12. Lombardi G, Sorbo AR, Guida G, La Brocca L, Fenici R, Brisinda D. Magnetocardiographic classification and non-invasive electro-anatomical imaging of outflow tract ventricular arrhythmias in recreational sport activity practitioners. J Electrocardiol. 2018;51(3):433–9.
13. Cohen D. Shielded facility for low level magnetic measurements. J Appl Phys. 1967;38:1295.
14. Cohen D, Chandler L. Measurements and a simplified interpretation of magnetocardiograms from humans. Circulation. 1969;39(3):395–402.
15. Bardeen J, Cooper LN, Schrieffer JR. Microscopic theory of superconductivity. Phys Rev. 1957;106(1):162–4. https://link.aps.org/doi/10.1103/PhysRev.106.162.
16. Cohen D, Edelsack EA, Zimmerman JE. Magnetocardiograms taken inside a shielded room with a superconducting point-contact magnetometer. Appl Phys Lett. 1970;16:80–278. https://doi.org/10.1063/1.1653195.
17. Cohen D, Norman JC, Molokhia F, Hood W. Magnetocardiography of direct currents: S-T segment and baseline shifts during experimental myocardial infarction. Science. 1971;172(3990):1329–33.
18. Cohen D, Kaufman LA. Magnetic determination of the relationship between the S-T segment shift and the injury current produced by coronary artery occlusion. Circ Res. 1975;36(3):414–24. http://www.ncbi.nlm.nih.gov/pubmed/1111998.
19. Fenici R, Romani GL, Barbanera S, Zeppilli P, Carelli P, Modena I. High resolution magnetocardiography. Non-invasive investigation of the His-Purkinje system activity in man. G Ital Cardiol. 1980;10(10):1366.
20. Brockmeier K, Comani S, Erné SN, Di Luzio S, Pasquarelli A, Romani GL. Magnetocardiography and exercise testing. J Electrocardiol. 1994;27(2):137–42.
21. Hailer B, Van Leeuwen P, Lange S, Wehr M. Spatial distribution of QT dispersion measured by magnetocardiography under stress in coronary artery disease. J Electrocardiol. 1999;32(3):207–16.
22. Tavarozzi I, Comani S, Del Gratta C, Romani GL, Di Luzio S, Brisinda D, et al. Magnetocardiography: current status and perspectives. Part I: Physical principles and instrumentation. Ital Heart J. 2002;3(2):75–85. http://www.ncbi.nlm.nih.gov/pubmed/11926016.
23. Erné SN, Fenici RR, Hahlbohm H-D, Lehmann HP, Trontelj Z. Beat to beat surface recording and averaging of His-Purkinje activity in man. J Electrocardiol. 1983;16(4):355.
24. Barbanera S, Carelli P, Fenici R, Leoni R, Hadena I, Romani GL. Use of a superconducting instrumentation for biomagnetic measurements performed in a hospital(x). IEEE Trans Magn. 1981;17(1):849.
25. Mooney JW, Ghasemi-Roudsari S, Banham ER, Symonds C, Pawlowski N, Varcoe BTH. A portable diagnostic device for cardiac magnetic field mapping. Biomed Phys Eng Express. 2017;3(1):015008. http://stacks.iop.org/2057-1976/3/i=1/a=015008?key=crossref.2cec5aa bd79a18710f03f6459b94f27d.
26. Zhu K, Shah A, Berkow J, Kiourti A. Miniature coil Array for passive magnetocardiography in non-shielded environments. IEEE J Electromagn RF Microwaves Med Biol. 2020;44:1–19.
27. Fenici R, Mashkar R, Brisinda D. Performance of miniature scalar atomic magnetometers for magnetocardiography in an unshielded hospital laboratory for clinical electrophysiology. Eur Heart J. 2020;41(Suppl_2) https://doi.org/10.1093/ehjci/ehaa946.0386.

28. Seki Y, Kandori A, Kumagai Y, Ohnuma M, Ishiyama A, Ishii T, et al. Unshielded fetal magnetocardiography system using two-dimensional gradiometers. Rev Sci Instrum. 2008;79(3):36103–6.
29. Stroink G. Forty years of magnetocardiology. In: IFMBE proceedings; 2010.
30. Rogalla H, Kes PH, editors. 100 Years of superconductivity. Boca Raton: CRC Press; 2012.
31. Fenici R, Brisinda D, Nenonen J, Morana G, Fenici P. First {{}MCG{}} multichannel instrumentation operating in an unshielded hospital laboratory for multi-modal cardiac electrophysiology: preliminary experience. Biomed Tech Eng. 2001;46(s2):219–22. https://doi.org/10.1515/bmte.2001.46.s2.219.
32. Fenici R, Brisinda D. First 36-channel system for clinical magnetocardiography in unshielded Hospital Laboratory for Cardiac Electrophysiology. Int J Bioelectromagn. 2003;5(1):80–3.
33. Fenici R, Brisinda D. Predictive value of rest magnetocardiography in patients with stable angina. Int Congr Ser. 2007;1300:737–40.
34. Tavarozzi I, Comani S, Del Gratta C, Di Luzio S, Romani GL, Gallina S, et al. Magnetocardiography: current status and perspectives. Part II: Clinical applications. Ital Heart J. 2002 [cited 2017 Feb 20];3(3):151–65. http://www.ncbi.nlm.nih.gov/pubmed/11974660.
35. Tolstrup K, Madsen BE, Ruiz JA, Greenwood SD, Camacho J, Siegel RJ, et al. Non-invasive resting magnetocardiographic imaging for the rapid detection of ischemia in subjects presenting with chest pain. Cardiology. 2006;106(4):270–6. http://www.ncbi.nlm.nih.gov/pubmed/16733351.
36. Jurkko R, Mäntynen V, Tapanainen JM, Montonen J, Väänänen H, Parikka H, et al. Non-invasive detection of conduction pathways to left atrium using magnetocardiography: validation by intra-cardiac electroanatomic mapping. Europace. 2009;11(2):169–77.
37. Thiel F, Schnabel A, Knappe-Grüneberg S, Burghoff M, Drung D, Petsche F, et al. The 304 SQUIDs vector magnetometer system for biomagnetic measurements in the Berlin magnetically shielded room 2. Biomed Tech. 2005;50:169.
38. Wikswo J, Fairbank W. Application of superconducting magnetometers to the measurement of the vector magnetocardiogram. IEEE Trans Magn. 1977;13(1):354–7.
39. Nousiainen JJO, Tech D, Lekkala JO, Tech D, Malmivuo JAV. Comparative study of the normal vector magnetocardiogram and vector electrocardiogram. J Electrocardiol. 1986;19(3):275–90. http://www.sciencedirect.com/science/article/pii/S0022073686800371.
40. Burghoff M, Schleyerbach H, Drung D, Trahms L, Koch H. A vector magnetometer module for biomagnetic application. IEEE Trans Appl Supercond. 1999;9(2):4069–72.
41. Kominis IK, Kornack TW, Allred JC, Romalis MV. A subfemtotesla multichannel atomic magnetometer. Nature. 2003;422(6932):596–9. http://www.nature.com/doifinder/10.1038/nature01484.
42. Weis A, Wynands R, Fenici R, Bison G. Dynamical MCG mapping with an atomic vapor magnetometer. Neurol Clin Neurophysiol. 2004;2004:38.
43. Pena ME, Pearson CL, Goulet MP, Kazan VM, DeRita AL, Szpunar SM, et al. A 90-second magnetocardiogram using a novel analysis system to assess for coronary artery stenosis in Emergency department observation unit chest pain patients. Int J Cardiol Heart Vasc. 2020;26:100466. https://doi.org/10.1016/j.ijcha.2019.100466.
44. McCaig LF, Burt CW. National Hospital Ambulatory Medical Care Survey: 1999 emergency department summary. Adv Data. 2001;320:1–34.
45. Januzzi JL, McCarthy CP. Evaluating chest pain in the Emergency Department: searching for the optimal gatekeeper. J Am Coll Cardiol. 2018;71(6):617–9.
46. Hsia RY, Hale Z, Tabas JA. A national study of the prevalence of life-threatening diagnoses in patients with chest pain. JAMA Intern Med. 2016;176(7):1029–32.
47. Amsterdam EA, Kirk JD, Bluemke DA, Diercks D, Farkouh ME, Garvey JL, et al. Testing of low-risk patients presenting to the emergency department with chest pain: a scientific statement from the American Heart Association. Circulation. 2010;122(17):1756–76.

48. Montalescot G, Sechtem U, Achenbach S, Andreotti F, Arden C, Budaj A, et al. 2013 ESC guidelines on the management of stable coronary artery disease. Eur Heart J. 2013;34(38):2949–3003.

49. Roffi M, Patrono C, Collet JP, Mueller C, Valgimigli M, Andreotti F, et al. 2015 ESC guidelines for the management of acute coronary syndromes in patients presenting without persistent st-segment elevation: task force for the management of acute coronary syndromes in patients presenting without persistent ST-segment elevation of. Eur Heart J. 2016;37(3):267–315.

50. Wikswo JPJ, Barach JP. Possible sources of new information in the magnetocardiogram. J Theor Biol. 1982;95(4):721–9.

51. Roth BJ, Wikswo JP. Electrically silent magnetic fields. Biophys J. 1986;50(4):739–45.

52. Irimia A, Swinney KRWJ. Partial independence of bioelectric and biomagnetic fields and its implications for encephalography and cardiography. Phys Rev E Stat Nonlinear Soft Matter Phys. 2009;79:051908.

53. Dutz S, Bellemann ME, Leder U, Haueisen J. Passive vortex currents in magneto- and electrocardiography: comparison of magnetic and electric signal strengths. Phys Med Biol. 2006;51(1):145–51.

54. Brockmeier K, Schmitz L, De Jesus Bobadilla Chavez J, Burghoff M, Koch H, Zimmermann R, et al. Magnetocardiography and 32-lead potential mapping: repolarization in normal subjects during pharmacologically induced stress. J Cardiovasc Electrophysiol. 1997;8(6):615–26.

55. Agarwal R, Saini A, Alyousef T, Umscheid CA. Magnetocardiography for the diagnosis of coronary artery disease: a systematic review and meta-analysis. Ann Noninvasive Electrocardiol. 2012;17(4):291–8.

56. Camm AJ, Henderson R, Brisinda D, Body R, Charles RG, Varcoe B, et al. Clinical utility of magnetocardiography in cardiology for the detection of myocardial ischemia. J Electrocardiol. 2019;57:10–7.

57. Chaikovsky I, Hailer B, Sosnytskyy V, Lutay M, Mjasnikov G, Kazmirchuk A, et al. Predictive value of the complex magnetocardiographic index in patients with intermediate pretest probability of chronic coronary artery disease: results of a two-center study. Coron Artery Dis. 2014;25(6):474–84.

58. Wu Y-W, Lee C-M, Liu Y-B, Wang S-S, Huang H-C, Tseng W-K, et al. Usefulness of magnetocardiography to detect coronary artery disease and cardiac allograft vasculopathy. Circ J. 2013;77(7):1783–90. http://www.ncbi.nlm.nih.gov/pubmed/23603823.

59. Steinisch M, Torke PR, Haueisen J, Hailer B, Grönemeyer D, Van Leeuwen P, et al. Early detection of coronary artery disease in patients studied with magnetocardiography: an automatic classification system based on signal entropy. Comput Biol Med. 2013;43(2):144.

60. Kwon H, Kim K, Lee YH, Kim JM, Yu KK, Chung N, et al. Non-invasive magnetocardiography for the early diagnosis of coronary artery disease in patients presenting with acute chest pain. Circ J. 2010;74(7):1424–30.

61. Tao R, Zhang S, Huang X, Tao M, Ma J, Ma S, et al. Magnetocardiography-based ischemic heart disease detection and localization using machine learning methods. IEEE Trans Biomed Eng. 2019;66(6):1658–67.

62. Shin ES, Park SG, Saleh A, Lam YY, Bhak J, Jung F, Morita SBJ. Magnetocardiography scoring system to predict the presence of obstructive coronary artery disease. Clin Hemorheol Microcirc. 2018;70(4):365–73.

63. Savard P, Cohen D, Lepeschkin E, Cuffin BN, Madias JE. Magnetic measurement of S-T and T-Q segment shifts in humans. Part I: early repolarization and left bundle branch block. Circ Res. 1983;53(2):264–73.

64. Cohen D, Savard P, Rifkin RD. Magnetic measurements of S-T and T-Q segment shifts in humans. Part II: exercise-induced S-T segment depression. Circ Res. 1983;53(2):274–9.

65. Antzelevitch C, Yan GX, Ackerman MJ, Borggrefe M, Corrado D, Guo J, et al. J-wave syndromes expert consensus conference report: emerging concepts and gaps in knowledge. Europace. 2017;19(4):665–94.

66. Cohen D, Lepeschkin E, Hosaka H, Massell BF, Myers G. Part I: abnormal patterns and physiological variations in magnetocardiograms. J Electrocardiol. 1976;9(4):398–409.

67. Saarinen M, Karp PJ, Katila TE, Siltanen P. The magnetocardiogram in cardiac disorders. Cardiovasc Res. 1974;8(6):820–34. https://doi.org/10.1093/cvr/8.6.820.

68. Saarinen M, Siltanen P, Karp PJ, Katila TE. The normal magnetocardiogram: I morphology. Ann Clin Res. 1978;10(Suppl 2):1–43.

69. Awano I, Muramoto A, Awano N. An approach to clinical Magnetocardiology. Tohoku J Exp Med. 1982;138(4):367–81.

70. Karp PJ, Katila TE, Saarinen M, Siltanen P, Varpula TT. The normal human magnetocardiogram. II. A multipole analysis. Circ Res. 1980;47(1):117–30.

71. Green LS, Lux RL, Stilli D, Haws CW, Taccardi B. Fine detail in body surface potential maps: accuracy of maps using a limited lead array and spatial and temporal data representation. J Electrocardiol. 1987;20(1):21–6.

72. Tolstrup K, Brisinda D, Meloni AM, Cheung B, Siegel RJFR. Comparison of resting magnetocardiography with stress single photon emission computed tomography in patients with stable and unstable angina. J Am Coll Cardiol. 2006;47(4 Suppl 1):176.

73. Steinberg BA, Roguin A, Watkins SP, Hill P, Fernando D, Resar JR. Magnetocardiogram recordings in a nonshielded environment--reproducibility and ischemia detection. Ann Noninvasive Electrocardiol. 2005;10(2):152–60. http://www.ncbi.nlm.nih.gov/pubmed/15842427.

74. Park J-W, Hill PM, Chung N, Hugenholtz PG, Jung F. Magnetocardiography predicts coronary artery disease in patients with acute chest pain. Ann Noninvasive Electrocardiol. 2005 [cited 2017 Feb 20];10(3):312–23. http://www.ncbi.nlm.nih.gov/pubmed/16029382.

75. Bakharev AA. Ischemia identification, quantification and partial localization in MCG—EP 1 349 494 B1, vol. Bulletin 2; 2011. p. 1–20.

76. Erné SN, Fenici RR, Hahlbohm H-D, Jaszczuk W, Lehmann HP, Masselli M. High-resolution isofield mapping in magnetocardiography. Nuovo Cim D. 1983;2(2):291.

77. Nenonen JT. Solving the inverse problem in magnetocardiography. IEEE Eng Med Biol Mag. 1994;13(4):487–96.

78. Hänninen H, Takala P, Mäkijärvi M, Montonen J, Korhonen P, Oikarinen L, et al. Detection of exercise-induced myocardial ischemia by multichannel magnetocardiography in single vessel coronary artery disease. Ann Noninvasive Electrocardiol. 2000;5(2):147–57.

79. Hänninen H, Takala P, Mäkijärvi M, Montonen J, Korhonen P, Oikarinen L, et al. Recording locations in multichannel magnetocardiography and body surface potential mapping sensitive for regional exercise-induced myocardial ischemia. Basic Res Cardiol. 2001;96(4):405–14. http://www.ncbi.nlm.nih.gov/pubmed/11518197.

80. Van Leeuwen P, Hailer B, Lange S, Gronemeyer D. Spatial distribution of repolarization times in patients with coronary artery disease. Pacing Clin Electrophysiol. 2003;26(8):1706–14.

81. Van Leeuwen P, Hailer B, Lange S, Klein A, Geue D, Seybold K, et al. Quantification of cardiac magnetic field orientation during ventricular de- and repolarization. Phys Med Biol. 2008;53(9):2291–301. https://doi.org/10.1088/2F0031-9155/2F53/2F9/2F006.

82. Park JW, Jung F. Qualitative and quantitative description of myocardial ischemia by means of magnetocardiography. Biomed Tech (Berl). 2004 [cited 2017 Feb 20];49(10):267–73. http://www.ncbi.nlm.nih.gov/pubmed/15566075.

83. Park J-W, Leithäuser B, Hill P, Jung F. Resting magnetocardiography predicts 3-year mortality in patients presenting with acute chest pain without ST segment elevation. Ann Noninvasive Electrocardiol. 2008;13(2):171–9. http://doi.wiley.com/10.1111/j.1542-474X.2008.00217.x.

84. Kandori A, Ogata K, Miyashita T, Takaki H, Kanzaki H, Hashimoto S, et al. Subtraction magnetocardiogram for detecting coronary heart disease. Ann Noninvasive Electrocardiol. 2010;15(4):360–8.

85. Tsukada K, Miyashita T, Kandori A, Mitsui T, Terada Y, Sato M, et al. An iso-integral mapping technique using magnetocardiogram, and its possible use for diagnosis of ischemic heart disease. Int J Card Imaging. 2000;16(1):55–66. http://www.ncbi.nlm.nih.gov/pubmed/10832626.

86. Shiono J, Horigome H, Matsui A, Terada Y, Watanabe S, Miyashita T, et al. Evaluation of myocardial ischemia in Kawasaki disease using an isointegral map on magnetocardiogram. Pacing Clin Electrophysiol. 2002;25(6):915–21. http://www.ncbi.nlm.nih.gov/pubmed/12137343.

87. Gapelyuk A, Schirdewan A, Fischer R, Wessel N. Cardiac magnetic field mapping quantified by Kullback{\textendash}Leibler entropy detects patients with coronary artery disease. Physiol Meas. 2010;31(10):1345–54. https://doi.org/10.1088/2F0967-3334/2F31/2F10/2F004.

88. Wu YW, Lin LC, Tseng WK, Bin LY, Kao HL, Lin MS, et al. QTc heterogeneity in rest magnetocardiography is sensitive to detect coronary artery disease: in comparison with stress myocardial perfusion imaging. Acta Cardiol Sin. 2014;30(5):445–54.

89. Fenici R, Brisinda D, Meloni AM, Sternickel K, Fenici P. Clinical validation of machine learning for automatic analysis of multichannel magnetocardiography. FIMH. 2005;3504:143–52.

90. Tantimongcolwat T, Naenna T, Isarankura-Na-Ayudhya C, Embrechts MJ, Prachayasittikul V. Identification of ischemic heart disease via machine learning analysis on magnetocardiograms. Comput Biol Med. 2008;38(7):817–25. http://linkinghub.elsevier.com/retrieve/pii/S001048250800070X.

91. Kwon H, Kim K, Kim JM, Lee YH, Lim HK, Kim TE, et al. Classification of magnetocardiographic parameters based on the probability density function. J Korean Phys Soc. 2006;48(5 I):1114–6.

92. Park J-W, Shin E-S, Ann SH, Gödde M, Park LS-I, Brachmann J, et al. Validation of magnetocardiography versus fractional flow reserve for detection of coronary artery disease. Clin Hemorheol Microcirc. 2015;59(3):267–81. http://www.ncbi.nlm.nih.gov/pubmed/25480934.

93. Shin E-S, Lam Y-Y, Her A-Y, Brachmann J, Jung F, Park J-W. Incremental diagnostic value of combined quantitative and qualitative parameters of magnetocardiography to detect coronary artery disease. Int J Cardiol. 2017;228:948–52. http://linkinghub.elsevier.com/retrieve/pii/S0167527316336257.

94. Hosaka H, Cohen D, Cuffin BN, Horacek BM. Part III the effect of the torso boundaries on the magnetocardiogram. J Electrocardiol. 1976;9(4):418–25. http://www.sciencedirect.com/science/article/pii/S0022073676800428.

95. Ogata K, Kandori A, Watanabe Y, Suzuki A, Tanaka K, Oka Y, et al. Repolarization spatial-time current abnormalities in patients with coronary heart disease. Pacing Clin Electrophysiol. 2009;32(4):516–24.

96. Haberkorn W, Steinhoff U, Burghoff M, Kosch O, Morguet A, Koch H. Pseudo current density maps of electrophysiological heart, nerve or brain function and their physical basis. Biomagn Res Technol. 2006;4:5.

97. Kandori A, Ogata K, Miyashita T, Watanabe Y, Tanaka K, Murakami M, et al. Standard template of adult magnetocardiogram. Ann Noninvasive Electrocardiol. 2008;13(4):391–400.

98. Kandori A, Kanzaki H, Miyatake K, Hashimoto S, Itoh S, Tanaka N, et al. A method for detecting myocardial abnormality by using a total current-vector calculated from ST-segment deviation of a magnetocardiogram signal. Med Biol Eng Comput. 2001;39(1):21–8. http://www.ncbi.nlm.nih.gov/pubmed/11214269.

99. Ikefuji H, Masahiro N, Nakaya Y, Mori T, Kondo N, Ieishi K, et al. Visualization of cardiac dipole using a current density map: detection of cardiac current undetectable by electrocardiography using magnetocardiography. J Med Investig. 2007;54(1–2):116–23.

100. Hailer B, Van Leeuwen P, Chaikovsky I, Auth-Eisernitz S, Schafer H, Gronemeyer D. The value of magnetocardiography in the course of coronary intervention. Ann Noninvasive Electrocardiol. 2005;10(2):188–96.

101. Smith WE, Dallas WJ, Kullmann WH, Schlitt HA. Linear estimation theory applied to the reconstruction of a 3-D vector current distribution. Appl Opt. 1990;29(5):658–67.

102. Kullmann WH. Separation of sources of neuromagnetic examinations. Physiol Meas. 1993;14(4A):A27–34. https://doi.org/10.1088/2F0967-3334/2F14/2F4a/2F005.

103. Leder U, Haueisen J, Huck M, Nowak H. Non-invasive imaging of arrhythmogenic left-ventricular myocardium after infarction. Lancet. 1998;352(9143):1825.

104. Fenici R, Brisinda D, Pesola K, Nenonen J. Validation of magnetocardiographic current density imaging with a non-magnetic stimulation catheter. In: Proceedings of 12th international conference on biomagnetism; 2001. p. 839–42. http://citeseerx.ist.psu.edu/viewdoc/download?doi=10.1.1.5.7244&rep=rep1&type=pdf.

105. Nenonen J, Pesola K, Feneici R, Lauerma K, Mäkijärvi M, Katila T. Current density imaging of focal cardiac sources. Biomed Tech Eng. 2009;46(s2):50–3.

106. Goernig M, Haueisen J, Schreiber J, Leder U, Hänninen H, Mäkelä T, et al. Comparison of current density viability imaging at rest with FDG-PET in patients after myocardial infarction. Comput Med Imaging Graph. 2009;33(1):1–6.

107. Chaikovsky I, Primin M, Nedayvoda I, Verba A, Mjasnikov G, Kazmirchyk A, et al. GW28-e0524 Magnetocardiographic polar map image reveal regional wall motion abnormalities: comparison study with stress-echocardiography. J Am Coll Cardiol. 2017;70(16):C88. https://doi.org/10.1016/j.jacc.2017.07.309.

108. Sosnytskyy VN, Stadnyuk LA, Sosnytska TV, Kozhukhov SN, Miasnikov GV. Value of current density dispersion alternans assessed by magnetocardiography mapping in patients with ischemic heart disease and ventricular arrhythmias. Eur Heart J. 2017;38(Suppl_1):P5502. https://doi.org/10.1093/eurheartj/ehx493.P5502.

109. Zhao C, Jiang S, Wu Y, Zhu J, Zhou D, Hailer B, et al. An integrated maximum current density approach for noninvasive detection of myocardial infarction. IEEE J Biomed Heal informatics. 2018;22(2):495–502.

110. Nakai K, Kazui T, Okabayashi H, Hayashi R, Fukushima A, Suwabe A. Development of three-dimensional analysis of current density distribution by 64-ch magnetocardiography and clinical application. Rinsho Byori. 2008;56(12):1118–24.

111. Nenonen J, Pesola K, Hänninen H, Lauerma K, Takala P, Mäkelä T, et al. Current-density estimation of exercise-induced ischemia in patients with multivessel coronary artery disease. J Electrocardiol. 2001;34(Suppl):37–42. http://www.ncbi.nlm.nih.gov/pubmed/11781934.

112. Park J-W, Leithäuser B, Vrsansky M, Jung F, et al. Clin Hemorheol Microcirc. 2008;39(1–4):21–32. http://www.ncbi.nlm.nih.gov/pubmed/18503107.

113. Kwong JSW, Leithäuser B, Park J-W, Yu C-M. Diagnostic value of magnetocardiography in coronary artery disease and cardiac arrhythmias: A review of clinical data. Int J Cardiol. 2013;167(5):1835–42. https://doi.org/10.1016/j.ijcard.2012.12.056.

114. Hailer B, Chaikovsky I, Auth-Eisernitz S, Schäfer H, Steinberg F, Grönemeyer DHW. Magnetocardiography in coronary artery disease with a new system in an unshielded setting. Clin Cardiol. 2003;26(10):465–71.

115. Fenici R, Brisinda D, Meloni AM. Effects of filtering on computer-aided analysis for detection of chronic ischemic heart disease with unshielded rest magnetocardiography mapping. Neurol Clin Neurophysiol. 2004;2004:7.

116. Brisinda D, Meloni AM, Fenici R. First 36-channel magnetocardiographic study of CAD patients in an unshielded laboratory for interventional and intensive cardiac care. Funct Imaging Model Heart. 2003;LNCS 2674:122–31.

117. Brisinda D, Meloni AM, Nenonen J, Giorgi A, Fenici R. First 36-channel magnetocardiographic study of patients with coronary artery disease in an unshielded laboratory. Biomed Tech. 2004;Band 48(Ergänzungsband 2):134–6.

118. Brisinda D, Meloni AM, Nenonen J, Fenici R. Unshielded stress multichannel magnetocardiography of patients with coronary disease and normal subjects with standard ergometer. Comparison with ECG. Biomed Tech. 2004;48(2):137–9.

119. Endt P, Hahlbohm HD, Kreiseler D, Oeff M, Steinhoff U, Trahms L. Fragmentation of bandpass-filtered QRS-complex of patients prone to malignant arrhythmia. Med Biol Eng Comput. 1998;36(6):723–8.

120. Korhonen P, Husa T, Tierala I, Väänänen H, Mäkijärvi M, Katila T, et al. Increased intra-QRS fragmentation in magnetocardiography as a predictor of arrhythmic events and mortality in patients with cardiac dysfunction after myocardial infarction. J Cardiovasc Electrophysiol. 2006;17(4):396–401.

121. Gapelyuk A, Wessel N, Fischer R, Zacharzowsky U, Koch L, Selbig D, et al. Detection of patients with coronary artery disease using cardiac magnetic field mapping at rest. J Electrocardiol. 2007;40(5):401–7.

122. Iwakami N, Aiba T, Kamakura S, Takaki H, Furukawa TA, Sato T. Identification of malignant early repolarization pattern by late QRS activity in high-resolution magnetocardiography. Ann Noninvasive Electrocardiol. 2020;25:e12741.

123. Kardesch M, Hogancamp CE, Bing RJ. The effect of complete ischemia on the intracellular electrical activity of the whole mammalian heart. Circ Res. 1958;6(6):715–20. http://circres.ahajournals.org/cgi/doi/10.1161/01.RES.6.6.715.

124. Holland RP, Brooks H. Precordial and epicardial surface potentials during myocardial ischemia in the pig: a theoretical and experimental analysis of the TQ And ST segments. Circ Res. 1975;37:471–80.

125. Spach MS, Barr RC, Johnson EA, Kootsey JM. Cardiac extracellular potentials. Analysis of complex wave forms about the Purkinje networks in dogs. Circ Res. 1973;33(4):465–73.

126. Hänninen H, Takala P, Mäkijärvi M, Korhonen P, Oikarinen L, Simelius K, et al. ST-segment level and slope in exercise-induced myocardial ischemia evaluated with body surface potential mapping. Am J Cardiol. 2001;88(10):1152–6.

127. Takala P, Hänninen H, Montonen J, Korhonen P, Mäkijärvi M, Nenonen J, et al. Heart rate adjustment of magnetic field map rotation in detection of myocardial ischemia in exercise magnetocardiography. Basic Res Cardiol. 2002;97(1):88–96. http://www.ncbi.nlm.nih.gov/pubmed/11998980.

128. Hänninen H, Takala P, Korhonen P, Oikarinen L, Mäkijärvi M, Nenonen J, et al. Features of ST segment and T-wave in exercise-induced myocardial ischemia evaluated with multichannel magnetocardiography. Ann Med. 2002;34(2):120–9. http://www.ncbi.nlm.nih.gov/pubmed/12108575.

129. Takala P, Hanninen H, Montonen J, Makijarvi M, Nenonen J, Oikarinen L, et al. Magnetocardiographic and electrocardiographic exercise mapping in healthy subjects. Ann Biomed Eng. 2001;29(6):501–9.

130. Kanzaki H, Nakatani S, Kandori A, Tsukada K, Miyatake K. A new screening method to diagnose coronary artery disease using multichannel magnetocardiogram and simple exercise. Basic Res Cardiol. 2003;98(2):124–32.

131. Lim HK, Kwon H, Chung N, Ko Y-G, Kim J-M, Kim I-S, et al. Usefulness of magnetocardiogram to detect unstable angina pectoris and non-ST elevation myocardial infarction. Am J Cardiol. 2009;103(4):448–54. http://linkinghub.elsevier.com/retrieve/pii/S0002914908018766.

132. Shin E-S, Ann SH, Brachmann J, Lam Y-Y, Jung F, Park J-W. Noninvasive detection of myocardial ischemia: a case of magnetocardiography. Clin Hemorheol Microcirc. 2015;60(1):163–9. http://www.medra.org/servlet/aliasResolver?alias=iospress&doi=10.3233/CH-151945.

133. Kawakami S, Takaki H, Hashimoto S, Kimura Y, Nakashima T, Aiba T, et al. Utility of high-resolution magnetocardiography to predict later cardiac events in nonischemic cardiomyopathy patients with normal QRS duration. Circ J. 2017;81(1):44–51.

134. Korhonen P, Vaananen H, Makijarvi M, Katila T, Toivonen L. Repolarization abnormalities detected by Magnetocardiography in patients with dilated cardiomyopathy and ventricular arrhythmias. J Cardiovasc Electrophysiol. 2001;12(7):772–7. https://doi.org/10.1046/j.1540-8167.2001.00772.x.

135. Flüg M, Achenbach S, Moshage W, Schubert J, Bachmann K. [Bicycle ergometric stress in healthy probands: differences between magnetocardiography (2-plane measurement) and electrocardiography]. Biomed Tech (Berl). 1997;42(Suppl):241–2.

136. On K, Watanabe S, Yamada S, Takeyasu N, Nakagawa Y, Nishina H, et al. Integral value of JT interval in magnetocardiography is sensitive to coronary stenosis and improves soon after coronary revascularization. Circ J. 2007;71(10):1586–92.

137. Morguet AJ, Behrens S, Kosch O, Lange C, Zabel M, Selbig D, et al. Myocardial viability evaluation using magnetocardiography in patients with coronary artery disease. Coron Artery Dis. 2004;15(3):155–62. http://www.ncbi.nlm.nih.gov/pubmed/15096996.
138. Zhao C, Chen Y, Zhao D, Wang J, Chen Q. Comparison between magnetocardiography and myocardial perfusion imaging in the diagnosis of myocardial ischemia in patients with coronary artery disease. Int J Clin Exp Med. (ISSN : 1940-5901). 2019;12(11):13127–34.
139. Gibbons RJ, Balady GJ, Bricker JT, Chaitman BR, Fletcher GF, Froelicher VF, et al. ACC/AHA 2002 guideline update for exercise testing: summary article: a report of the American College of Cardiology/American Heart Association Task Force on Practice Guidelines (Committee to Update the 1997 Exercise Testing Guidelines). Circulation. 2002;106(14):1883–92.
140. Hendel RC, Berman DS, Di Carli MF, Heidenreich PA, Henkin RE, Pellikka PA, et al. ACCF/ASNC/ACR/AHA/ASE/SCCT/SCMR/SNM 2009 appropriate use criteria for cardiac radionuclide imaging: a report of the American College of Cardiology Foundation Appropriate Use Criteria Task Force, the American Society of Nuclear Cardiology, the American College of Radiology, the American Heart Association, the American Society of Echocardiography, the Society of Cardiovascular Computed Tomography, the Society for Cardiovascular Magnetic Resonance, and the Society of Nuclear Medicine. Circulation. 2009;119(22):e561–87.
141. Fenici R, Brisinda D, Nenonen J, Fenici P. Phantom validation of multichannel magnetocardiography source localization. Pacing Clin Electrophysiol. 2003;26(1 Pt 2):426–30.
142. Fenici R, Nenonen J, Pesola K, Korhonen P, Lötjönen J, Mäkijärvi M, et al. Nonfluoroscopic localization of an amagnetic stimulation catheter by multichannel magnetocardiography. Pacing Clin Electrophysiol. 1999;22(8):1210–20.
143. Oikarinen L, Paavola M, Montonen J, Viitasalo M, Mäkijärvi M, Toivonen L, et al. Magnetocardiographic QT interval dispersion in postmyocardial infarction patients with sustained ventricular tachycardia: validation of automated QT measurements. Pacing Clin Electrophysiol. 1998;21(10):1934–42.
144. Gödde P, Agrawal R, Müller HP, Czerki K, Endt P, Steinhoff U, et al. Magnetocardiographic mapping of QRS fragmentation in patients with a history of malignant tachyarrhythmias. Clin Cardiol. 2001;24(10):682–8.
145. Mäkelä T, Pham QC, Clarysse P, Nenonen J, Lötjönen J, Sipilä O, et al. A 3-D model-based registration approach for the PET, MR and MCG cardiac data fusion. Med Image Anal. 2003;7(3):377–89.
146. Huang X, Hua N, Tang F, Zhang S. Effectiveness of magnetocardiography to identify patients in need of coronary artery revascularization: a cross-sectional study. Cardiovasc Diagn Ther. 2020;10(4):831–40.
147. Tamaki W, Tsuda E, Hashimoto S, Toyomasa T, Fujieda M. Magnetocardiographic recognition of abnormal depolarization and repolarization in patients with coronary artery lesions caused by Kawasaki disease. Heart Vessel. 2019;34(10):1571–9.
148. Tamaki W, Tsuda E, Hashimoto S, Toyomasa T, Fujieda M. Correction to: Magnetocardiographic recognition of abnormal depolarization and repolarization in patients with coronary artery lesions caused by Kawasaki disease. Heart Vessel. 2019;34(10):1580.
149. Brisinda D, Meloni AM, Fenici R. Magnetocardiographic study of ventricular repolarization in hypertensive patients with and without left ventricular hypertrophy. Neurol Clin Neurophysiol. 2004;2004:13.
150. Brisinda D, Meloni A, Fenici P, Fenici R. Unshielded multichannel magnetocardiographic study of ventricular repolarization abnormalities in patients with mitral valve prolapse. Biomed Tech. 2004;48(2):128–30.
151. Shiono J, Horigome H, Matsui A, Terada Y, Miyashita T, Tsukada K. Detection of repolarization abnormalities in patients with cardiomyopathy using current vector mapping technique on magnetocardiogram. Int J Cardiovasc Imaging. 2003;19(2):163–70.
152. Sosnytskyy V, Chaikovsky I, Stadnyuk L, Miasnykov G, Kazmirchyk A, Sosnytska T, et al. Magnetocardiography capabilities in myocardium injuries diagnosis. World J Cardiovasc Dis. 2013;03(05):380–8.

153. Boeddinghaus J, Nestelberger T, Koechlin L, Wussler D, Lopez-Ayala P, Walter JE, et al. Early diagnosis of myocardial infarction with point-of-care high-sensitivity cardiac troponin I. J Am Coll Cardiol. 2020;75(10):1111–24.

154. Escalona-Vargas D, Bolin EH, Lowery CL, Siegel ER, Eswaran H. Recording and quantifying fetal magnetocardiography signals using a flexible array of optically-pumped magnetometers. Physiol Meas. 2021;41(12):125003. https://doi.org/10.1088/1361-6579/abc353.

155. Desai L, Wakai R, Tsao S, Strasburger J, Gotteiner N, Patel A. Fetal diagnosis of KCNQ1-variant long QT syndrome using fetal echocardiography and magnetocardiography. Pacing Clin Electrophysiol. 2020;43(4):430–3.

156. Guida G, Sorbo AR, Fenici R, Brisinda D. Predictive value of unshielded magnetocardiographic mapping to differentiate atrial fibrillation patients from healthy subjects. Ann Noninvasive Electrocardiol. 2018;23(6):e12569.

157. Somarajan S, Muszynski ND, Olson JD, Bradshaw LA, Richards WO. Magnetoenterography for the detection of partial mesenteric ischemia. J Surg Res. 2019;239:31–7.

158. Ghasemi-Roudsari S, Al-Shimary A, Varcoe B, Byrom R, Kearney L, Kearney M. A portable prototype magnetometer to differentiate ischemic and non-ischemic heart disease in patients with chest pain. PLoS One. 2018;13(1):1–10. https://doi.org/10.1371/journal.pone.0191241.

159. Goodacre S, Walters SJ, Qayyum H, Coffey F, Carlton E, Coats T, et al. Diagnostic accuracy of the magnetocardiograph for patients with suspected acute coronary syndrome. Emerg Med J. 2020; https://doi.org/10.1136/emermed-2020-210396.

160. Zheng W, Su S, Zhang G, Bi X, Lin Q. Vector magnetocardiography measurement with a compact elliptically polarized laser-pumped magnetometer. Biomed Opt Express. 2020;11(2):649.

161. Li Y, Che Z, Quan W, Yuan R, Shen Y, Liu Z, et al. Diagnostic outcomes of magnetocardiography in patients with coronary artery disease. Int J Clin Exp Med. 2015;8(2):2441–6.

162. Park JW, Hill PM, Chung N, Hugenholtz PG, Jung F. Magnetocardiography predicts coronary artery disease in patients with acute chest pain. Ann Noninvasive Electrocardiol. 2005;10(3):312–23. https://doi.org/10.1111/j.1542-474X.2005.00634.x.

163. Leithäuser B, Park J-W, Hill P, Lam Y-Y, Jung F. Magnetocardiography in patients with acute chest pain and bundle branch block. Int J Cardiol. 2013;168(1):582–3. http://www.sciencedirect.com/science/article/pii/S0167527313003148.

164. Fenici R, Brisinda D. Bridging noninvasive and interventional electroanatomical imaging: role of magnetocardiography. J Electrocardiol. 2007;40(1 Suppl):47–52.

165. Fenici R, Brisinda D. From 3D to 4D imaging: is that useful for interventional cardiac electrophysiology? Annu Int Conf IEEE Eng Med Biol Soc. 2007;2007:5996–9. https://doi.org/10.1109/IEMBS.2007.4353714.

166. Lau S, Petković B, Haueisen J. Optimal magnetic sensor vests for cardiac source imaging. Sensors (Switzerland). 2016;16(6):1–17.

167. Yang Y, Xu M, Liang A, Yin Y, Ma X, Gao Y, et al. A new wearable multichannel magnetocardiogram system with a SERF atomic magnetometer array. Sci Rep. 2021;11(1):1–12.

168. Burghoff M, Nenonen J, Trahms L, Katila T. Conversion of magnetocardiographic recordings between two different multichannel SQUID devices. IEEE Trans Biomed Eng. 2000;47(7):869–75.

# Disposition from the Short Stay Unit

**Jason P. Stopyra**

## 1 Chest Pain Unit Patient Entry: Appropriate Patient Selection

Appropriate initial patient selection is one of the most critical determinants of success of the disposition process from a chest pain unit (CPU). In most cases, patients with a chief complaint of chest pain are placed in a CPU by an emergency physician after initial patient evaluation. A history, physical examination, 12-lead electrocardiogram (ECG), and initial serum cardiac biomarker measurement is assumed to be performed before entry into a CPU. The basic information obtained through this process should help to identify either a) patients at such high risk for acute coronary syndrome (ACS) or adverse events that inpatient admission is indicated without further testing or b) patients with syndromes that are clearly noncardiac in origin where initiation of a clinical pathway to rule out ACS would not be appropriate. In addition, before entry into the CPU, practical and logistical factors that prevent safe discharge of the patient from the hospital should be assessed. Early identification of this type of patient will enable the CPU to run more efficiently and prevent final patient disposition problems. This is particularly important in a setting where shift changes between physicians, advanced practice providers (APPs), and nurses will lead to the transfer of patient care. There must be a clearly delineated set of disposition possibilities if and when shift change occurs.

J. P. Stopyra (✉)
Department of Emergency Medicine, Wake Forest University School of Medicine, Winston-Salem, NC, USA
e-mail: jstopyra@wakehealth.edu

© The Author(s), under exclusive license to Springer Nature Switzerland AG 2022
M. Pena et al. (eds.), *Short Stay Management of Chest Pain*, Contemporary Cardiology, https://doi.org/10.1007/978-3-031-05520-1_18

## 1.1 Exclusion of Patients at High Risk for Acute Coronary Syndrome

Clearly, patients having grossly abnormal vital signs (e.g., hypotension, respiratory instability), unstable cardiac rhythms, diagnostic ischemic changes on ECG, or elevations of serum cardiac markers in a diagnostic range for significant myocardial injury should not be entered into a CPU pathway. These patients are at high risk based on initial physician assessment and should be admitted to the hospital not be placed in the CPU. The diagnostic component of the observation process will, in most cases, only delay hospital admission and more definitive care. The exclusion of unstable patients and patients with ACS from the CPU is at the cornerstone of a unit that maintains the highest quality, efficiency, and safety [1].

## 1.2 Exclusion of Patients at Very Low Risk of Acute Coronary Syndrome

Although the diagnosis of subtle or even occult ACS can be difficult, it is occasionally possible to make a definitive non-ACS diagnosis in the patient with signs or symptoms associated with ACS such as chest pain or dyspnea. The emergency department (ED) evaluation to identify the very low risk patient should focus on a validated ED chest pain risk stratification tool and the identification of common cardiopulmonary processes like pneumonia and pulmonary embolism that can be proven through readily available ED testing [2].

The practical advantage of excluding patients with very low-risk scenarios lies primarily in reducing the over utilization of observation resources. Patients with very low pretest probabilities of ACS (<1%) will be more likely to have false-positive ECG and cardiac marker results than actual ACS [3]. Applying the CPU testing strategy to these patients will increase the number of false-positive results, unnecessary imaging or invasive testing, cost, as well as risk to patients [4]. However, while some patients can have ACS excluded due to the definite diagnosis of an alternative process, many cannot, and physicians should not overreach this strategy. For example, although gastroesophageal reflux disease (GERD) is common in ED patients with atraumatic chest pain, it cannot be definitively proven in the ED. This difficulty creates a common pitfall for physicians who would like to make a clinical diagnosis of a common disease such as GERD while ignoring the possibility of a subtle ACS. In all cases, the evaluating physician must carefully entertain the possibility that ACS can occur concurrently with ACS mimics [5].

### *1.3 Exclusion of Patients with Logistical and Nonmedical Barriers to Safe Discharge*

Before a patient enters into an observation pathway, a realistic logistic assessment of whether or not a patient can be discharged if all testing is negative is warranted. Frequently nonmedical barriers to safe discharge from the hospital are present and easily recognizable. The initial physician should determine these factors before entry to the CPU, and these barriers must be addressed before signing out the care of a patient to another provider. Some patients presenting to the ED who previously lived independently may be judged to now need additional care on a full- or part-time basis. Common reasons for this change in status include progressive or previously unrecognized lack of mobility or cognitive impairment that inhibits the patient's ability to carry out activities of daily living. If no immediate outpatient caregivers can be identified for these patients, appropriate steps should be taken to admit the patient to the hospital. Entry into the CPU will only delay this inevitable "social" admission.

## 2  Indications for Hospitalization from the Short Stay Unit: Admission Triggers

During the observation period of the CPU stay, the primary goal of the clinical pathway to identify the ACS patient is achieved through the continual collection of data aimed at providing further risk assessment. This new information—both objective and subjective—can either establish a low-risk status of a patient in the CPU or change the assessment of the patient's risk from low/intermediate for ACS into a higher range that would likely require hospital admission and possibly acute intervention.

Any clinical pathway for the observation of patients being evaluated for possible ACS should have defined admission triggers—clinical or diagnostic endpoints that, if found, result in hospital admission with or without acute intervention (Table 1). While the activities of the patient undergoing observation are passive, those of the health-care providers are active and include frequent reassessments. The core diagnostic elements of a CPU pathway should consist of the following: regular measurement of vital signs, assessment of patient symptoms, serial 12-lead ECGs, and serial serum cardiac marker determination. Another role of the CPU pathway is to allow for more time beyond a patient's initial evaluation to observe for disease progression such that the clinician may entertain and definitively make alternative diagnoses during the allotted time. Thus, the actual time in observation is another tool of significant value in the CPU process. Consideration of alternative diagnoses adds accuracy and efficiency to the overall diagnostic process.

**Table 1** CPU admission triggers

| Clinical factors |
| --- |
| Unexplained bradycardia or tachycardia |
| Hypotension |
| Severe hypertension |
| Progressive or persistent dyspnea |
| Intractable or recurring ischemic chest pain |
| Severe decrement in patient's functional capacity at baseline |
| New diagnosis warranting hospitalization |
| Diagnostic factors |
| New or dynamic ischemic ECG changes |
| New significant elevations of serum cardiac markers |
| Abnormalities on immediate provocative testing |

## *2.1  Assessment of Clinical Factors*

The assessment of clinical factors is of paramount importance during observation in the CPU. Clinical factors include simple measurement of vital signs and reassessment of patients' symptoms. Repeated, routine measurement of vital signs will help to detect early signs of clinical decompensation. These should be scheduled by protocol and recorded diligently. As a general rule, the development of abnormal vital signs in a patient undergoing an observation protocol in the CPU requires explanation and management. In the absence of a benign cause, patients may require admission to the hospital for further evaluation and management.

### 2.1.1  Heart Rate

Unexplained bradycardia or tachycardia should always be addressed as they may represent significant physiologic impairment. Bradycardia may be an early sign of ischemia or infarction of the conduction system, especially if it involves the atrioventricular (AV) node; worsening degrees of AV nodal block may indicate the progression of an infarction. Tachycardia in the CPU patient has many possible implications. Rhythm identification in the newly tachycardic patient is essential. Sinus tachycardia may be the only clinical sign of underlying clinical decompensation or early shock. If the underlying etiology is cardiac ischemia, sinus tachycardia may indicate left ventricular dysfunction or a new hemodynamic lesion (e.g., acute mitral regurgitation from papillary muscle dysfunction). Increased adrenergic tone related to ischemia and pain is also a common cause of sinus tachycardia in the ACS patient. The clinician must always have a high index of suspicion for alternative non-ACS diagnosis in the CPU patient that suddenly develops tachycardia. Sepsis, pneumonia, and pulmonary embolism are common diseases that may initially present with relatively normal vital signs and diagnostic studies. New rhythms other than sinus tachycardia should be identified and treated appropriately.

Iatrogenic causes for abnormal heart rates in the CPU are common and must be considered. The clinician must consider the influence of cardioactive medications (e.g., beta-blockers, calcium channel blockers, and other AV nodal agents) that are commonly used in the treatment of cardiac patients. Reflex sinus tachycardia may result as a reflex from the use of vasodilators such as nitrates and hydralazine, and can also be related to volume depletion resulting from diuretic administration. Vasovagal episodes related to things such as phlebotomy may cause transient brady-cardia and hypotension. These episodes are self-limited and should not be overly concerning or affect CPU disposition. The treating CPU clinicians are the most appropriate personnel to determine the significance of any alteration in heart rate or other clinical data as well as make further diagnostic and management decisions.

### 2.1.2   Blood Pressure

Much like heart rate abnormalities, unexplained hypotension is an ominous sign that should alert the clinician to the possibility of either severe cardiac dysfunction or the presence of a non-ACS diagnosis. Except for iatrogenic hypotension from commonly used medications and vasovagal episodes, patients experiencing hypo-tension in the CPU should be considered for admission. Hypertension, on the other hand, is a much less reliable indicator of acute illness or decompensation. Judicious treatment of hypertension should be considered. Rarely, extreme, isolated hyperten-sion requires hospital admission in the appropriately screened CPU patient.

### 2.1.3   Respiratory Distress and Hypoxia

Unexplained tachypnea, increased work of breathing at rest and/or hypoxia may indicate recurrent ischemia or other conditions such as a pulmonary embolus or the development of pulmonary edema. Elderly patients, in particular, commonly pres-ent with dyspnea as an anginal equivalent [6]. An immediate, careful reexamination of the patient should be performed by the treating clinician if respiratory distress or hypoxia develops. The clinician should strongly consider expanding their differen-tial diagnosis, reimage the chest with the most appropriate imaging modality, and proceed with other pertinent diagnostic studies.

### 2.1.4   Recurrent Symptoms

The reoccurrence of a patient's symptoms during the period of observation affords the clinician an opportunity to reevaluate for ACS versus non-ACS. Constant intrac-table pain that is not associated with ECG changes or elevated troponin levels after several hours is far less likely to be of cardiac origin than if the pain is episodic and recurrent. However, brief episodes of chest pain or anginal equivalent symptoms due to cardiac ischemia may not result in ECG changes or serum cardiac marker elevations. The determination of the etiology of a patient's chest pain is the diagnostic challenge that has brought them to the CPU, and the very nature of the process may take hours and further evaluation and testing to identify.

## *2.2　Abnormal ECG and Serum Cardiac Marker Testing*

### 2.2.1　Dynamic ECG Changes

Rhythm monitoring and repeated 12-lead ECGs based on additional clinical changes are essential parts of observation. Admission triggers related to the ECG assume that the initial ECG has been nondiagnostic (normal, nonspecifically abnormal, or unchanged from previous tracings) with a stable rhythm (Table 2).

### 2.2.2　Continuous ECG Rhythm Monitoring

Patients may be placed on continuous ECG rhythm monitoring while undergoing the rule-out acute myocardial infarction (AMI) procedure. This step aims to detect new arrhythmias with particular attention to ventricular arrhythmias and high-grade AV nodal blocks. If these are identified, they should result in hospital admission. Atrial arrhythmias like atrial fibrillation/flutter and other supraventricular tachycardias occur with some frequency and may redirect the evaluation and provide a reasonable alternative diagnosis to ACS.

### 2.2.3　ST Segment Changes

With changes in symptoms, serial or continuous 12-lead ECG monitoring is performed to detect diagnostic ST-segment changes that cannot be found through standard telemetry systems (i.e., single or multilead rhythm monitoring). Specifically, dynamic ST-segment elevation or depression greater than or equal to 1 mm as compared to the baseline ECG should warrant concern for ACS, immediate patient reevaluation, and cardiology consultation as indicated.

**Table 2** Diagnostic ECG triggers for admission

| Dynamic ST changes |
| --- |
| ST depression |
| ST-elevation |
| New bundle branch block—not rate-related |
| New arrhythmias |
| New second or third AV nodal block |
| Ventricular tachycardia |
| Excessive ventricular ectopy |

### 2.2.4  T-Wave Changes

T-wave inversions and flattening are less specific changes than ST-segment deviation for acute ischemia but may still be associated with increased mortality risk [7]. In the CPU, dynamic T wave changes should be looked at with some skepticism before making an admission decision. One potentially helpful aspect of the inverting T-wave is summarized as such: as the depth of the T-wave inversion increases, the rate of ACS also increases [8]. A common pitfall that may occur over the course of hours spent in the CPU that can result in T-wave inversions or flattening include different ECG techniques between baseline and repeat 12-lead ECGs. Changes in body position were once thought to significantly influence T-wave appearance, but this has recently been challenged [9]. A patient sitting upright or lying in the lateral decubitus position can have changes in the heart's anatomical position inside the thorax. Likewise, changes in lead position can significantly impact ECG appearance [10, 11]. The CPU staff should be aware that the different ECG manufacturers may use different software filters that aid in the generation of the tracing. These data processing differences can result in slight variations in ECG appearance. Ideally, all 12-lead ECGs for each patient should be performed in the same semiupright position, using the same machine and leads throughout the observation process for consistency.

Another potential confounder of apparent dynamic ECG findings is the presence of a significant electrolyte disturbance, particularly involving potassium, calcium, and magnesium [12]. It is common practice in the CPU to correct these abnormalities during the observation period, so it would be expected that the ECG appearance may change as well. The CPU clinicians should be careful not to overreact to the normalization of the ECG after the electrolyte corrections. In any case, T-wave changes should be used as one part of the patient's clinical picture in making hospital admission decisions.

### 2.2.5  Abnormal Cardiac Markers

The use of serum cardiac markers for ACS diagnosis and prognostication is discussed more extensively elsewhere in this text. This discussion is focused on using these cardiac markers as a basis for hospital admission from the CPU.

Contemporary cardiac troponin assays (cTnI or cTnT) as well as high sensitivity cardiac troponin assays (hs-cTnI or hs-cTnT) can detect tiny concentrations of circulating troponin [13, 14]. As a result, a significant percentage of patients in a CPU environment will have detectable troponin levels. Many low-risk patients are included in this population, but these troponin elevations may not be associated with ACS. In fact, these troponin elevations may be related to other cardiac, non-ACS conditions such as decompensated heart failure and hypertensive urgencies/emergencies among the most common. While these alternative conditions may not represent true ACS, troponin elevations have been associated with increased mortality and short-term adverse outcome rates and deserve appropriately aggressive care [15].

To improve the accuracy of admission decisions for ACS based on serum troponin elevations, two strategies can be incorporated into the CPU guidelines.

(a) Determine a diagnostic cutoff that will be respected at your institution.

With assistance from the local laboratory and/or assay manufacturer, cardiologists and emergency physicians should agree on an established diagnostic cutoff level or change in serial samples that, once met on a single sample, should result in admission. These diagnostic levels should not define AMI or ACS but do provide a posttest odds assessment such that ACS is highly probable [16].

(b) Measure troponin trends to look for peaking patterns versus plateaus.

Troponin concentrations below the predetermined diagnostic cutoff and above the lower level of detection should be addressed through careful patient reassessment and serial measurements. Going back to the bedside with the added knowledge of an indeterminate troponin elevation can sometimes yield new information from the physical examination or patient history that was not previously discerned. Serial measurements are performed to distinguish trends as well as to detect analytic false positives. The timing between sample collections in the CPU should be in the range of every 1–4 h [17]. If a clinical answer is not apparent from reevaluation, then repeat testing for trend analysis is appropriate.

Trend analysis of nondiagnostic troponin levels will yield three patterns: peaking, declining, or a plateau. Peaking patterns are highly specific for acute processes, and in the appropriately selected CPU patient, ACS is the most common of these. Both declining and plateau patterns commonly indicate subacute non-ACS processes, the detection of a prior recent ACS which is resolving, or analytical errors [18]. In summary, patients with peaking troponin patterns should generally be hospitalized, but those with plateauing patterns should have individualized treatment and disposition, taking into consideration their clinical presentation.

## 2.3 *Provocative Testing and Advanced Imaging*

The integration of advanced imaging and provocative testing into the CPU protocol is determined mainly by local factors, especially resource availability, institutional preference, and expertise. Specific aspects of various advanced testing modalities appear elsewhere in this text. Admission criteria based on positive results of these advanced tests should focus on the intention to treat ACS and the need for further invasive testing (i.e., coronary angiography). Most patients with positive tests will require hospital admission, but the demonstration of coronary artery disease alone does not dictate admission if the patient is clinically at low risk for ACS. (See the section below on outpatient strategies for patients with known coronary artery disease.)

## 2.4 Reassessment of Functional Status at the End of the Chest Pain Unit Protocol

After the patient has stabilized and serial cardiac marker and ECGs are nondiagnostic, basic functional status can easily be assessed. A CPU walk or "road test" can be a powerful maneuver to help determine appropriateness for discharge [19]. The CPU staff can assist the patient with low-level exercise by simply having the patient walk inside the unit and in the hallways for 1 or 2 min. Efforts to reproduce the patient's home conditions should be made with baseline supplemental oxygen and mobility aids such as a walker or a cane. This exercise test occasionally results in recurrent ischemic symptoms, respiratory distress, and/or significantly abnormal blood pressure or heart rate responses not present at rest. A positive finding on this simple evaluation prior to the arrangement of provocative testing therefore uncovers the patient at high risk for discharge who will now necessitate hospital admission.

## 2.5 Situations When Outpatient Medical Management Strategies for Patients with Known Coronary Artery Disease Are Appropriate

Patients with coronary artery disease (CAD) will become symptomatic at times and present for evaluation. It is impractical to exclude all patients with preexisting CAD from observation protocols because of their CAD history. A careful assessment of the presenting symptoms can help identify patients at low-intermediate versus high risk for ACS. These low-intermediate risk patients with known CAD will have specific diagnostic and therapeutic goals. Since CAD is already known in this subset of patients, the immediate diagnostic goals are to exclude AMI and determine if the patient's chest pain is ischemic in nature. Therapeutic goals should include stabilization and optimization of medical management of myocardial oxygen delivery, oxygen demand, and platelet inhibition (e.g., aspirin).

A few specific scenarios involving patients with known CAD are commonly seen in the CPU and may result in outpatient care rather than admission. In some cases, patients with known severe, inoperable, or nonintervenable CAD will have been previously evaluated by their physicians. After careful deliberation between doctor and patient, a long-term plan for medical management may be determined. When these patients present for evaluation with limited ischemic symptoms, they may be discharged home after successfully completing an observation protocol to rule out AMI. As mentioned previously, recurrent ischemia in the CPU is an indication for hospital admission, including this patient population. Medical therapy can be optimized with the help of the patient's primary team of physicians, and close follow-up can be established. These patients should be made aware of the long-term risk of coronary events associated with their disease.

Medication noncompliance is one of the most common reasons for ischemic symptoms in the patient with established CAD. Patients who are noncompliant with antianginals and antihypertensives are relatively straightforward. Ischemic symptoms result from a reversible supply–demand mismatch and do not represent an acute coronary event (i.e., plaque rupture or thrombosis). After AMI is excluded, a simple resumption of medications and referral back to the patient's cardiologist or primary care physician may be sufficient. However, it is important to keep in mind that patients that become symptomatic after noncompliance with antiplatelet agents have a higher risk of acute coronary thrombosis, especially if coronary stents are in place. These patients may have a more significant short-term risk for ACS and may need to be admitted for more aggressive anticoagulation and platelet inhibition even if they rule out for AMI [20, 21].

Finally, some patients with known CAD, yet low–intermediate ACS risk, will be successfully ruled out for AMI by ECG and serial cardiac markers, but will need assessment for inducible ischemia to further guide therapy. In contrast to the "medical management only" subset, these patients would potentially be eligible for surgery or percutaneous coronary intervention (PCI) if indicated. The CPU process allows for cardiology consultation as well as immediate or outpatient testing of these patients once they have successfully completed the CPU protocol without any subjective or objective concerns. The outpatient strategy assumes that the patient is compliant with medical instructions, follow-up appointments, and precautions.

# 3 Indications for Safe Discharge from the Chest Pain Unit

## 3.1 Clinical Criteria

The patient should meet a set of clinical criteria prior to discharge from the chest pain unit. The most obvious are a negative cardiac test such as a stress test or cardiac computed tomography angiography (cCTA) and negative or nonrising serial cardiac troponins. These findings are the primary focus for whether a patient can be safely discharged. In addition, patients must also have acceptable vital signs, the ability to tolerate a diet and perform activities of daily living with available resources. Finally, as mentioned previously, it is wise to reassess a patient after they take a short walk around the unit to identify any subtle abnormalities brought on by ambulation.

## 3.2 Shared Decision-Making

Shared decision-making is an approach that providers can employ when patients have nontraditional requests, and different management and disposition options are fairly equivalent [22–25]. This is most commonly used prior to discharge for patients who choose not to undergo immediate cardiac testing and request an outpatient testing approach. Providers and patients in these situations may together evaluate the available options. Whenever differing opinions exist, the patient's opinion of the next steps in chest pain evaluation should be addressed and incorporated into decision-making. A discussion of risks, benefits and patient preference needs to occur in an honest and open environment with the goal of reaching the best option for the patient.

It should be noted that each center needs to decide on the balance it strikes between medical paternalism and a patient's responsibility for their own care. If patients have access to outpatient care, lack nonmedical barriers to follow-up, and are given specific scheduled instructions for follow-up, immediate provocative testing of low-risk patients, although convenient, may not be medically necessary [26, 27].

## 3.3 Discharge Planning and Establishment of Follow-Up

The patient should be involved in the discharge planning process so that they are aware of the process completed, understand their test results, are comfortable with the treatment and discharge plan, and have the opportunity to ask questions. The final step in the CPU disposition process is the arrangement of outpatient follow-up. Patients should leave the CPU with firm plans for close follow-up with a primary care physician (PCP) or cardiologist—that is, days, not weeks. Cardiac risk factor modification and general reassessment will be the focus of the next outpatient visit.

One of the major determinants of compliance with follow-up plans is access to care. It is strongly recommended that the CPU have procedures in place for direct lines of referral with participating primary care clinics and/or cardiologists who will accept CPU referred patients. An on-call or referral list of outpatient clinic options is frequently available for new patients presenting to hospital-based EDs. It is reasonable to use these connections to ensure patients are not lost to follow-up.

It is particularly critical to address access to outpatient-care issues in settings where outpatient provocative testing is offered or encouraged [28]. Both immediate and delayed provocative testing models are in use today, although data supporting the safety of delayed testing is sparse [29]. Integrating immediate provocative testing or coronary imaging into CPU guidelines for patients with no access to scheduled outpatient testing due to payer status or other nonmedical barriers may be necessary. Despite the resultant costs in CPU length of stay and increased hospital admission rates, patient safety must come first. The most elegant plan for outpatient care will fail if the patient cannot logistically fulfill it.

Finally, it is essential that the patient is not given the impression that their medical care is complete; rather, it should be stressed that they have successfully completed one step in their evaluation and treatment. Predischarge education and discharge documents should clearly explain that while they do not appear to be having ACS at this time, they need to comply with follow-up instructions to help prevent future cardiac events.

## 4    Summary

Utilization of the short stay CPU for the evaluation of patients with possible ACS is only effective if there is a clear understanding of the various disposition outcomes that are possible. Clarifying specific admission triggers and discharge criteria is essential to maintain an efficient process that improves early recognition and treatment of ACS and accuracy of admissions. A clinical pragmatism is currently required when designing the necessary clinical pathways for admission or discharge because in many critical areas related to observation medicine, the level of evidence present in the literature is not strong or does not correlate with the real-world undifferentiated patient population that inevitably presents in the acute-care setting. Local solutions that emphasize patient safety and realistic resource utilization should always be sought, and the chosen methods should be refined over time through sound process improvement activities.

## References


1. Conley J, Bohan JS, Baugh CW. The establishment and management of an observation unit. Emerg Med Clin North Am. 2017;35:519–33.
2. Stopyra J, Snavely AC, Hiestand B, Wells BJ, Lenoir KM, Herrington D, Hendley N, Ashburn NP, Miller CD, Mahler SA. Comparison of accelerated diagnostic pathways for acute chest pain risk stratification. Heart. 2020;106:977–84.
3. Mahler SA, Riley RF, Hiestand BC, Russell GB, Hoekstra JW, Lefebvre CW, et al. The HEART pathway randomized trial: identifying emergency department patients with acute chest pain for early discharge. Circ Cardiovasc Qual Outcomes. 2015;8(2):195–203.
4. Riley RF, Miller CD, Russell GB, Harper EN, Hiestand BC, Hoekstra JW, Lefebvre CW, Nicks BA, Cline DM, Askew KL, Mahler SA. Cost analysis of the history, ECG, age, risk factors, and initial troponin (HEART) pathway randomized control trial. Am J Emerg Med. 2016;35(1):77–81.
5. Hollander JE, Robey JL, Chase MR, Brown AM, Zogby KE, Shofer FS. Relationship between a clear-cut alternative non-cardiac diagnosis and 30-day outcome in emergency department patients with chest pain. Acad Emerg Med. 2007;14:210–5.
6. Kayani WT, Khan MR, Deshotels MR, Jneid H. Challenges and controversies in the management of ACS in elderly patients. Curr Cardiol Rep. 2020;22:51.
7. Istolahti T, Lyytikäinen LP, Huhtala H, Nieminen T, Kähönen M, Lehtimäki T, Eskola M, Anttila I, Jula A, Rissanen H, Nikus K, Hernesniemi J. The prognostic significance of T-wave inversion according to ECG lead group during long-term follow-up in the general population. Ann Noninvasive Electrocardiol. 2020;26:e12799.
8. Lin KB, Shofer FS, McCusker C, Meshberg E, Hollander JE. Predictive value of T-wave abnormalities at the time of emergency department presentation in patients with potential acute coronary syndromes. Acad Emerg Med. 2008;15:537–43.
9. Markendorf S, Lüscher TF, Gerds-Li JH, Schönrath F, Schmied CM. Clinical impact of repolarization changes in supine versus upright body position. Cardiol J. 2018;25:589–94.
10. Adams MG, Drew BJ. Body position effects on the ECG: implication for ischemia monitoring. J Electrocardiol. 1997;30:285–91.
11. Nelwan SP, Meij SH, van Dam TB, Kors JA. Correction of ECG variations caused by body position changes and electrode placement during ST-T monitoring. J Electrocardiol. 2001;34(Suppl):213–6.

12. El-Sherif N, Turitto G. Electrolyte disorders and arrhythmogenesis. Cardiol J. 2011;18:233–45.
13. Wu AH, Jaffe AS. The clinical need for high-sensitivity cardiac troponin assays for acute coronary syndromes and the role for serial testing. Am Heart J. 2008;155:208–14.
14. Mueller C, Giannitsis E, Christ M, Ordóñez-Llanos J, deFilippi C, McCord J, Body R, Panteghini M, Jernberg T, Plebani M, Verschuren F, French J, Christenson R, Weiser S, Bendig G, Dilba P, Lindahl B, TRAPID-AMI Investigators. Multicenter evaluation of a 0-hour/1-hour algorithm in the diagnosis of myocardial infarction with high-sensitivity cardiac troponin T. Ann Emerg Med. 2016;68(1):76–87.e4.
15. Jia X, Sun W, Hoogeveen RC, Nambi V, Matsushita K, Folsom AR, Heiss G, Couper DJ, Solomon SD, Boerwinkle E, Shah A, Selvin E, de Lemos JA, Ballantyne CM. High-sensitivity troponin I and incident coronary events, stroke, heart failure hospitalization, and mortality in the ARIC study. Circulation. 2019;139:2642–53.
16. Thiruganasambandamoorthy V. Using single sex-specific high-sensitivity cardiac troponin cut-off values for ruling out myocardial infarction - are we there yet? CJEM. 2019;21:7–8.
17. Summers SM, Long B, April MD, Koyfman A, Hunter CJ. High sensitivity troponin: the Sisyphean pursuit of zero percent miss rate for acute coronary syndrome in the ED. Am J Emerg Med. 2018;36:1088–97.
18. Sajeev JK, New G, Roberts L, Menon SK, Gunawan F, Wijesundera P, The AW. High sensitivity troponin: does the 50% delta change alter clinical outcomes in chest pain presentations to the emergency room? Int J Cardiol. 2015;184:170–4.
19. Beatty AL, Schiller NB, Whooley MA. Six-minute walk test as a prognostic tool in stable coronary heart disease: data from the heart and soul study. Arch Intern Med. 2012;172(14):1096–102.
20. McFadden EP, Stabile E, Regar E, Cheneau E, Ong AT, Kinnaird T, Suddath WO, Weissman NJ, Torguson R, Kent KM, Pichard AD, Satler LF, Waksman R, Serruys PW. Late thrombosis in drug-eluting coronary stents after discontinuation of antiplatelet therapy. Lancet. 2004;364:1519–21.
21. Waters RE, Kandzari DE, Phillips HR, Crawford LE, Sketch MH. Late thrombosis following treatment of in-stent restenosis with drug-eluting stents after discontinuation of antiplatelet therapy. Catheter Cardiovasc Interv. 2005;65:520–4.
22. Elwyn G, Frosch D, Rollnick S. Dual equipoise shared decision making: definitions for decision and behaviour support interventions. Implement Sci. 2009;4:75.
23. Elwyn G, Edwards A, Kinnersley P, Grol R. Shared decision making and the concept of equipoise: the competences of involving patients in healthcare choices. Br J Gen Pract. 2000;50:892–9.
24. Stiggelbout AM, Weijden TV, Wit MPTD, Frosch D, Légaré F, Montori VM, Trevena L, Elwyn G. Shared decision making: really putting patients at the centre of healthcare. BMJ. 2012;344:e256.
25. Probst MA, Kanzaria HK, Schoenfeld EM, Menchine MD, Breslin M, Walsh C, Melnick ER, Hess EP. Shared decision making in the emergency department: a guiding framework for clinicians. Ann Emerg Med. 2017;70:688–95.
26. Roifman I, Han L, Koh M, Wijeysundera HC, Austin PC, Douglas PS, Ko DT. Clinical effectiveness of cardiac noninvasive diagnostic testing in patients discharged from the emergency department for chest pain. J Am Heart Assoc. 2019;9:e013824.
27. Roifman I, Han L, Koh M, Wijeysundera HC, Austin PC, Douglas PS, et al. Use of cardiac noninvasive testing after emergency department discharge: Association of Hospital Network Testing Intensity and Outcomes in Ontario, Canada. J Am Heart Assoc. 2020;9(21):e017330.
28. Kite TA, Gaunt H, Banning AS, Roberts E, Kovac J, Hudson I, Gershlick AH. Clinical outcomes of patients discharged from the rapid access chest pain clinic with non-anginal chest pain: a retrospective cohort study. Int J Cardiol. 2020;302:1–4.
29. Natsui S, Sun BC, Shen E, Wu YL, Redberg RF, Lee MS, Ferencik M, Zheng C, Kawatkar AA, Gould MK, Sharp AL. Evaluation of outpatient cardiac stress testing after emergency department encounters for suspected acute coronary syndrome. Ann Emerg Med. 2019;74:216–23.

# Examples of Chest Pain Accelerated Decision Pathways, Rule-Out ACS/ACS Protocols, Order Sets, and Discharge Instructions


**Damian Stobierski, Yue Jay Lin, Yitzchak Weinberger, and Christopher Caspers**


Chest pain protocols have been developed and in use in ED observation units since the 1980s [1]. These protocols include risk stratification with serial EKG and troponin testing and, if negative, may progress to provocative testing or coronary imaging [2]. These protocols will differ regionally and institutionally based on availability and expertise in modality of stress testing (nuclear versus echocardiography), coronary CTA, and diagnostic and interventional coronary angiography.

Prior prospective, randomized, controlled trials have demonstrated the benefits of protocol-based chest pain care [3]. In general, these studies have found that protocol-based chest pain care is associated with shorter length of stay, lower costs, improved quality, improved patient experience, and ultimately higher value [4–9].

Below are examples of chest pain and ACS protocols and order sets, as well as discharge instructions.


D. Stobierski · Y. J. Lin · Y. Weinberger · C. Caspers (✉)
Ronald O. Perelman Department of Emergency Medicine, NYU Langone Health, New York, NY, USA
e-mail: Christopher.Caspers@nyulangone.org



© The Author(s), under exclusive license to Springer Nature Switzerland AG 2022

M. Pena et al. (eds.), *Short Stay Management of Chest Pain*, Contemporary Cardiology, https://doi.org/10.1007/978-3-031-05520-1_19

# 1 Accelerated Decision Pathway for Chest Pain Evaluation

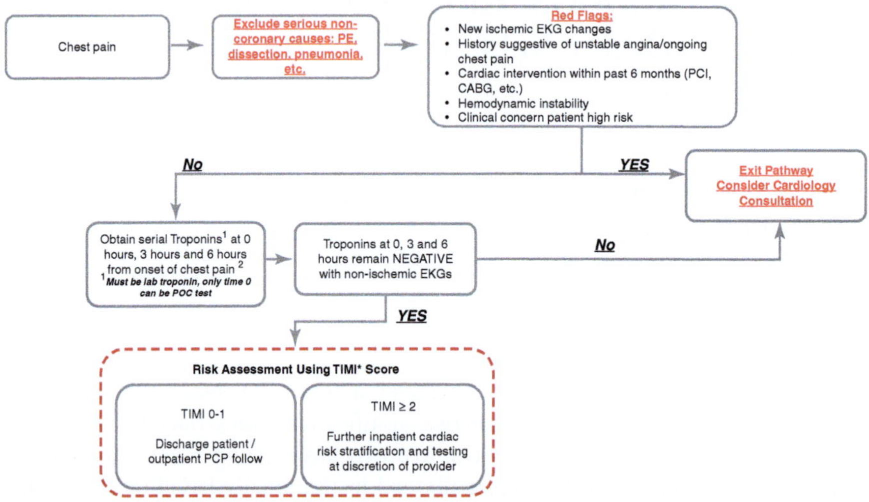


[2] Amsterdam E.A., Wenger N.K., Brindis R. G., et al. 2014 ACC/AHA guideline for the management of patients with non-ST-elevation acute coronary syndromes: A report of the American College of Cardiology/American Heart Association Task Force on Practice Guideline. *Journal of the American College of Cardiology.*` 2014;54(24):e139–e228.

## High Sensitivity Troponin Evaluation Workflow

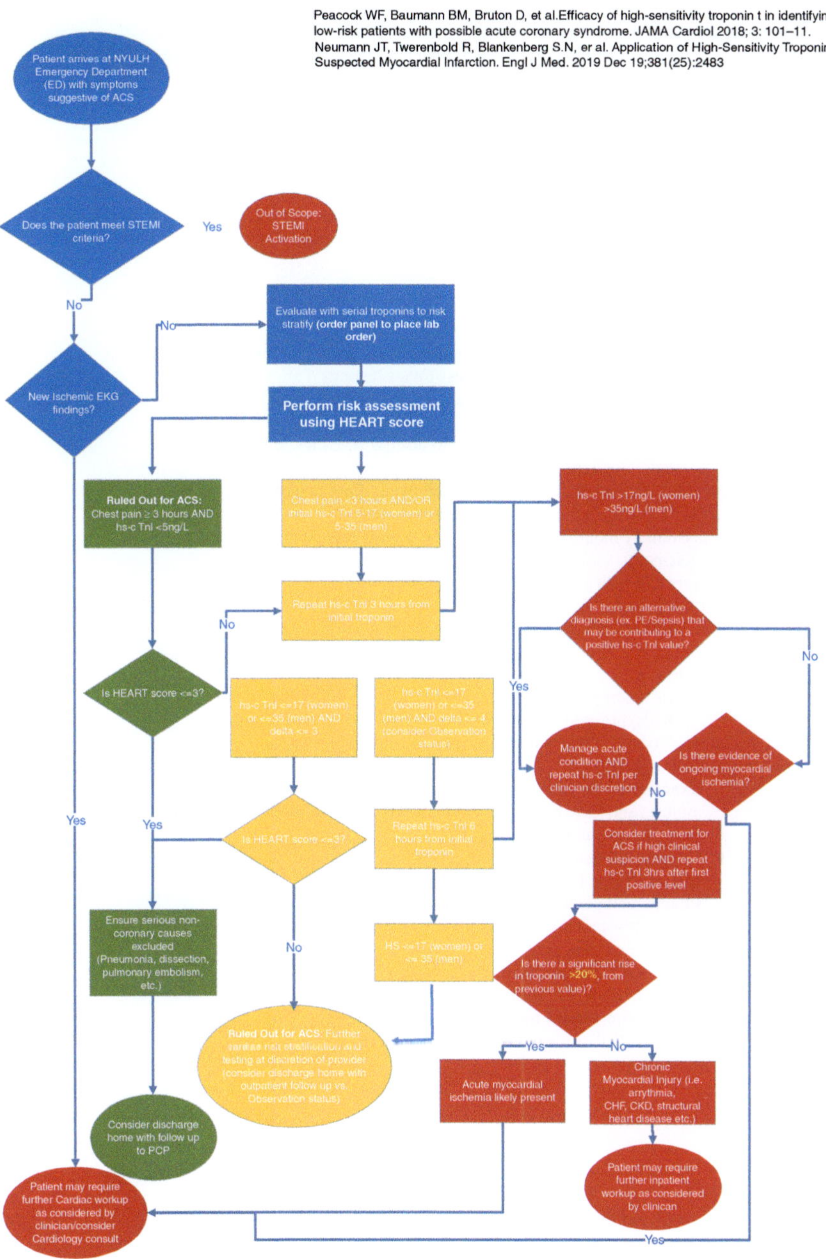

# Chest Pain Obs Protocol

**Inclusion criteria**: Chest pain with evaluation to rule-out ACS (low probability, with or without known CAD); other non-cardiac causes of pain have been adequately addressed

**Protocol-Specific Exclusion criteria**: positive troponin, refractory chest pain, need for nitroglycerin drip, EKG with acute ischemic or dynamic changes (T-wave or ST-segment changes on serial EKGs during the **current** ED visit)

*Note*: Baseline EKG changes noted on present EKG when compared to an old EKG from a prior visit do not preclude placement in the Observation Unit; consider consultation with Cardiology if clarification desired on how to further evaluate patient (ie. stress test vs non-emergent catheterization)

**Intervention:**

1. Verify patient's cardiologist (PCP if no cardiologist) is aware of Observation Unit status and care plan (ie. type of cardiac stress/image testing)
   a. If patient has known CAD, document discussion with cardiologist/PCP regarding stress test selection
      i. Consult cardiology if unable to discuss stress test selection with cardiologist/PCP
2. ASA non-enteric 325 mg po, chewed and swallowed, if not taken within the past 12 hours or in ED (or document reason why not given)
3. Replete potassium by mouth prior to stress test if level less than 3.5 mEq/L
4. Continuous telemetry
5. EKG at 6 hours and with any recurrent chest pain
6. Troponin at 6 hours after first troponin
   a. Note: if the initial troponin is performed 6 hours or more since the most recent episode of chest pain resolved, the patient may proceed directly to stress testing
      i. (ie. chest pain ended at 2a, patient's initial troponin negative at 830a, proceed to stress test)
7. Cardiac testing* (write "Observation Unit patient" and Observation PA phone number in EPIC order)
   A. **Exercise stress test** (preferred; patient able to walk briskly for 10 minutes and raise heart rate and no STD, TWI, or LBBB on baseline EKG; lowest sensitivity for CAD)
   B. **Exercise nuclear stress test** (patient able to exercise as above, but has baseline STD, TWI or higher sensitivity desired)
   C. **Pharmacologic nuclear stress test** (patient unable to exercise sufficiently and baseline STD, TWI, LBBB, or patient unable to exercise and increased sensitivity desired)
   D. **Coronary CTA** (medium probability patient, see separate detailed protocol, can be performed after first negative troponin)
   E. **Stress Echo should not be ordered** unless specifically requested by patient's PCP or the patient is receiving a stress test on Saturday

# Coronary CTA Protocol

**Eligibility (all must be true):**

1. No known CAD
2. TIMI Score 0-2 (1 point each for Age ≥ 65 years, ≥ 3 CAD Risk Factors, ASA Use in Past 7 days, or Severe Angina [2 or more episodes within last 24 hours])
3. Able to receive beta-blocker; if beta-blocker contraindicated (ie. severe asthma, COPD, CHF), pt must then be able to receive calcium-channel blocker; if unable to receive either, pt is excluded from this protocol
4. First troponin negative
5. No dynamic changes on ECG
6. No new ischemic changes on ECG
7. No active chest pain
8. No contraindications to IV contrast (e.g. GFR<45, allergy to IV contrast)
9. No contraindication to nitroglycerin (e.g. sildenafil use)
10. No recent cocaine use
11. Not pregnant
12. No pacemaker
13. Normal mental status
14. Normal sinus rhythm with little or no ectopy
15. BMI < 40
16. Calcium score <400 (on unenhanced acquisition to be performed at time of CT angiogram)

**Protocol:**

1. Verify plan for Coronary CTA (CCTA) has been discussed with patient's cardiologist or PCP
2. 18G IV catheter placed in the right antecubital fossa (left antecubital fossa permissible if contraindication to the right exists or if IV access cannot be obtained on the right; 20G IV permissible if 18G cannot be placed)
3. Provider (MD/PA) will coordinate study timing with CT Tech
4. If heart rate is > 70 bpm, administer metoprolol to lower heart rate < 70 bpm

     a. Metoprolol recommendations:
        i. If HR 70-75, provider (MD or PA[*] in consultation with the Attending) will give metoprolol 5 mg IV
        ii. If HR 75-90, give metoprolol 50 mg PO
        iii. If HR >90, give metoprolol 100 mg PO

# Non-STEMI Center ED STEMI Protocol

**"DOOR" TO "EXIT" (GOAL <25 MINUTES)**

- ☐ STEMI identified in ED
- ☐ Provider notifies ESA to activate STEMI protocol
- ☐ ESA notifies ALS ambulance crew to prepare to transport STEMI, confirms destination with ALS crew and prepares transfer documentation for transport with patient (EMTALA requirement)
- ☐ ESA calls STEMI notification line at STEMI receiving hospital
- ☐ RN initiates STEMI Recognition tool, places patient on monitor, places PIV, draws labs for Basic Metabolic Panel, CBC and Troponin
- ☐ MD orders medication per ACS/STEMI protocol
- ☐ MD writes standing orders for transport (at sending MD's discretion) and ensures EMS crew has MD contact # for patient updates/additional orders en route
- ☐ EMS crew departs with patient as soon as patient prepared to depart ED and transports per EMS protocol without delay
- ☐ Patient leaves and "Exit" time is documented on STEMI Recognition Tool (SRT).  SRT is photocopied, copy remains at ED and original copy travels with patient.
- ☐ ED RN calls receiving hospital RN and gives handoff (this step does not delay transport)

**Receiving Center 1 (RC1) workflow: STEMI being transported to Receiving Center 1 Hospital Cath Lab:**

- ☐ ED ESA calls RC1 Hospital at (***) ***-**** and indicates a STEMI is being transferred from ED and obtains receiving MD name.
- ☐ Receiving Center Hospital ED activates STEMI code
- ☐ ED ESA faxes EKG to RC1 CATH LAB FAX: (***) ***-****
- ☐ ALS arrives in RC1 Hospital ED

**Backup workflow: in event transport time anticipated to be prolonged (ie. traffic) or Receiving Center 1 unable to accept.  STEMI is instead transported to Receiving Hospital 2 (RC2) Cath Lab:**

- ☐ MD at ED calls RC2 Cath Lab at (***) ***-*** and states "STEMI alert at ED is being activated" (triggers RC2 Cath lab to activate Cath Lab STEMI workflow) and ED MD documents handoff upon speaking to Cath Lab
- ☐ RC2 Cath Lab staff notifies Cath fellow and RC2 Nurse Administrator
- ☐ CH MD must place orders for "Left Heart Cath with Possible PCI" and "Transfer to Procedure Area"
- ☐ ALS ambulance transports to RC2 Hospital Cath Lab and arrives at Amblance Drop-off Area of Main Lobby at RC2 Hospital
- ☐ Cath Lab RN calls CH RN and verbal report is given (this step does not delay transport)

*Adapted from NYU Langone Health STEMI Guidelines*

## <u>EMS Direct to Cath Lab: STEMI Guideline and Checklist</u>

**STEMI checklist for direct cath lab transfer:**

Eligible patients: Those that have pre-hospital notification of STEMI and if FDNY ECG is transmitted to Cardiology Team
Patient is awake, alert, and consentable by EMS history
Cardiology Team (Fellow or Attending) is present prior to the arrival of the patient.
Cardiology Team notifies Cath Lab and confirms Cath Lab is ready for direct transport.

1. Cardiology team will respond to ambulance bay and and ask triage nurse which Attending is next for critical activation.
2. Cards Team will approach attending and discuss activation of Direct to Cath lab Guideline.
3. Patient Arrival and Mini-Reg by Mini-Reg Clerk.  Obtains ID/paperwork for complete registration that can be performed later.
4. Patient left on EMS Stretcher, EMS Monitor, EMS Oxygen source and nasal canula.
5. Brief history and exam by ED Team (Attending and PGY3/2).  Brief concurrent exam by Cardiology Fellow
6. Vital signs checked and stable
7. If IV access established by EMS confirm functionality.  If not present, Cardiology STEMI box will contain EZ – IO access kit.
8. Defibrillator pads on and attached to defibrillator
9. Cardiology STEMI Transfer Box will contain emergency medications.  (Lidocaine, Epinephrine, Atropine, ASA, Pavix, SLNTG, Heparin Load, Prasugrel).
10. **Verbal hand off from ED Resident or Attending to Cardiology Fellow**
11. **If at any point the impression is not STEMI and/or confounding history or exam is identified (ie. aortic dissection) the workflow can be terminated by the ED Resident, Attending, or Cardiology Team and the patient will follow the standard ED Resucitation Room Protocol.**
12. ED Resident and Attending complete brief ED Initial Note and Disposition Note.
13. Cardiology Team completes STEMI note.
14. Triage Nurse completes Brief Triage Note as ESI level 2 with chief complaint, related s/s, onset of symptoms, initial vital signs, prior to admission meds administered by FDNY, any allergies, significant PMHx (if known) and presenting cardiac rhythm.
15. STAT elevator paged by Triage Nurse/ Clerk Ext. **** "Ground Floor to Cath Lab"

**Patients not eligible for direct transport:**
Unresponsive cardiac arrest patients
Patients intubated in the field
Patients requiring IV medications for hemodynamic instability

*Adapted from NYU Langone Health STEMI Guidelines*

# STE-ACS Provider Role Checklist

**Purpose:** To promote a coordinated, efficient team effort to maximize outcomes and provide early interventional therapies for acute STE-ACS.

## Role Checklist:

**RN #1:** Assessment/Documentation; accompanies pt to cath lab

**RN #2:** Line & Labs, places pt on 2L O2 by NC

**RN #3:** gives meds (ste-acs pack)

**PCT #1**: does ECG if not already done; if previous ECG is done then a second ECG is not needed; portable O2 under stretcher

**PCT #2:** places patient on transport monitor with BP cuff, undresses pt if time permits

**EM Resident:** takes H and P, places all orders; documents visit

**EM Attending:** supervises team and encourages move to cath lab; discourages interventions that will delay time to cath lab

**Charge Nurse:** allocates additional nursing resources as needed; monitors STE-ACS time sheet and reviews with attending post event; assists ESA in contacting STE-ACS alert and on call cardiology attending and fellow; responsible for post STE-ACS time sheet with critique of event; assigns who will be RN 1 and 2 above, also pct 1 and 2 above

**ESA:** initiates a STE-ACS alert; also pages the on call interventional cardiologist for the ED; faxes copy of ECG to cath lab.

*Adapted from NYU Langone Health STEMI Guidelines*

**<u>CARDIOLOGY ADMITTING GUIDELINES</u>**

**<u>CLINICAL CONTEXT AND PURPOSE:</u>**

The following guidelines specify which inpatient service is primarily responsible for accepting patients based on certain diagnoses. The list of diagnoses is not a complete one and guidelines are intended to be used flexibly as described. In all cases, the Emergency Department (ED) physician is expected to conduct an evaluation sufficient to ascertain the need for admission, to determine the appropriate admitting service, and to identify significant medical comorbidities if present. Furthermore, the ED physician has discretion to interpret the guidelines in a way that best serves the patient. Discussions about the appropriate service should never take place in front of the patient and decisions should be made collaboratively, professionally, and in a patient centered manner.

**<u>GUIDELINE RECOMMENDATIONS:</u>**

**STEMI:** Patients with concern for an acute STEMI should be admitted to cardiology upon evaluation by the cardiac catheterization teams at each site.

**Cardiac Diagnoses/Conditions Requiring Intermediate or Critical Level of Care:** Patients who require intermittent or critical level of care may require evaluations by Intermediate ICU/MICU (****) or CCU (****)

- need for invasive monitoring (e.g., arterial, central, or PA pressure)
- need for cardiac device (e.g., intra-aortic balloon pump, impella device, LVAD)
- need for select continuous IV drips *** (refer to local hospital practices and floor capabilities)
- congestive heart failure with significant respiratory distress requiring bipap/CPAP/HFNC/intubation
- unstable cardiac arrhythmia, including sustained ventricular tachycardia (VT) or VT storm
- heart block requiring transvenous or external pacing
- cardiac tamponade not requiring CT surgery operative intervention
- post-cardiac catheterization patients with femoral arterial sheaths or venous introducers

Post-cardiac arrest patients on hypothermia protocol generally should be admitted to MICU all sites (though some may be eligible for CCU post-catheterization).  Patients with acute cardiac pathologies secondary to acute medical problems (e.g., metabolic derangement, malignancy) or in setting of multiple primary active medical diagnoses who require ICU level of care may be better served on MICU instead of CCU.

***Continuous IV drips: refer to local site practices and floor capabilities based on individual medication drip (e.g., nitroglycerin, furosemide, antiarrhythmics, BP/rate control, inotropic support).  Certain medications not requiring active titration may be appropriate for acute cardiology on telemetry.

# 2  Chest Pain Order Set for Observation Unit

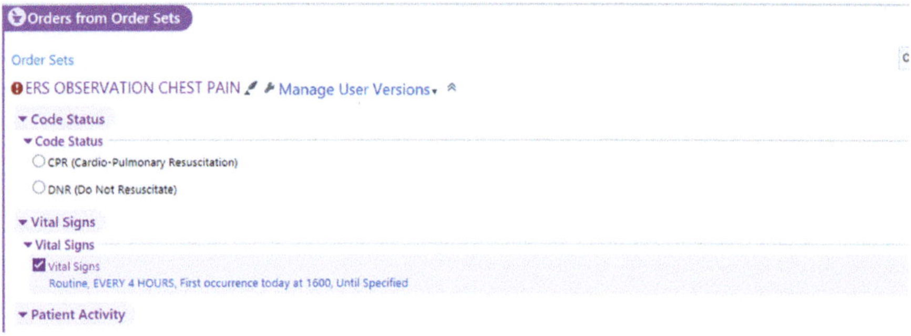

**⊙ Orders from Order Sets**

Order Sets

**❶ ERS OBSERVATION CHEST PAIN** ✎ ⚲ Manage User Versions ▾ ⌃

▾ **Code Status**
  ▾ Code Status
    ○ CPR (Cardio-Pulmonary Resuscitation)
    ○ DNR (Do Not Resuscitate)

▾ **Vital Signs**
  ▾ Vital Signs
    ☑ Vital Signs
      Routine, EVERY 4 HOURS, First occurrence today at 1600, Until Specified

▾ **Patient Activity**

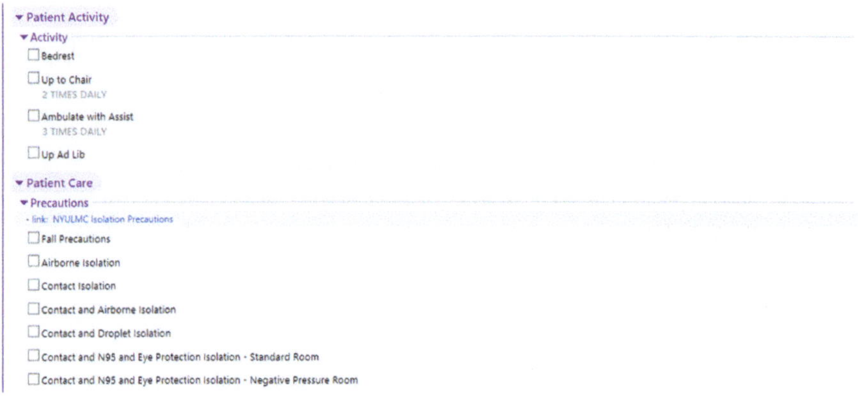

▾ **Patient Activity**
  ▾ Activity
    ☐ Bedrest
    ☐ Up to Chair
      2 TIMES DAILY
    ☐ Ambulate with Assist
      3 TIMES DAILY
    ☐ Up Ad Lib

▾ **Patient Care**
  ▾ Precautions
    - link: NYULMC Isolation Precautions
    ☐ Fall Precautions
    ☐ Airborne Isolation
    ☐ Contact Isolation
    ☐ Contact and Airborne Isolation
    ☐ Contact and Droplet Isolation
    ☐ Contact and N95 and Eye Protection Isolation - Standard Room
    ☐ Contact and N95 and Eye Protection Isolation - Negative Pressure Room

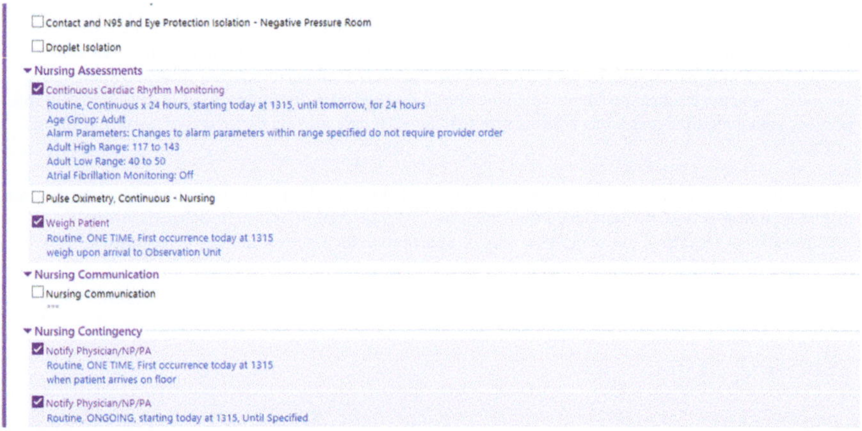

    ☐ Contact and N95 and Eye Protection Isolation - Negative Pressure Room
    ☐ Droplet Isolation
  ▾ Nursing Assessments
    ☑ Continuous Cardiac Rhythm Monitoring
      Routine, Continuous x 24 hours, starting today at 1315, until tomorrow, for 24 hours
      Age Group: Adult
      Alarm Parameters: Changes to alarm parameters within range specified do not require provider order
      Adult High Range: 117 to 143
      Adult Low Range: 40 to 50
      Atrial Fibrillation Monitoring: Off
    ☐ Pulse Oximetry, Continuous - Nursing
    ☑ Weigh Patient
      Routine, ONE TIME, First occurrence today at 1315
      weigh upon arrival to Observation Unit
  ▾ Nursing Communication
    ☐ Nursing Communication
      ***
  ▾ Nursing Contingency
    ☑ Notify Physician/NP/PA
      Routine, ONE TIME, First occurrence today at 1315
      when patient arrives on floor
    ☑ Notify Physician/NP/PA
      Routine, ONGOING, starting today at 1315, Until Specified

▾ Education

☐ Education - Tobacco Cessation and Second Hand Smoke Avoidance

▾ ❶ Nutritional Services

▾ ❶ Diet

☐ Diet NPO

☐ Diet Clear Liquid

☐ Diet Full Liquid

☐ Diet Regular

☐ Diet Diabetes

☐ Diet Heart Healthy

☐ Diet Renal

▾ IV Fluids

▾ Saline Lock

☑ Saline Lock

    Saline Lock
    Routine, ONE TIME, First occurrence today at 1315

▾ Medications

▾ Pain Medication

☐ acetaminophen (TYLENOL) tablet
    1,000 mg, Oral, Every 6 Hours PRN, Mild pain (1-3), Fever > 100.4 F

☑ lidocaine (LMX) 4 % cream
    Topical, Every 6 Hours PRN, Other, for Procedures including phlebotomy and IV starts, Starting today at 1302, For 30 days
    Apply Lidocaine (LMX) to intact, uncleaned skin 20-30 minutes prior to procedures

☐ morphine sulfate injection
    0.5 mg, Intravenous, Once PRN, Severe pain (7-10), Starting 5/21/21, for 1 dose

☐ nitroGLYCERIN (NITROSTAT) SL tablet
    0.4 mg, SubLingual, Every 5 Min PRN, Chest pain, Starting 5/21/21, for 3 doses, notify provider when administed; HOLD for Systolic BP less than 90 mmHg

▾ Anticoagulation

*For heparin protocol, please use heparin protocol order set.

*Aspirin should be administered within 24 hours of arrival and prescribed upon discharge.  If not given, please document reason.

☐ warfarin (COUMADIN) tablet
    Oral, Once (warfarin), Indication for anticoagulation: (Anticoagulation Indications:20276:a) Warfarin goal range INR: (Goal Range INR:20279:a) HIGH ALERT MEDICATION

☐ aspirin tablet
    325 mg, Oral, Once, if not administered in ED

☐ Reason for no aspirin at arrival

▾ VTE Prophylaxis

▾ ❶ VTE Prophylaxis

◯ Patient with additional risk factor(s) for VTE: prior DVT, obesity, active cancer, known hypercoagulable state, IBD, recent prolonged immobilization

◯ Patient with NO additional risk factors

▾ Laboratory

▾ Panels

☑ Lipid Panel
    Routine, ONE TIME, First occurrence today at 1315

☐ Hemoglobin A1c

☑ Troponin I
    Routine, ONE TIME, First occurrence today at 1315
    3 hours after first Troponin

☑ Troponin I
Routine, ONE TIME, First occurrence today at 1315
6 hours after first Troponin

▾ Imaging
▾ Computed Tomography

☐ CT Angio Coronary Arteries and Pulmonary Veins with IV Contrast panel

▾ Procedures/Diagnostic Tests
▾ Cardiology

*For CTA, please use CCTA Panel above.

*Generally Echo Stress with Exercise, wall motion analysis is only used on Saturdays or by specific request of cardiologist

*Patient requires an EKG at 3 and 6 hours following the first EKG. Please time the EKG orders appropriately

▾ Consults
▾ Consults

☐ IP Consult to Social Work

☐ IP Consult to Cardiology

☐ IP Consult to Decompensated Heart Failure Management Team

☐ IP Consult to Electrophysiology

☐ IP Consult to Palliative Care

☑ EKG 12-Lead
Routine, ONE TIME, First occurrence today at 1315
Indication: Chest Pain
Release to patient: Immediate
3 hours after first EKG

☑ EKG 12-Lead
Routine, ONE TIME, First occurrence today at 1315
Indication: Chest Pain
Release to patient: Immediate
6 hours after first EKG

☐ Echocardiogram Transthoracic Complete

☐ Stress Test Exercise Adult

☐ NM Nuclear Cardiology Stress Test Exercise

☐ NM Nuclear Cardiology Stress Test Pharmacologic

☐ Echocardiogram Stress with Exercise
wall motion analysis

☐ Echocardiogram Dobutamine Stress
wall motion analysis

*Adapted from NYU Langone Health Guidelines*

## 3    Stemi Order Set

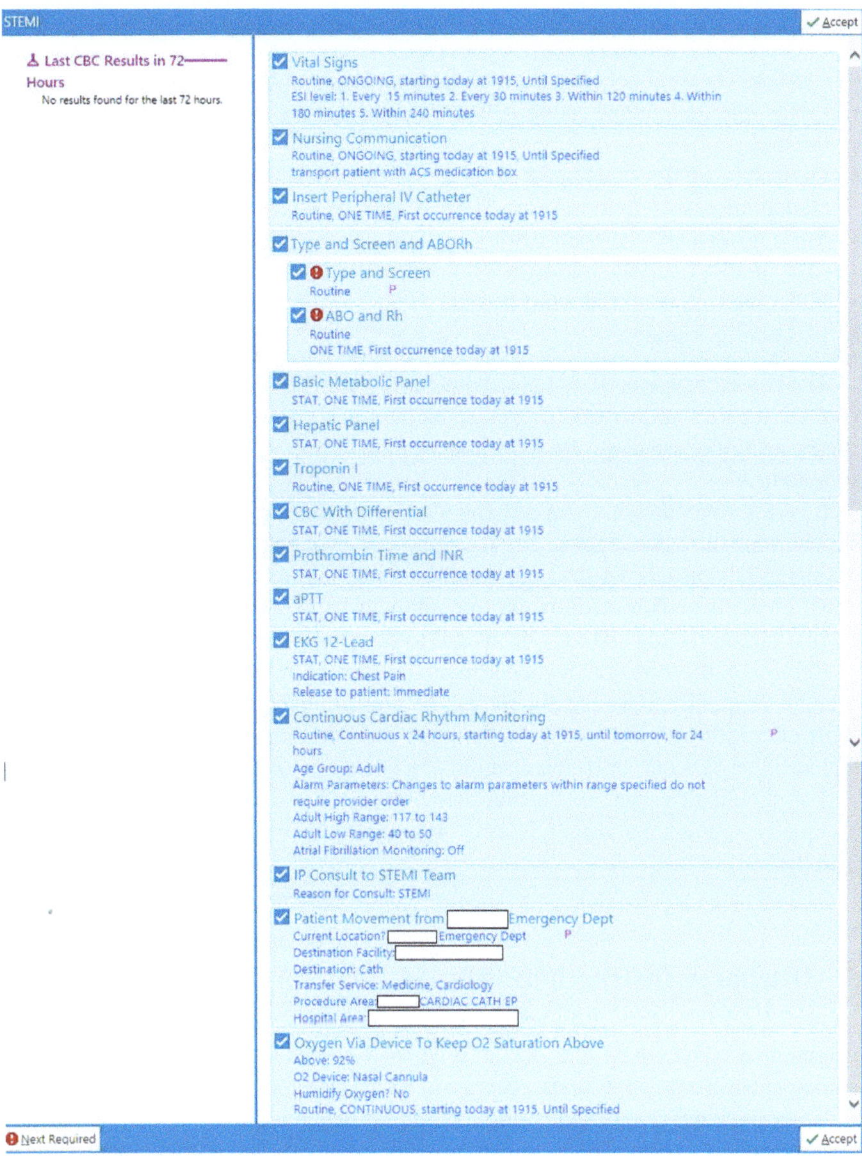



*Adapted from NYU Langone Health Guidelines*

## 4    Discharge Instructions: Chest Pain

Chest pain can occur for many reasons. These include the following.

- Cardiac—heart attack, myocarditis (inflammation of the heart)
- Lung—pneumothorax (collapsed lung), pulmonary embolism (blood clot of the lung)
- Gastrointestinal—esophageal reflux, gastritis, pancreatitis, liver disease, gall bladder disease
- Musculoskeletal—costochondritis (inflammation of the rib cartilage), broken ribs, sprained muscle, overworked muscle
- Infectious—pneumonia, viral illness
- Psychiatric—anxiety

The emergency department physician has determined that a dangerous cause for your chest pain is unlikely. However, sometimes a dangerous diagnosis is in its early stages and may develop, so it is important that you continue to monitor your symptoms.

It is recommended that you rest and avoid strenuous activity for 24 h. After that, slowly return to your regular activity. Take any medications that your emergency physician has prescribed for you. Also, continue taking all of your prior medications. Please schedule a follow-up appointment with your primary care doctor to discuss further testing that may be needed to determine the cause of your chest pain.

Return to the emergency department if your pain becomes more severe or changes in quality, if your pain spreads to your arm/shoulder/jaw, if you become short of breath or have trouble walking around due to difficulty breathing, if you feel weak or pass out, or if you develop any other new or concerning symptoms.

You should also speak to a health-care provider if you develop cough productive of bloody sputum, persistent fevers, or swelling in one leg that is worse than the other.

## 5    Discharge Instructions: Angina

Angina is a type of pain that occurs in your chest when your heart muscle is not getting enough oxygen. It often occurs when you are exerting yourself, such as with exercise, walking, or even with emotional upset. Angina often feels like a crushing pain inside your chest. The pain can move to your shoulder, arm, or jaw, and can lead to a sensation of shortness of breath as well. While angina is a sign of coronary artery disease, there are management strategies you can use for the pain. You can also improve your heart's health with some lifestyle changes.

## 5.1   Managing Angina

Angina often occurs with exertion. If you feel the pain starting, it is important that you sit down and rest from whatever you were doing, as this may help the pain improve. This may also include attempting to relax and removing yourself from any stressful situations.

If the pain does not improve with rest, call 911, as you may be experiencing not only angina but a heart attack.

Your doctor may have prescribed you nitroglycerin to manage your angina. Nitroglycerin helps by dilating the blood vessels near your heart. If he/she did, please keep your nitroglycerin with you at all times as you do not know when you may experience angina.

When you experience an episode of angina, sit down and take 1 table of nitroglycerin under your tongue. Do not take it standing up as you may pass out. Do not chew or swallow the tablet.

Your pain should improve within a few minutes of taking the nitroglycerin. If you do not notice any improvement within 5 min, you should call 911, as you may be experiencing not just angina but a heart attack. If your pain partially resolves and you have discussed it with your doctor, you may take a second dose of nitroglycerin five minutes after the first. You can repeat this for up to three times.

If your chest pain goes away completely after the nitroglycerin, remain seated for five minutes, and then slowly return to your activity. Take note of when you experience angina and when you use nitroglycerin to improve your symptoms and share this log with your physician.

## 5.2   Managing Risk Factors

### 5.2.1   Diet

Your health-care provider may talk to you about making dietary changes to improve your heart health.

Some changes that may be effective include the following.

- Eat less sodium.
- Eat less processed sugars.
- Eat less fatty/greasy food.
- Eat more vegetables and fruits.
- Eat lean proteins instead of red meat.
- Limit sweets and processed foods.
- Limit sodas and high-calorie foods
- Limit fried foods.

### 5.2.2  Physical Activity

Your health-care provider may have recommended an exercise program for you. It is often beneficial to exercise vigorously (such that you feel your heart rate increasing) for 30 min/day, 5 days/week. Any exercise that elevates your heart rate is appropriate. Some examples including walking briskly, jogging, biking, swimming, hiking, dancing, and martial arts. Discuss any drastic changes in your exercise plan with your health-care provider.

### 5.2.3  Weight Management

If you are overweight, your health-care provider may recommend losing weight. A good goal to aim for is to lose 5–10 lbs in 6 months. Making the diet and exercise changes listed above will be helpful in attaining this goal.

### 5.2.4  Smoking

If you smoke cigarettes, use electronic cigarettes, or chew tobacco, it is recommended that you quit or at least cut back on your use. Quitting can be difficult, and you should discuss how to increase your chances of success with your health-care provider. Some patients find being part of a support group helpful. Nicotine gum and nicotine patches can be bridges on the road to quitting. There are also medications that can be prescribed to help with cravings.

## 5.3  When to Call 911

Because you have coronary artery disease that causes your angina, you are at risk of having a heart attack. These are some symptoms you should watch out for that may indicate you are having a heart attack. If you experience any of these, please call 911 or go to an emergency department immediately.

- Chest pain that is more severe than usual.
- Chest pain that moves to a different location than usual (arm, shoulder, jaw).
- Chest pain that comes with shortness of breath and/or sweating.
- Chest pain that comes with a sensation that you may pass out.
- Chest pain that lasts longer than normal.
- Chest pain that is brought on by less exercise than normal.
- Chest pain that is not improved with nitroglycerin.

# 6    Discharge Instructions: Heart Attack

You had a heart attack (myocardial infarction). This occurs when a blood vessel on the surface of your heart that brings blood to your heart muscle is suddenly blocked entirely. This causes that portion of your heart to not receive oxygen and function more poorly.

You may have had an intervention such as a stent performed at the hospital, or you may have had your medications changed to better manage your coronary artery disease. Either way, it is very important for you to take all of your medications as prescribed. You are at risk of a blockage forming in your coronary blood vessels again and having another heart attack. This risk will be lowered if you take your medications.

It is also important that you follow up with your cardiologist and your other doctors as recommended. You may need to have your medications adjusted at these follow-up visits.

Recovery from a heart attack can take time. Take it easy for the first few weeks after you leave the hospital. Recovery may be easier as part of a cardiac rehabilitation program. These are programs that help patients who have survived heart attacks or cardiac surgery to regain strength in their heart muscle and safely reenter their daily lives after these health issues were acutely addressed. Cardiac rehab programs can also assist with dietary modifications, smoking cessation, or other health issues that may be affecting your heart.

Your doctor may have recommended lifestyle changes that would help prevent your heart from accumulating further damage. These may include the following.

## 6.1    Diet

Your health-care provider may talk to you about making dietary changes to improve your heart health.

Some changes that may be effective include the following.

- Eat less sodium.
- Eat less processed sugars.
- Eat less fatty/greasy food.
- Eat more vegetables and fruits.
- Eat lean proteins instead of red meat.
- Limit sweets and processed foods.
- Limit sodas and high-calorie foods.
- Limit fried foods.

## 6.2 Physical Activity

Your health-care provider may have recommended an exercise program for you. It is often beneficial to exercise vigorously (such that you feel your heart rate increasing) for 30 min/day, 5 days/week. Any exercise that elevates your heart rate is appropriate. Some examples including walking briskly, jogging, biking, swimming, hiking, dancing, and martial arts. Discuss any drastic changes in your exercise plan with your health-care provider.

## 6.3 Weight Management

If you are overweight, your health-care provider may recommend losing weight. A good goal to aim for is to lose 5–10 lbs in 6 months. Making the diet and exercise changes listed above will be helpful in attaining this goal.

## 6.4 Smoking

If you smoke cigarettes, use electronic cigarettes, or chew tobacco, it is recommended that you quit or at least cut back on your use. Quitting can be difficult, and you should discuss how to increase your chances of success with your health-care provider. Some patients find being part of a support group helpful. Nicotine gum and nicotine patches can be bridges on the road to quitting. There are also medications that can be prescribed to help with cravings.

## References


1. Farkouh ME, Smars PA, Reeder GS, et al. A clinical trial of a chest-pain observation unit for patients with unstable angina. N Engl J Med. 1998;339(26):1882–8.
2. Graff L, Joseph T, Andelman R, et al. American College of Emergency Physicians information paper: chest pain units in emergency departments – a report from the short-term observation services section. Am J Cardiol. 1995;76:1036–9.
3. Anderson RT, Montori VM, Shah ND, et al. Effectiveness of the chest pain choice decision aid in emergency department patients with low-risk chest pain: study protocol for a multicenter randomized trial. Trials. 2014;15:166.
4. Gaspoz JM, Lee TL, Weinstein MC, et al. Cost-effectiveness of a new short-stay unit to "rule out" acute myocardial infarction in low-risk patients. J Am Coll Cardiol. 1994;24:1249–59.
5. Borawski JB, Graff LG, Limkakeng AT. Care of the patient with chest pain in the observation unit. Emerg Med Clin North Am. 2017;35(3):535–47.
6. Than M, Flaws D, Sanders S, et al. Development and validation of the emergency department assessment of chest pain score and 2 h accelerated diagnostic protocol. Emerg Med Australas. 2014;26(1):34–44.

7. Huis In't Veld MA, Cullen L, Mahler SA, et al. The fast and the furious: low-risk chest pain and the rapid rule-out protocol. West J Emerg Med. 2017;18(3):474–8.
8. Than M, Cullen L, Aldous S, Parsonage WA, et al. 2-Hour accelerated diagnostic protocol to assess patients with chest pain symptoms using contemporary troponins as the only biomarker: the ADAPT trial. J Am Coll Cardiol. 2012;59(23):2091–8.
9. Ross MA, Hockenberry JM, Mutter, et al. Protocol-driven emergency department observation units offer savings, shorter stays, and reduced admissions. Health Aff. 2013;32(12):2149–56.

# Correction to: Risk Scoring Systems: Are They Necessary?

Jaron Raper, Laura Goyack, and Matthew DeLaney

**Correction to:**
**Chapter 10 in: M. Pena et al. (eds.), *Short Stay Management of Chest Pain*, Contemporary Cardiology, https://doi. org/10.1007/978-3-031-05520-1_10**

An author's name was incorrectly printed in Chapter 10 (Risk Scoring Systems: Are They Necessary?) as Laurie Goyak.

It has now been corrected to **Laura Goyack** in Chapter 10 (two occurrences on page 105), Table of Contents, and Contributors List.

---

The updated original version of this chapter can be found at
https://doi.org/10.1007/978-3-031-05520-1_10


M. Pena et al. (eds.), *Short Stay Management of Chest Pain*, Contemporary
Cardiology, https://doi.org/10.1007/978-3-031-05520-1_20

# Index

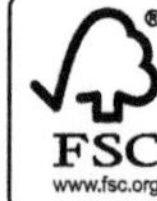

MIX
Papier aus verantwortungsvollen Quellen
Paper from responsible sources
**FSC® C105338**

FSC
www.fsc.org

If you have any concerns about our products,
you can contact us on
**ProductSafety@springernature.com**

In case Publisher is established outside the EU,
the EU authorized representative is:
**Springer Nature Customer Service Center GmbH**
**Europaplatz 3, 69115 Heidelberg, Germany**

Printed by Libri Plureos GmbH
in Hamburg, Germany